The Complete Home Guide to Herbs, Natural Healing, and Nutrition

The Complete Home Guide to Herbs, Natural Healing, and Nutrition

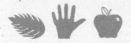

Jill Rosemary Davies

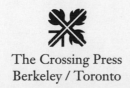

The Crossing Press
Berkeley / Toronto

The Crossing Press
P.O. Box 7123
Berkeley, California 94707
www.tenspeed.com

Distributed in Australia by Simon and Schuster Australia, in Canada by Ten Speed Press
Canada, in New Zealand by Southern Publishers Group, in South Africa by Real Books, and
in the United Kingdom and Europe by Airlift Book Company.

Cover design by Nancy Austin
Text design by Valerie Brewster
Tree dressing illustration and line drawings of plants by Toby Driver
Illustrations of culinary equipment by Stephen Sturgess

LIBRARY OF CONGRESS CATALOGING-IN-PUBLICATION DATA
Davies, Jill.
    The complete home guide to herbs, natural healing, and nutrition / Jill Rosemary Davies.
    p. cm.
    "First published in the United Kingdom by Gill & Macmillan" — T.p. verso.
    Includes bibliographical references and index.
    ISBN 1-58091-145-5 (pbk.)
    1. Herbs — Therapeutic use. 2. Naturopathy. 3. Nature, Healing power of. 4. Nutrition.
    I. Title.
    RM666.H33D378 2003
    615'.321 — dc22   2003016395

First printing, 2004

Printed in the United States of America

1 2 3 4 5 6 7 8 9 10 — 08 07 06 05 04

Contents

❧ 6 ❧

Cleansing and Detoxification   78

❧ 7 ❧

Immunity   103

❧ 8 ❧

Life Stage   122

❧ 9 ❦
Body Systems   150

❧ 10 ❦
Diseases   183

❧ 11 ❦
First Aid   268

Acknowledgments

I dedicate this book with love and gratitude to the memory of Dr. John Christopher for all his work and teaching and to Dr. Richard Schulze for keeping this herbal legacy alive and moving it on and into the twenty-first century. It is also dedicated to all herbalists worldwide for keeping safe and sharing the knowledge in the face of constant threats, legislation, and land ravaging.

I may have written a book about natural healing and herbalism, but I am certainly not a natural writer and so, in effect, this book would not have become a reality without my friend Ruth Butterfield, whose patience, intelligence, and organizational and editing skills have completed this work. Huge thanks also go to Alick and Kevin at Gateway Books for their gentle encouragement and support and to Deirdre Greenan and Michael Gill of Gill & Macmillan. For this American edition I would like to thank all those at Crossing Press whose very stringent editing skills have impressed me immensely; thank you, Meghan, and team. For "life" support during the writing of this book I would like to thank Dr. Shamim Daya, Professor Linda Fellows, Ray Hill from the British Holistic Medical Association, Anna Piper, Debs Chater, Andrea Stainsby, Jack Silverstone, Melanie and Abigail, and also my wonderful family, Nityananda, Lorna, and Jasmine.

My thanks go to all the practitioners, colleagues, and students who have shaped the information in this book—in Britain, the United States, France, Spain, and India. I wish I could list you all, but I can't; so many thanks, even to those unmet whose books have taught and inspired me.

Caution

In many cases small quantities of herbs are therapeutic, given at the correct dose and in correct proportion of herb within a formula. In larger doses they are often highly dangerous, for example coltsfoot *(Tussilago farfara)*, goldenseal *(Hydrastis canadensis)*, licorice *(Glycyrrhiza glabra)*, and pokeweed *(Phytolacca americana)*. I also never advise combining drugs and herbal medicines as their interactions are unpredictable.

For formulas that are very similar to the ones described in this book, that are safely sold over the counter to many millions of people all over the United States since 1979 by mail order, contact:

> The American Botanical Pharmacy
> 4114 Glencoe Avenue
> Marina del Rey, CA 90292
> Tel: 800-Herb-Doc
> Website: http://www.800herbdoc.com

For British and European equivalent formulas contact Herbs Hands Healing Ltd. (see address and details below).

In general, no parts of formulas nor doses have been given for the herbal formulas and herbs. Neither have the contraindications of herbs been included, as they are numerous and specific, those pregnant and breastfeeding being in the highest category to avoid certain herbs. A very comprehensive list of herb contraindications and drug interactions, plus more information on dosage, is available on the Internet at www.herbshandshealing.co.uk and from:

> Herbs Hands Healing Ltd.
> Station Warehouse
> Station Road, Pulham Market
> Norfolk IP21 4XF, United Kingdom
> Tel: 011-44-0137-9608201
> Email: info@herbshandshealing.co.uk

The books *Herb Contraindications and Drug Interactions* by Francis Brinker and American Herbal Products Association's *Botanical Safety Handbook* edited by Michael McGuffin, Christopher Hobbs, Roy Upton, and Alicia Goldberg can provide alternative information. For added information see also *The United States Pharmacopeia* and *American Herbal Pharmacopoeia* by Roy Upton. For more details on the above books contact American Botanical Council at 800-373-7105.

All of the herbs mentioned in this book can be used by qualified herbalists and the majority can be sold over the counter in line with laws varying from country to country.

Introduction

The stars of this book are the plants, trees, and flowers themselves. They are endearing, beautiful, mysterious, fundamental, and primitive. The delight and uses of their seeds, roots, bark, color, and form are phenomenal and, set among the rest of the intricate web of nature, they are truly miraculous. This book is not only about the plants, however, it is also about a combination of natural healing methods, healthy lifestyle, and the use of herbs as potent tools for natural healing. Were this simply a book on herbal medicine, it would be dangerously easy to see plants as a direct substitute for conventional drugs. But although it is often possible gently and carefully to substitute one for the other, on the whole it is best to use herbs as an integral part of life, combining them with a wealth of other lifestyle choices and thus preventing and balancing disorders or diseases.

Plant healing is deeply ingrained in our ancestry, yet the privilege of healing our own bodies has been increasingly taken away from us and put into the hands of doctors and conventional medicine. It is not surprising that night calls to doctors have doubled in the past few years, pill taking has soared, and the skills of home nursing have diminished. Many people tend to view ill health as a "supermarket affair," demanding quick answers with the cry, "Give me a pill and make it go away, now!" Others, however, feel a desperate yearning to know more about natural home-healing skills, combined with herbs. So this book has been written with the understanding that herbalism and natural healing should be restored to the home as safely and effectively as possible. All practitioners insist that if there is any doubt about the cause of a patient's condition, a doctor's diagnosis should be sought. From this diagnosis you, and perhaps your local herbalist, can work on your body naturally until you regain full health.

This book also explains the philosophy and ethos behind herbalism and natural healing. Perhaps you are not ill but just want to learn how to look after yourself. Knowing how to prevent ill health by understanding your body and having some practical insight into ways to look after it is all part of the ethos of natural healing. By gaining this knowledge, you will learn how to return some of the responsibility for your health to where it should be. The need to do so becomes especially urgent when one considers that 50 percent of the forty-six thousand patient deaths in Britain every year from iatrogenic (doctor-involved) ailments are associated with operations performed as a result of diagnostic errors.

Many of the natural healing programs in this book require the cleansing of the body by consuming special foods. This is called *detoxification* and it is fundamental to the natural healing process. Its basic importance rests on the fact that the human body has the ability to regenerate itself using its own genetic blueprint. Until recently it was believed that it took two years for the individual cells of the liver to regenerate and thus create a new liver; now it is believed to take just a few months. This possibility offers phenomenal hope for so many people. Of course, the health of each new blood cell and thus each new organ reflects what it is created from—that is to say, if we feed our bodies nutritionally deficient or toxic food, we cannot expect to create healthy organs. However, with the correct directives and input, repairing our bodies is possible. Three groundbreaking healers of the twentieth and twenty-first centuries—Dr. John Christopher, Dr. Richard Schulze, and Dr. Deepak Chopra—have proved this and continue to teach this inspiring thought for many years.

Other methods, which will be explained, include the use of water: to heat or cool the body in order to encourage circulation, to support and nurture, to destagnate, to cleanse, and to provoke. As you read the chapter on diseases, you will see how vigorous some of the programs need to be in order to get results. You may be tempted to follow only part of a program and to leave out some of the harder tasks, but if you are seriously ill, it is imperative that you carry out the treatment as directed. If your condition is not chronic, or if the treatment is simply a preventative, you may use cleanses, such as a bowel or liver cleanse, specifically suited to your needs. It is no coincidence that one of the most important health quests of the twenty-first century is the understanding of the immune and hormone systems, which are now being tested and punished in a myriad of ways. We must, therefore, ask more questions, and herbs are very good at providing some of the answers.

Why Try Herbalism?

Medical science took a big leap forward in the United States and Europe after World War II with the introduction of a whole collection of drugs, including beta-blockers, anesthetics, antidepressants, steroids, and antibiotics, to name but a few. Some remain extremely useful, especially the anesthetics, some painkillers, and antibiotics, when used in highly selective situations. Medical technology also took a big leap and, although some discoveries are now readily accepted as being useful and noninvasive, much new technology seems to have been designed simply to make lots of money for the manufacturers, while some is positively destructive, invasive, and life-threatening.

Robert Mendelsohn, MD, says in his book *Confessions of a Medical Heretic*,

> I believe that modern medicine treatments for disease are seldom effective and that they are often more dangerous than the diseases they are designed to treat. I believe the dangers are compounded by the widespread use of dangerous procedures for non-diseases. I believe that more than 90 percent of modern medicine could disappear from

the face of the earth—doctors, hospitals, drugs, equipment—and the effect on our health would be immediate and beneficial. I believe that modern medicine has gone too far, by using, in everyday situations, extreme treatments designed for critical conditions!

We need to become more discerning about medical treatment and to ask for what we want instead of simply accepting whatever current medical development is thrust upon us. Most of all, we need to avoid becoming one of 100,000 yearly U.S. citizens killed by the orthodox medical profession itself.

Some natural healing methods may initially appear to be drastic, time-consuming, old-fashioned, and crude. You may not have met anyone who has used them and be asking yourself whether they really work. A few of us, the recipients and facilitators of these methods, know that they do work and have kept the knowledge alive. Now more than ever, people need to be enlightened with the knowledge and ability to heal themselves. According to the World Health Organization, the number of cancers is expected to double in most countries over the next twenty-five years. The reason is that we have an ever-increasing population that is living longer—but in a sicklier state. With this in mind, it is important for every household to have a clearer understanding of healthy daily living and self-help methods, and to be aware that little problems need not become large ones if they are dealt with early enough. Because of the overuse of antibiotics, vaccinations, poor nutrition, and pollution, our children are becoming sicker and weaker with more persistent allergies than ever. We need to redress this widespread problem.

All too often we are scared away from herbs, regarding them as being the exclusive province of the professionals, but herbs furnish us with our own natural healing laboratories in our own kitchens. Herbs are potent, and their benefits are usually felt quite quickly.

In previous times, herbalists used only the plants in their own terrain, but personal territory has dwindled everywhere. As a means of sharing these resources and enriching our knowledge, plants from luxuriant rain forests, spacious mountains, and spartan deserts are now as easily available as those obtainable from the local garden center. Yet though we now have access to an incredible repertoire of healing plants, we actually have all we need on our doorstep, with everyday weeds capable of taking care of a host of viruses, bacteria, parasites, and much more.

The Roots of Herbalism

Archaeological evidence tells us that during their time as hunter-gatherers, humans collected and consumed approximately one hundred to two hundred different plant species in any one year. The diverse chemical compounds in these plants would have greatly protected the immune system and stimulated digestion more efficiently than does our modern diet. Not only did human-kind flourish on this diet, but so did the animals that people subsequently consumed. Sadly, the same cannot be said of the "animal foods" of today.

Modern people's normal dietary range of plants is generally only be-tween twenty and forty species. These include carrots, cabbages, potatoes, parsnips, onions, apples, bananas, strawberries, peaches, lettuce, tomatoes, peas, broccoli, beans, wheat, blackberries, zucchini and other squashes, oil made from sunflower seeds or olives, lemons, garlic, chiles, and rice. Super-markets, on average, stock thirty to thirty-five species. It is an unfortunate fact that many of these plants are also genetically engineered. Their chem-ical composition today is far removed from that of the wild plants they once were, which is an important health consideration. Interestingly, a herbalist's materia medica is normally in the range of one hundred to two hundred plants, some of which are used frequently, some less so, while others are used very rarely—very much as the historical range of food species would have been used. Herbs give us back the diversity of plants in our lives, their complex chemistries mixing to form patterns as individual and necessary as those taking place in every human being.

The Chinese, like many other peoples, spend a lot of time considering the correlation between our bodies and our entire existence, recognizing that we are in fact part of the sun, stars, moon, earth, and nature. Their di-agnostic work also takes into consideration the effect of geography on our impressionable bodies—of heat, cold, damp, high or low altitude, and how they correspond to the temperatures of our own bodies, which consist mostly of water and minerals. Native Americans, Russians, and peoples of many other cultures have used these systems, which show a high degree of simi-larity in technique and wisdom. Tibetans have similar, yet unique, forms of understanding disease, which have stemmed from their experience of day-to-day life on their harsh, barren mountainsides. The monks of these Tibetan mountains were often the primary healers in the scattered villages. Among other things, they were excellent at reading the eye, its color, markings, and depths, with each area of the eye giving clues about particular parts of the body, genetic tendencies, emotional predispositions, and so on. A modern-day version of this therapy is now called iridology; it remains a brilliant tool for assessing constitutional and genetic tendencies. Indian Ayurvedic med-icine pays great attention to the clues of body structure, voice timbre, and vital energy levels, right down to the color of the saliva on the tongue.

In fact, all traditional cultures have their own ways of tracking the roots of disease, but those ways overlap and arrive at the same destination via dif-ferent routes. What they have in common is their attention to detail; watching, feeling, seeing, remembering, and experiencing; noticing the small alongside the large and the whole. These diagnostic and assessment methods are merely an extension of everyday life.

My Influences

As a natural healer, my aim is to empower and reeducate people within the home, using nature in all her forms, with her foods and herbs as allies, in order to remedy disease and rebalance the system. It is always very exciting to find "like" spirits; I have met them in many countries, including Britain, the United States, all over Europe, and India. These people and places have all shaped and molded me, but I was perhaps most greatly influenced by Dr. John Christopher, who for his time was a pioneer of modern herbalism and helped instigate and shape the American herbal renaissance of the 1970s, 1980s, and 1990s.

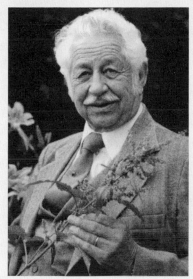

Dr. Christopher

Not a week goes by without my thoughts and gratitude going out to him. I am especially grateful that I am legally allowed to practice as a herbalist in Britain as a direct legacy of laws passed by Henry VIII and, more recently, through the work of the Medicines and Healthcare products Regulatory Agency (MHRA), the British Herbal Medicine Association (BHMA), and the European Herbal Practitioners Association.

Life for my American teachers (herbalists) has not been so easy. Dr. Richard Schulze, a colleague and main apprentice to Dr. Christopher, has had to suffer the financial loss and indignity of having his herb stores smashed, despoiled, and confiscated by the U.S. Food and Drug Administration. Similarly, Dr. Christopher was thrown into jail many times, but he still healed many thousands of people and started up clinic after clinic — each after the last one had been shut down. In France, Spain, Belgium, Greece, Italy, and other countries, herbalism is illegal unless you are a qualified medical doctor. Nevertheless, plant usage is very much alive among the ordinary people in those countries, and I have had the honor of learning a great deal from European herbalists, particularly those of the older generation who used only the herbs found growing around them, maybe fifteen or twenty varieties in total, to treat a wide range of diseases. Germany, the Netherlands, Sweden, Denmark, and Britain remain among the few nations in Europe where herbalism can be practiced legally by practitioners.

In developing countries, by contrast, plants are still the main source of medicine. According to the World Health Organization, as many as 80 percent of the world's people rely for their primary health care on traditional medicine, most types of which use remedies made from plants. In fact, the use of traditional medicine in developing countries is increasing. The reason is that populations are increasing, and governments want to encourage indigenous forms of medicine rather than rely on imported drugs.

In summer 2002, the British Department of Health discussed the possibility and desire to integrate herbal practitioners into the National Health Service—in other words, within its hospitals and the medical community at large. It hopes to go ahead with this idea if and when Statutory Self Regulation has been accomplished, perhaps by 2006. Britain has been running many training courses in herbal medicine, providing more qualified practitioners as each year goes by. Additionally, the Medicines and Healthcare products Regulatory Agency (the British equivalent to the U.S. Food and Drug Administration) is regulating over-the-counter sales of herbal medicines to make sure that quality is safeguarded. This is a European-led policy and it is hoped that a more uniform approach throughout Europe will be the outcome, helping to ensure that safety and quality are priorities. Certainly the new labeling will allow greater information for the purchaser—from the product's usage to daily dose, adverse reactions, and so on.

Dr. Christopher's style of herbalism is particularly suited to home use, partly because he was always working outside the law and, therefore, employed methods that could be safely used at home. His favorite saying was, "There should be a herbalist in every home, a practitioner in every town." He often treated those who couldn't afford medical insurance, and used many revolutionary approaches for home health care and first aid that work simply, cheaply, and efficiently. These methods were subsequently upgraded by his apprentice, Dr. Schulze, to suit modern life and its diseases. Much of the style of natural healing and herbalism described in this book owes its origins to these two men. It has also been influenced by the teachings of Dr. Shyam Singha, an Ayurvedic practitioner, acupuncturist, osteopath, and natural healer with whom I also served an apprenticeship. These people and others have been my inspiration and guides, both in my life and in my practice, which I first established in 1982.

On a historical note, Ezra Suggett, a herbal apothecary in Beccles, Suffolk, was my great-great-grandfather. He inspired me through the wonderful tales of his work that were told to me as a child by my grandmother. His dispensary and clinic was similar to many of its kind in the mid nineteenth century. His materia medica would have included at least 40 percent herbs imported from America, such as slippery elm, goldenseal, and sarsaparilla, with the other 60 percent coming from Europe, mostly from Britain, and a few from Asia. Many would have been collected locally (by knowledgeable gatherers), and many remedies would have included these local plants—for instance, sea holly root from the beaches, or fennel, burdock, and plantain from the hedges and meadows. His clientele would have visited his dispensary and bought herbs after a quick chat or lengthier consultation, or alternatively he would have made a house call on his horse, carrying a saddlebag large enough to hold his traveling medicine bag and poisons box (which I still have). One story passed down was that upon being called out in the middle of the night, he rode twelve miles to a cottage deep in the fens to assist. He found a worried mother and a screaming baby. He simply undressed the baby and removed the diaper pin, which was pricking the baby's tummy! He then rode twelve miles home again.

The large building that once housed his thriving business is now a bank, but his love and use of herbs live on. It is believed that when the apothecaries came under fire from the medical profession, Suggett joined the National Institute of Medical Herbalists, which was founded to safeguard their profession. To this date it is one of the largest and oldest herbal associations in Britain.

Ill Health, the Greatest Teacher

My teacher, Dr. Christopher, was in and out of a wheelchair for most of his early life. His illnesses included serious spleen and liver disease and a crumbling spine resulting from chronic arthritis and rheumatism, all of which became progressively worse. When he was thirty-five years old it was predicted that he would not reach his fortieth birthday, and it was probably this close brush with death that became a turning point in his life. He rediscovered herbs, along with food and water treatments, and finally examined his long-buried negative feelings about being abandoned by his original parents. Most of all he rebelled against the fate assigned to him, married, had many children, and went on to live to the age of eighty-two. He established flourishing clinics and taught herbalism, while continually learning himself from Native American healers and inspiring many others. He proved that a man who was once virtually a skeleton in a wheelchair could dramatically change the quality and direction of his life, transforming it through positive thought and action combined with natural healing methods. Read his book *A Herbal Legacy of Courage* for his full and spellbinding life story, which was often beset with legal problems, fines, and jail sentences, as well as his main text, *The School of Natural Healing*.

Another teacher, Dr. Schulze, watched both his parents die of heart attacks, leaving him orphaned by the age of fourteen. By the time he was sixteen, he had himself begun to experience chest pains, which became increasingly painful and consistent. His consultant diagnosed angina and, as time went by, open-heart surgery was recommended as his only hope, his combined parental gene package having now bequeathed him a life-threatening situation. Yet Schulze felt there were many other methods and ways to treat his problem. At first he talked to a monk who suggested that he should not consume any meat or alcohol, and he felt a little better for these dietary restrictions. He went on to exclude fats (especially from cakes and pastries), fish, and sugar. Someone else suggested that he should take plenty of exercise and, all in all, he began to feel a great deal better. Nevertheless, at the age of nineteen, he was scheduled for major open-heart surgery. On discovering, however, that a friend of a similar age had died on the operating table undergoing the same surgery just the day before, he literally fled the hospital and continued his self-healing quest. To this day he remains healthy and more alive than almost anyone I know, having used no drugs or surgery at any point in his life. His successful clinic, treating many thousands of terminally sick (and other) patients, was closed down by the U.S. Food and Drug Administration (FDA) in 1994, but his work lives on ever stronger through his books, seminars, videos, teaching tapes, and his herbal medicine company, the American Botanical Pharmacy, in California.

My major personal experience of ill health started at the age of eighteen. It took the form of intense knifelike pains on my right side, sometimes lasting hours or days. I saw twelve bowel consultants, yet gained no insight or advice. When I was nineteen years old, my stomach was cut open because it was suspected that I might have cancer. The doctors found nothing, but removed my healthy appendix. I couldn't walk properly for months, and I couldn't wear a bikini! But after a while, I discovered yoga and the effects of its general balancing and internal massage, which started healing my problems. Eventually, I discovered healing foods, cleanses, herbs, and colon health care, through Dr. Christopher and other teachers.

Book List

Common Sense Health and Healing by Dr. Richard Schulze (Santa Monica, California: Natural Healing Publications, 2002)

Confessions of a Medical Heretic by Robert Mendelsohn, MD (Chicago: Contemporary Books, 1990)

A Herbal Legacy of Courage by David Christopher (Springville, Utah: Christopher Publications, 1993)

The School of Natural Healing by Dr. John Christopher (Springville, Utah: Christopher Publications, 1976)

⊰ 1 ⊱

Our Bodies, Our Health

The Clues to Health and Sickness

It is a great blessing if your body can transport you through life without too many recurring breakdowns. Being unaware of the body's warning signs is part of a more general loss of many primal and gut instincts. When things do go wrong, there is a tendency to curse your body, treating it as something separate from yourself—an entity that has failed in its service to you. What people often fail to realize is that this reaction is the result of an ever-increasing disconnection with the body, and that the physical breakdown is the conclusion to a long series of unheeded warnings, which the body has been trying to communicate. These communications can be as simple as an awareness that you have not felt quite right for a while, that you have been unusually terse with loved ones or simply the feeling that you can't cope any more. They can also take a more physical form, like a headache or indigestion—symptoms often suppressed with a pill, when you should be addressing the cause and questioning the reason for them. Sometimes, as with so many children nowadays, ill health becomes a way of life. Allergies, digestive disorders, and overuse of antibiotics are all too common.

Listening to your body, observing and asking how and why you react to situations the way you do, can tell you an awful lot about yourself. With physical symptoms, what is often required is a process of seeing the external signs and tracing them back to the inside. Initially, there may be just a jumble of clues and tidbits of information, great and small. Every sensory ability has to be thrown into feeling more and gathering information. Approach the problem like a great detective novel; it will invariably contain many false trails that must be patiently tracked by applying all available wisdom. Drawing conclusions too quickly is as dangerous as overcomplexity and tunnel vision. Simplicity and common sense should be your primary focus. A practitioner can often make sense of all the pieces for you and design a helpful route back to health.

In many cases of ill health, a disease progresses for some years before severe symptoms set in. The further advanced a disease is, the harder it is to find the source or to locate the actual moment, or moments, when the initial disharmony spawned the illness. So seeing and being aware of yourself is a habit you can begin at any age and is a lesson that it is never too early or too late to learn. In many ways it is a very natural process. Some may find comfort in knowing that their ill health is their destiny. What is certain is that what counts is the course of action that follows.

The Basics That Can Be Achieved at Home

Nutrition: Eat good foods, avoiding those that contain pesticides, hormones, and any other additives or contaminants. Instead, concentrate on foods that are organic, if available, and rich in vitamins, minerals, and other desirable constituents. An occasional checkup on the body through food cleanses is important. Today, digestive problems are rife and are at the bottom of much ill health. Weak digestive juices are often the cause.

Medicinal nutrition: Use healing plants to tone, support, and stimulate.

Herbalism: Use plant oils, tinctures, infusions, poultices, syrups, compresses, fomentations, and decoctions.

Hydrotherapy: This healing method can be practiced in the bathroom. Showering, soaking, and steaming are just a few ways in which water can be used to circulate blood and massage internal organs and systems—giving them more oxygen and nourishment in order to avoid or dispel congestion and stagnation.

Exercise: Keep the body moving, flexing, circulating, pumping, inhaling, exhaling, and detoxifying. Yoga and breathing exercises are especially good for all of these requirements and for those with limited movement.

Body contact: Massage, yoga, reflexology, tai chi, and other movement therapies help the body stay healthy or, if necessary, heal.

Celebrating Nature's Alchemy and Fragrance

"While the plant is growing, an enormous amount of electrical or vital energy is absorbed into the different parts of the plant. It is first generated by the sun, diffused through the atmosphere, the water and the earth; and the plants select what they need to build acids, alkalines, phosphates, carbonates, chlorides, glycerides, oils, fats, waxes and so forth.

In this profoundly wonderful vegetable kingdom that covers the earth with beauty, perfume and flavor, there is every conceivable requirement for every living creature, even to the breath of life. Plants arrange themselves into families, choose their own habitation and select their own food. Through long study of the chemistry of soil and plants we are able to predict what we shall find stored away in the leaves, roots, barks and fruits of particular plants for the purpose of supplying our own bodies with the specific material and specific energy we require."

— Dr. Edward E. Shook, *Advanced Treatise on Herbology*

There are many ways to make contact with nature. Anyone who has spent time communing with it will understand and feel its unseen gifts and potential as much as the more visible ones. The rocks, the earth, the many greens of foliage, and the rainbow colors of the blossoms and fruits speak for themselves. A flower, when you stare into it, can heal by its color and form alone, while its vibration and essence are something else.

Nature can respond like a true friend or lover, as events have shown time and again. The Findhorn Project in northern Scotland continues to provide a wonderful experience and revelation of the power of love and tuning into nature, showing that plants are intelligent, responsive, and emotional, lacking only, perhaps, the power of movement in an otherwise full spectrum of humanlike abilities. On stony soil under windy conditions, unbelievable plants, fruits, and vegetables have been produced at Findhorn, proving that really relating to nature can produce some surprising results—such as double-size fruits and vegetables with no pests. This vibrational attunement with nature could produce even more wonderful benefits for world food production. Indeed, we are all going to need to reassess our methods as time goes by. Perhaps we need to recall times when our relationship with growing things was founded on more simple gratitude and celebration.

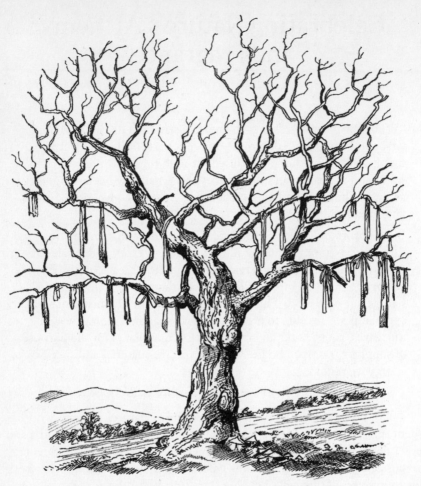

Traditional "tree dressing" in the winter months

All over the world in earlier times, trees were "dressed" using ribbons or small toys tied on in the winter, in order to thank the tree for the splendor of its greenness and the joy of its blossom in spring and summer. In fact, there were hundreds of ancient rituals for celebrating nature. Well dressing was another, to thank the springwater for providing the basis for life.

Access to nature was, luckily, something I grew up with, and it has affected my life ever since. My mother produced homemade wine, and I gathered for her the wild yellow broom flowers, nettle tops, blackberries, elder flowers, elderberries, dandelion flowers, and birch sap required. Spending hours and hours over years and years with these colorful plants gave me something that is very much a part of myself. Camping and traveling have given me an accumulated love of mountains, rivers, streams, woods, and valleys; sun, rain, thunder, wind, cold, and heat. Sometimes too tired to put a tent up, I have lain in powder-dry ploughed fields, the odd ditch, or under a sheltering tree. Moonlight, darkness, firelight, and stars have become familiar and friendly. It is there for us all to be touched by.

The Sweet Smell of Nature

The scent of plants on a wet early spring morning; the smell of newly mown grass; the first roses of summer; the hot, dry, arid herbs on a scorched mountain—these are just a few of the many sweet smells of nature.

Smell is one of the most evocative memory joggers. Not only does it stop you at the time, helping you to extend and savor all that is present, but it also has a beautiful way of reviving memories to sweeten the present. When we remember someone, we very often remember their scent. We smell their individual pheromones (from the Greek *pherein* meaning "to carry," and *hormon* meaning "to excite"). Pleasant odors make us feel happy, while noxious ones can irritate or depress. So whether you like the smell of tar, bergamot essential oil, or the latest chemical perfume is for you to decide, but the sensation will change your own body chemistry. It does this through a portion of the brain that controls emotional well-being, which is originally triggered by the nerves of the olfactory organ—the nose.

Essential oils come from all parts of plants and trees: bark, berries, seeds, leaves, and flowers. They all basically work to balance our sympathetic and parasympathetic nervous systems, relaxing and bringing harmony and equilibrium, clarity and awareness. This is why they were, and still are, burned in so many temples around the world in the form of incense: myrrh and frankincense from Africa and western Asia, sage from the Western Hemisphere, and lavender from south Europe.

Nature and Its Health

Pollution has already affected half of Britain's trees. Visible symptoms like sparse foliage, broken tops, bare branches, or trees to which autumn seems to come early are the outward signs of complex internal problems. A survey done in 1991 showed that 56.7 percent of British trees had lost more than a quarter of their leaves. Britain ranks worst out of the whole of Europe: even heavily polluted Poland and the Czech Republic have relatively healthier trees. A combination of pollution and drought, with ensuing infestations of insects and fungi, seems to be the problem, resulting in the trees' natural defense systems becoming weaker and weaker. This problem mirrors humans' own alarming global rise in immune-system diseases and allergy problems.

Much open land is being lost to development; it has fallen victim to money and an increase in population. Historically, common land in Britain was often unlawfully sold off by the crown and the church; more recently, footpaths have been plowed up by farmers and other landowners. Land has been given over to intensive farming, industry, and housing. But many Britons are now dedicated to reopening footpaths and preserving what little countryside we have left; some churchyards and cemeteries are now a haven for nature. Spending time out in nature will inspire us to save and create more. We should also remember that trees and plants are intelligent enough to adapt to changes in the environment, responding with new reactions in order to survive, protecting themselves from or transforming pollution. As major oxygenators, trees are very important. Thus replanting is essential in order to keep the earth's atmosphere, and all who live off it, healthy.

Something that has increasingly struck me is that calcium-depleted soils produce sickly, weak trees that are prone to disease, while calcium-rich soils produce the opposite. Trees flourish in mineral- and nutrient-rich soils, the larger-leafed deciduous trees needing more nutrients than coniferous varieties. It is possible that we are in need of another ice age, in which the rocks and earth are moved and crushed to replenish nutrients the soil. Unfortunately, glaciers can take nine hundred centuries to remineralize the earth, and then a few more centuries would be needed to warm the ground up enough to grow anything again! But general loss of nutrient-rich, undisturbed soils is certainly a huge factor in the loss of tree health. Interestingly enough, calcium is one of the most needed minerals for our own bodies—another similarity we have to plants. Like all things, trees and humans are part of the same blueprint of nature.

Plant Aid

Although some trees and plants are being killed off by humankind's pollution, this faithful flora continues to step in to help with the mess we have gotten ourselves into! In evolutionary terms, humans developed only because of the presence of the plant kingdom.

In the past fifty years, Britain has suffered the destruction of 97 percent of its wildflower meadows, 75 percent of its open heath, 96 percent of its lowland peat bogs, and 190,000 miles of hedgerow—enough to circle the earth seven times. Studies have shown that plants seem to provide the simplest and easiest way for combating the effects of airborne pollution; for instance, trees that have large areas of leaves with fairly rough or hairy surfaces are effective pollution traps. Hawthorn, with its open and branching shape, is a good "trapper," using its canopy like a net. Dust that settles on the edge of a denser canopy, like that provided by a lime or poplar, is much more likely to be blown away. Rough-fissured bark can also trap, and trees planted in groups, with their increased ability to slow down passing air, help likewise. In effect, they are acting as air filters. There is also some research to show that trees "lock up" in their tissues pollutants such as sulfur and nitrogen dioxide from car exhaust. A single mature beech tree can lock up nearly four and a half pounds of carbon dioxide within one hour on a sunny day.

One problem close to my heart is that many playgrounds are unprotected by trees. Toddlers, infants, and schoolchildren spend time playing in open sun traps, often at times of the day when the sun is at its most fierce. A few trees planted would give the shade vital to protecting them from harmful ultraviolet radiation. An average six-foot sapling costs very little; ten fast-growing trees could pretty quickly make a huge difference to a playground. Plants and trees also provide noise barriers. Individual leaves absorb and reflect sound while the branches and foliage scatter the sound waves, making noises duller and softer.

Allowing and Sustaining Nature as Much as Possible

Permaculture, or forest gardening, is something practiced naturally by the native peoples of North America, the rain forests, and other places. These old cultures simply made or found tiny clearings and worked with the forest canopy, dew, sun, earth, light, and so on to grow fruits, vegetables, and other natural commodities, planting for their grandchildren and great-grandchildren as well as themselves. Forest gardening, as a system, works with nature and allows her to do as much of the work as possible. One of its most important principles is maximum observation with minimal interference. Permaculture takes into account the wind, sun, slope, climate, microclimates, and water flow, and uses a minimal amount of machinery, so as to change or destroy as little as possible of this natural tapestry.

There is increasing interest in leaving nature alone and trying to learn from her instead of trying to master her. Such endeavors include the Permaculture Association based in Devonshire, a vegan community with similar interests in Cornwall, and organic farming schemes in Britain run in association with the highly successful "box system," whereby organic fruits and vegetables are delivered to customers' doorsteps weekly. The famous Alternative Technology Centre in Wales is another encouraging enterprise.

Plantlife is an organization of paramount importance to herbalists in Britain because it addresses issues relating to local herbs. Plantlife is Britain's only national plant conservation organization working to protect and conserve Britain's wild flora in its natural habitats. It takes a strong lead in the quest to understand and change the causes for the loss of wild plants and the symptoms of destruction. It actually conserves threatened species of plants (including fungi), of which 232 are on the British government's "danger list." Some of the country's most respected botanists are involved. Plantlife now owns more than nineteen nature reserves that cover nearly five hundred acres.

In Spain and other European countries where nature reserves exist, herbs are gathered under strict supervision and care. This harvest has a twofold benefit: it provides an income for the reserve, and it provides much-needed organic and wild-crafted herbs for herbalists and the general public. This model could eventually be adopted elsewhere.

Horticultural practices in general are trying to help our "Green push" by using sustainable wood products for plant potting and packaging. Instead of pots made from peat (from disappearing peat bogs), moss (declining with the disappearance of boggy regions), or plastics (which cause pollution), wood wool, root cloths, coconut fiber, and more are coming into use. Key reasons for choosing certain materials are that they are sustainable, abundant, or recyclable.

Pesticides or Not

A problem arising from so-called monoculture (growing a single crop in the same soil year after year) concerns the use of chemical sprays. For years, because of the general gardening practices I employ, I have had no problem with slugs, whiteflies, or other pests. If I have the odd aphid, I spray successfully using strong herbal teas or a minute dilution of lavender and other essential oils in water. In so doing, I use something the insects find off-putting to deter them. Another method, called companion planting, uses plant chemistry to keep pests at bay. For example, wormwood will produce a toxic chemistry that is effective at keeping invasive plants such as nettles away from desired plants; this practice of using the natural relationships between certain plants has often been applied to forest gardening.

The idea of using essential oils and toxic plant chemistry is now being researched and is becoming more accepted, while the even more desirable technique of always keeping a balance is being rediscovered by farmers and gardeners. A few farmers now plant strips of wildflowers around fields of sweet corn or, in some cases, between batches of sweet corn and other vegetables. In time, perhaps, more trees will creep into the picture, but for now, the presence of a few more wildflowers and grasses has certainly been found to help maintain the balance between crops and their plant and insect predators and parasites. Even Britain's largest producer of chemical insecticides and fertilizers, ICI, has said that all gardens should have a small quantity of wild plant species growing near cultivated ornamental plants, pointing out that these plants assist friendly insects. Lacewings and hoverflies, for example, lay their eggs on some weeds, and both destroy aphids. That's quite a quantum leap for a firm like ICI, but we need more leaps from them in many more positive directions.

Dr. Francis Brinker of the Eclectic Institute in Arizona tells us that certain chemicals in the prickly ash (*Zanthoxylum* species) act on houseflies, mosquito larvae, ticks, and several leaf-eating insects, as well as being an ovicide for body lice and toxic to yellow mealworms. There is a great deal of research being carried out into natural insecticides. For instance, where eucalyptus grows, not a single mosquito is to be seen!

Agricultural chemicals may be a problem for industrialized nations, but they have had even more serious consequences in developing economies. A ten-million-strong peasants' revolt in 1994 in India tried to reverse some of the worst aspects of the GATT international trade regulations. Rural farmers in India and other developing nations want it to be known that their very survival is at stake. These farmers are obliged to buy hybrid seeds from certain companies. Plants grown from these hybrid seeds do not set seed, and therefore seed cannot be gathered from them for sowing the following year. Thus the farmers have to buy more seeds from Western companies, at enormous expense. In addition, these genetically developed seeds actually depend on chemicals for growth. These farmers' very livelihood is being threatened, and now a legacy of destruction can be seen, with farms, farmers, and their families being forced into failure. This arrangement may be disgustingly brilliant for monopolistic agribusiness, but it is a threat to the survival of small farmers, their families, and indeed whole peoples. In fact, only a few very rich farmers will survive. Many people will continue to starve and become parted from their land, homes, lifestyle, and everything they have or care for. Their own collected seeds are the excellent result of centuries of improvement and adaptation to local conditions and are best suited for mixed sustainable agriculture. The imported "miracle" hybrid versions are already reported to be giving lower yields and to require excessive water, which is simply not available.

Get Closer to Nature and Make a Herbal Profile

Spending time in nature, where you can rediscover and hone gut instincts, can be given an extra purpose by making your own herbal profile. A herbal profile is an intensive study of a small number of plants that are common in your immediate surroundings. The process of creating a herbal profile will help you to appreciate that the trees and "weeds" that grow around you are capable of feeding and healing you. You'll realize only too clearly that the whole body can be balanced and maintained by using what is to be found commonly growing. (See appendix 3 for further instructions and guidance if you wish to make your own herbal profile.)

On the pages that follow, I give brief profiles of sixteen plants widely available in Britain; most are also common in the United States, or are similar to species grown there. Be aware that some of the herbs described here do carry contraindications.

BURDOCK (*ARCTIUM LAPPA*)

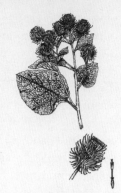

Parts used: root and seed

Burdock is used as a root vegetable in Japan. Highly nutritious, it will sustain the pancreas and spleen while balancing blood sugar levels. It is a strong general immune-boosting herb, rich in tumor-inhibiting chemistry. As a prime blood cleanser it will clear the skin, bloodstream, lymph, and colon of poisons. It is best used in combination with dandelion to safeguard the elimination of collected toxins.

DANDELION (*TARAXACUM OFFICINALE*)

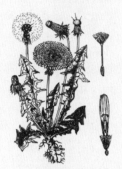

Parts used: flower, leaf, and root

This is a wonderful herb for the liver, heart, and kidneys. It helps stimulate liver function in general, aiding digestion as it does. It is also a prime kidney herb, helping to relieve water retention without exhausting the kidneys. It treats gallbladder problems, edema, high blood pressure, heart weakness, skin problems, and many other conditions.

ELDER (*SAMBUCUS NIGRA*)

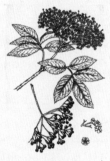

Parts used: fruit, flower, leaf, and bark

The elderberry is now recognized as a strong antiviral, though this knowledge has long been part of ancient Native American lore. The berries, leaves, and flowers are useful for treating fevers and inflammation, thanks to their anti-inflammatory chemistry. All parts of the plant clean and clear the bloodstream and aid the clearing of mucus from the lungs. When applied externally, the flowers and bark are useful for sore eyes, minor injuries, and skin problems such as eczema, psoriasis, warts, inflammation, and irritation.

HAWTHORN (*CRATAEGUS LAEVIGATA*, SOMETIMES CALLED *C. OXYACANTHA*)

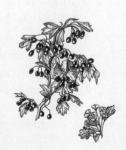

Parts used: flower, leaf, and berry

All parts of the hawthorn are very safe for use on the heart, and many heart patients regularly pick the leaves, berries, and flowers and make tea from them. It acts like a beta-blocker, blocking heart receptor cells and unblocking again as needed by the individual. It is a very clever herb, ideal for improving circulation and coronary blood flow, and for regulating heart rate and blood pressure. It also has antibacterial qualities.

LIME TREE (*TILIA EUROPAEA* OR *CORDATA*)

Part used: flower

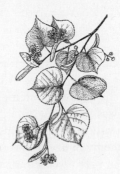

A wonderful musty and heady aromatic fragrance issues from the summer blossoms of the lime tree or linden (not the same as the citrus tree bearing green fruits). It is a good herb for the nervous system, sedating, calming, and relaxing. It relieves spasms, improves digestion, and often helps migraines and high blood pressure. It is also used for circulatory problems like hardening of the arteries, and for urinary infections and catarrh. It is commonly grown and used in France, Germany, and Britain.

MAHONIA (*MAHONIA AQUIFOLIUM*)

Parts used: root, root bark, and occasionally the fruit
This is a very common hedgerow plant found all over Britain. It is native to North America, where it grows prolifically. Native Americans used it to treat the liver and skin. Mahonia has the ability to inhibit the overproduction of skin cells associated with psoriasis and is used frequently in Germany for this purpose with great success. Whenever you see barberry (*Berberis*) mentioned in a formula, mahonia will often do just as well. It also has a beneficial effect on the bowel because, by stimulating bile flow, it helps stimulate peristalsis, which helps release toxins. If you don't want to dig the roots up, then just collect a bunch of the grapelike fruits in autumn. The yellow spring flowers bring attention to its use as a liver herb.

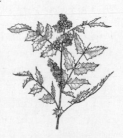

NETTLE (*URTICA DIOICA*)

Parts used: leaf and root
Nettles are rich in many vitamins, minerals, and trace elements, and are particularly high in available calcium, magnesium, and iron. Nettle is a wonderful blood cleanser and will greatly help anemia (along with any excess menstruation or hemorrhage). It is an old European rheumatism and arthritis remedy and

was originally brought to Britain by the Romans. British settlers brought it in turn to North America, where it has naturalized.

OAK (*QUERCUS ROBUR*)

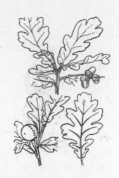

Parts used: bark, leaf, gall, and acorn
The oak is a bitter, astringent plant, rich in antiviral and antibacterial chemistry. Because of the strongly astringent qualities of its tannis, only small amounts can be taken internally. It is ideal for treating some types of diarrhea. It is also a wonderful treatment for the immune system. But it is mainly used for mouthwashes and as a gargle for sore throats and for gum and mouth problems. Relatives of this tree were a staple food source for many indigenous tribes around California, where the white oak still grows in profusion. Flour from the acorns really sustained these people, who often left the acorns in water for days to wash away the tannin and then crushed them. The resultant paste was very nutritious and good for boosting immunity.

PLANTAIN (*PLANTAGO MAJOR*)

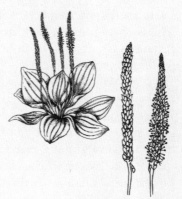

Parts used: leaf and juice
This roadside herb (not the banana relative) is a wonderful immune stimulant and can be taken internally for bacterial infection or put directly on wounds as a fresh poultice. It also has antihistaminic properties, which make it useful for treating allergies, insect bites, and so on. It cools, helps reduce inflammation, and acts as an efficient blood and lymph cleanser.

RED CLOVER (*TRIFOLIUM PRATENSE*)

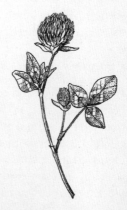

Part used: flower
Red clover is an unequaled blood cleanser used for degenerative diseases and specifically for cancers of the lymphatic system and bloodstream. It is also capable of relaxing spasms and will help release water retention and induce sweating when needed. Its red flower gives a huge clue to its blood-cleansing capabilities.

ST. JOHN'S WORT *(HYPERICUM PERFORATUM)*

Parts used: flower and top leaves

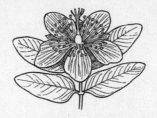

This yellow flower, which blooms at the summer solstice, has been used for a century in Europe for a wide variety of diseases, both internal and external. The list is impressive, and modern research is now able to support its older uses— externally for wounds, bruises, burns, and nerve pain (including dental), internally for liver and gallbladder complaints, bladder and lung problems, dysentery, worms, diarrhea, hysteria, and nervous complaints. Sales of St. John's wort outstrip those of Prozac in Germany because it has the ability to heighten serotonin levels in the brain. (St. John's wort should not be taken with drugs containing serotonin; it can also cause sensitivity to light in some individuals. It is advisable to seek professional advice before taking this herb.)

YARROW *(ACHILLEA MILLEFOLIUM)*

Parts used: flower and leaf

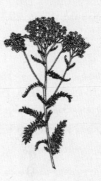

Yarrow is commonly found along road and field verges. Aromatic and bitter, it affects digestion favorably and lowers blood pressure. As a strong astringent it can staunch heavy blood loss. In Europe and North America, it has traditionally been used for fevers, colds, flu, and other viral diseases.

EUCALYPTUS (VARIOUS SPECIES)

Part used: leaf

Rich in rutin, this tree's leaves not only help strengthen the walls of the vascular system but, as a strong antiviral, make a wonderful tea for treating flu, colds, coughs, and more. It is used for the treatment of malaria all over the world.

JUNIPER (VARIOUS SPECIES)

Parts used: leaf and berry

This is another antimicrobial plant with a particular affinity to the urinary tract. The leaves of this shrub are used; make them up as a tea. A few juniper berries can also be used over a short term.

PINE (VARIOUS SPECIES)

Parts used: needle and resin

As a prime antioxidant, a cup of tea a day made from the needles will keep your body literally "alive." Pine is also a strong antiviral and anti-infection aid.

GINKGO (*GINKGO BILOBA*)

Part used: leaf
Favored for its ability to enhance brain and memory functions, ginkgo also has prime immunosupportive chemistry as well as vascular maintenance properties. A simple tea can be made at any time of year from the leaves, but late summer yellow-green ones are the best.

Book List

Advanced Treatise on Herbology by Dr. Edward E. Shook (Hastings, UK: Society of Metaphysicians Ltd., 1928)

A Field Guide to Western Medicinal Plants and Herbs by Steven Foster and Christopher Hobbs. The Peterson Field Guide Series (Boston: Houghton, Mifflin Co., 2002)

Forest Gardening by Robert Hart (Bideford, UK: Chelsea Green Publishing Co., 1996)

Herbal Medicine-Maker's Handbook by James Green (Berkeley, California: Crossings Press, 1996)

Herbal Renaissance: Growing, Using, and Understanding Herbs in the Modern World by Steven Foster (Layton, Utah: Gibbs Smith, Publisher, 1984)

Rolling Thunder by Doug Boyd (New York: Dell Publishing, 1974)

Tom Brown's Guide to Wild Edible and Medicinal Plants by Tom Brown Jr. (New York: Berkeley Books, 1985)

✤ 3 ✤

The Plants Themselves

Best-Quality Herbs

The best herbs to use for medicinal or culinary purposes are those collected from the wild, in areas where the plant is found growing naturally, away from contaminants. Unfortunately, the colossal increase in demand for herbs has meant that some of the time, they are being collected from unsuitable wild sources, such as roadside verges, and that wild sources are being overplundered.

The huge increase in demand and a belated desire for quality have led to an upsurge in organically grown herbs. Hundreds upon hundreds of acres of herbs are now being grown in parts of Europe (in particular Germany) and worldwide. Dr. John Christopher was a pioneer on the subject of organics. He insisted upon organic and wild-crafted herbs for medicinal purposes. So much of illness today is based upon allergies to pollution and toxicity levels that we don't want to add to it. Botanical herbalists know that plants growing in the wild will produce more "primitive" and original chemistry as they fight to survive selective pressures, resulting in some aggressive chemical variations. For instance, with the herb cascara sagrada *(Rhamnus purshiana)*, which is heavily harvested in the temperate rain forests of North America, demand instigated its cultivation in an area where it grows wild! This effort turned out to be unsuccessful, as the laxative effect of the cultivated variety was shown to be much less potent than that of the wild-harvested bark. However, in April 2002, the U.S. Fish and Wildlife Service listed cascara sagrada in CITES (Convention in Trade in Endangered Species) in their Appendix II category. This category houses species that are not threatened with extinction but may become so if international trade is not controlled. The monoculture of herbs will increase over time and, in the long term, could alter the chemistry of plants and eventually may even forever change them genetically. I have no personal answer to this problem, because we have a great need for herbs, we have diminished land, and we do not want to defoliate our wild areas. Many native U.S. medicinal plant species are being considered for inclusion into CITES Appendix III (a category which requires the cooperation of other countries to prevent unsustainable or illegal exploitation). These plants include black cohosh, echinacea, and osha *(Ligusticum porteri)*.

The question of good-quality herbs was always a vital one to herbalist John Christopher, and it was a treat to find his standard of excellence at a time that many people paid little attention to such details. He insisted on using only clean, wild-crafted or organic herbs, processing them in a way that retained their vibrancy and quality, much as earlier herbalists had done. Pesticides are a fact of modern farming methods, and "poisoned herbs" could be found in his day just as they are now. Dr. Christopher taught his students to choose carefully the sources from which they bought their herbs and to check how they were stored and later prepared. For this reason, he liked herbalists to prepare and even pick their own herbs, in order to make their own tinctures, ointments, and other preparations to a high standard.

He even went as far as to insist that anything prepared for external use should be of the same quality as that for internal use. His legacy of high standards lives on with many of his students, now excellent herbalists in their own right. To this day, herbal preparations vary in their quality and, sadly, I have met people who have not had beneficial experiences from some preparations. This is very likely due to the poor quality of the original herb or to the way it was prepared.

Twenty years ago it was hard to find organically grown herbs, so my personal choice was to grow my own as much as possible, to seek out organic herb growers in Britain, and to import from American wild-crafters when I needed to. Nowadays, needs and trends have changed dramatically, and access to good-quality herbs has become relatively easy. Nevertheless, my own experiences do not necessarily reflect the norm, so the whole issue deserves a closer look.

There is a recognized need for greater control on herb quality. As a result, rules and regulations have been put into place in Britain by the Medicines and Healthcare products Regulatory Agency (MHRA) which is addressing the quality, origins, storage, and preparation of herbs grown in or imported into Britain. The problem of quality has become more pressing in recent years as herbalism's popularity increased the need for herbs. To meet the ever growing demand, a few importers have become less fussy, and some herbs have been substituted or adulterated—as has been proved by laboratory testing.

Toxic metals have been found among some imported herbs. Fecal matter has been found among some crude herbs—where human feces have been used to fertilize fields. Radioactive waste has also been found, as some herbs are still collected in and around disaster areas, often by poor people who are eager to make a living and for whom herb collecting is still a way of life. Medical and other toxic wastes are buried or burned, and the fumes and leakages from these can contaminate the herbs in the area. Since the 1940s, there has been a thirty-three-fold increase in the use of pesticides, including insecticides, herbicides, fungicides, and other agents, with a tenfold increase in potency. Pesticide use on herbs is disastrous. According to the U.S. National Cancer Institute, cancer rates increase by seven or eight times through ingestion of pesticide-contaminated foods—not something that sits comfortably with herbs that are going to be used for medicine.

Sulfured herbs are now available; apricots and peaches are sulfured to keep their color and for storage, but do we want sulfured herbs as well? Rodents and insects are sometimes found among herbs. Microbes—for example fungi and bacteria—need to be kept to a minimum, but herbs are often sprayed in transit with noxious chemicals like ethylene oxide, thus causing them to become toxic. Bacteria such as *E. coli* and those causing typhus have been found in herbs, particularly low-growing plants, during monsoon seasons.

Some herbs are sprayed with antibiotics to bypass the need for expensive laboratory testing to determine toxicity and microbial levels (which are often unacceptably high). The resulting products are called pretreated and passed as "clean." Another way in which herb companies have sought to "clean up" herbs is by using autoclaving, a cleaning process that utilizes steam. Originally used solely for surgical tools, this sterilization technique is now used on herbs in an attempt to lessen severely the risk of contamination. Yet another method is to irradiate herbs, another controversial process that is routinely used on some foods. Very often the fact that the product has been irradiated is not put on the label, and recently some companies in Britain selling imported herbs were prosecuted for not disclosing this information.

In other cases the MHRA tested commonly sold, over-the-counter herbal remedies and some of the results were shocking though not surprising. Many were found to contain very little or almost no actual active herb ingredients. Often ash was the main constituent. This is what brings herbs into disrepute and fuels the "they don't work" problem which is common to Britain and worldwide. (For high quality U.S. herbs see the American Botanical Pharmacy on page xii.)

The bottom line is that organic (or clean, wild-collected) herbs have to become the only type of herb acceptable to the industry, which can happen if the public demands it. Exclusive use of such herbs needs to be coupled with procedures to analyze each plant's authenticity of species and with use of appropriate storage facilities, including storage of fresh tinctures or freeze-dried herbs, to ensure minimum spoilage and maximum potency.

Plants as Investments and Moneymakers

Plants are becoming an increasingly profitable investment. Europe, the United States, Japan, China, Brazil, and Mexico have been swept by a huge demand for herbs, which has led to an enormous increase in profits. In China, sales of traditional medicines more than doubled between 1998 and 2003, while India's booming export trade in medicinal plants rose almost threefold during the 1990s. In Germany, more than 80 percent of all physicians regularly use herbal products. In the United States, herbs and natural supplements were a $12 billion business in 1998, double the total in 1994. Britain, like everywhere else, is being swept along on the herb revival boom.

At the same time, pharmaceutical companies were not doing so well financially, and a lot of companies have swallowed up rivals in a bid to survive. In 1990, the pharmaceutical market profit was 15 percent; by 1994 it had fallen to 9 percent. In the West, this drop in revenue has halted research programs, as the money to fund them simply hasn't been available. Consequently, scientists were asked to be more creative! One idea they have developed is to focus on the older generation and the problems of aging. With the World Health Organization predicting that the incidence of cancer will double or triple as the number of older people increases, this age group would seem a likely target.

Another trend, already apparent in some areas of alternative medicine, is the move to bypass the doctor and sell more products directly to the public, either over the counter or through mail order. Pharmaceutical companies have begun "copying" herbs, and this trend should grow in the years to come. Several pharmaceutical companies are investigating methods for standardizing plant-based medicines. In the past, only single-molecule botanicals could be identified. Without proper identification, researchers could not prove the safety and efficacy of other plant agents, because there were batch-to-batch inconsistencies. Previously, pharmaceutical companies would not submit applications for herbal medicines because companies could not receive patents for them. However, recently a pharmaceutical company has developed the first pharmaceutical versions of multimolecule herbal medicines by standardizing the active molecules and their interactions. Meanwhile, other so-called herbal concoctions are now being sold by other pharmaceutical companies. A qualified herbal practitioner would not see these developments as herbs and certainly they must be treated as drugs, licensed as such, and their side effects given due heed.

Cuts have been made to research programs that study single herbs and try to isolate their "magic bullet" components. For years, pharmaceutical companies threw away the best bits of the plant while looking for that magic bullet. This problem was reflected in a lesson learned in 1995: flavonoids are a component of many plants, but these compounds had been regularly discarded for twenty years. Flavonoids are now known to be antioxidants—a now old buzzword among the more nutritionally aware. Antioxidants are known to inhibit and treat a wide range of illnesses and conditions including cancer, strokes, heart disease, emphysema, late-onset diabetes, rheumatism, arthritis, ulcers, cataracts, Crohn's disease, senility, arteriosclerosis, and old age; flavonoids do this by preventing our cells from "rusting" or aging. In hindsight, this lesson was indeed a bitter and costly one.

Now pharmaceutical companies are looking at multispecies herbal formulas, using many herbs in mixtures that are then tested. This is how herbalists have always worked! Our ancestors grazed plants in the days of hunting and gathering, ingesting a broad range of plant species, which kept them well. Now science is beginning to look down this avenue in the hope that its next billion lies at the end of it. It may well do, but I feel we can graze for ourselves. When some drugs come to the end of their patents and therefore their value as revenues expire (which will be soon, in some cases), the pharmaceutical industry will, no doubt, make an even greater investment in "natural" Green pills.

Plant Collecting and Drying

Plant chemistry varies according to the time of day and season. Traditionally, some plants were always collected prior to sunrise, and others were never collected after sunset. In all, plant harvesting practices included many important quirks, which are now being proved to be of value through scientific evaluation. It is possible to identify some basic guiding principles:

Leaves: Spring leaves are best because they have new sap in them. Their energy has not yet been drawn away to produce flowers or seeds.

Bark: Spring is the best time to collect bark, just as the sap rises. This is also when the newly formed bark is most easily cut off.

Flowers: These are at their peak just after they have opened.

Seeds: These are at their peak in late summer and early autumn.

Berries: Usually autumn is the best time to collect berries. Look for good, deep color and tight, glowing skin.

Roots, rhizomes, root bark, and tubers: Collect in late autumn when all the top foliage has died down, but before the nutrients stored in them are used during the winter and spring. Springtime is an option and will produce a slightly different chemistry, but spring collecting should be done before major foliage and stem production has begun.

Once harvested, the way in which herbs are dried and stored is of paramount importance. When a herb is picked, it immediately starts to decay; bacteria and fungi increase, and the plant's potency ebbs with its color, smell, and texture. It is vital to arrest this process as quickly as possible. The water content and type of fibrous material to be dried out varies for each plant, and some plants need to have their readily lost oils conserved very efficiently. Still others are more affected by the climate; for example, if it is constantly damp and rainy, fungal spores can completely destroy the plant. General rules for drying are to keep the plant out of direct sunlight and in constant aerated heat.

Basic Preparations of Herbs

A herb is sometimes used on its own or sometimes as part of a formula that contains several herbs. The latter, termed *polypharmacy*, employs a teamwork effect that is appropriate when the power of a single herb needs to be supplemented. Very often the formula consists of one main herb with others acting as support. The support team can be made up of one or two herbs, or even ten or twelve. The main herb may, for example, be required to soothe impaired tissue, while the others assist in nourishment, help eliminate toxins, assist in nerve or blood supply, or calm and sedate. These single or multiple herb choices can be prepared as teas (infusions), decoctions, tinctures, syrups, capsules, ointments, compresses, poultices, suppositories, pessaries, douches, essential oils, herbal oils, smudge sticks, or powders.

Differing forms of administering a herb or herbs are chosen for whether external or internal uses are needed. Also, a choice has to be made regarding by what means the specific beneficial chemistries are to be extracted. For instance, the main chemical constituents in ginkgo leaf are best extracted using water, and therefore a tea or decoction is ideal; whereas for echinacea root, alcohol is best, and therefore a tincture is ideal. Sometimes methods can be combined, thus taking advantage of all available chemistries. As mentioned before, all plants used in the basic preparation of herbs should be organic or wild-crafted. For information on the specific plants referred to by common name, see appendix 1.

HERBAL TEAS — INFUSIONS

Teas and infusions can be made using a specialized teapot, or if you wish to make tea in a mug or cup, then a tea sock is ideal. A tea sock is a simple cotton sock on a wire rim that holds the herbs and can be set into a mug, cup, or pot and left to infuse in boiling water.

Use ½ to 1 ounce of dried herbs or 1 to 2 ounces of fresh herbs to 3 cups of distilled water. Infuse the herbs in a mug or teapot for five to twenty-five minutes, then strain out the herbs and discard. Chamomile is the only exception—use ½ ounce of this herb to 3 cups of water and infuse for only five minutes.

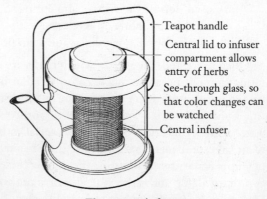

Teapot handle

Central lid to infuser compartment allows entry of herbs

See-through glass, so that color changes can be watched

Central infuser

The teapot infuser

Dosage Guide for a Seven-Minute Infusion

Adults:	3 cups a day
Children aged 3 to 12:	1½ cups a day
Children under 3:	¾ cup a day
Adults over 70:	1½ cups a day
Adults over 75:	¾ cup a day

You can mix many herbs together. In fact, it's better to do so, because that way you get a range of chemical properties and effects, and no one herb can dominate in either flavor or effect. Change your herb mixes regularly.

DECOCTIONS

A decoction is similar to a herbal tea but is designed for using the harder parts of herbs, such as nuts and hard seeds, barks, or rhizomes and roots. With these harder parts of plants, an infusion may not extract all the medicinal properties that are locked into them. Therefore, you need to heat them for a longer period of time.

A basic decoction is made by adding ½ ounce to 1 ounce (depending on how bulky the pieces are) of dried herbs to 3 cups of cold springwater (1 cup may evaporate during boiling). If you have the time, it is best to let the herbs soak and rehydrate in the water for up to twelve hours, and then slowly bring the mixture up to a boil. Let it simmer for between ten to thirty minutes.

Divide the resultant liquid (approximately 2 cups worth) into three glasses and drink at intervals throughout the day.

TINCTURES

These are mixtures in which the medicinal components of herbs have been extracted, ideally into organic grain alcohol or vinegar. To make a standard quantity of alcohol or vinegar tincture at home, use 8 ounces of dried roots, berries, leaves, or flowers, or 16 ounces of fresh material, with enough vodka to cover—a minimum of 32 fluid ounces (1 quart).

1. Place the chosen material in a blender or food processor and cover with vodka; standard 45-proof is effective, but 70- to 80-proof is even better. Blend the ingredients. If using berries, the mixture will be particularly stiff and hard, making it difficult for the blades to turn and requiring more vodka to get them to break down. Once the mixture is well blended, pour the tincture into a dark, airtight container—a dark glass jar with a rubber seal is ideal.

2. Shake well, label the jar carefully, then store it in a cool place out of direct sunlight.

3. After two days, measure the contents and add water. For dried berries, leaves, and flowers, add 20 percent of the volume if using 45-proof vodka, and 50 to 60 percent of the volume if using 70- to 80-proof vodka. Leave for two to four weeks, shaking at least twice a day.

4. Strain the mixture through a jelly bag, preferably overnight, until you have strained the last drop. For the best result, use a wine press.

5. Pour the resultant liquid into dark jars, label, and store in a cool, dark place. For personal use, decant into a 2-ounce tincture bottle.

Some herbalists like to plan the making of tinctures around the moon phases, using the gravitational waxing and waning of the moon to add power and energy as the old herb alchemists did. To do this, start the process when the moon is new, then strain and bottle at the full moon.

To keep tinctures over a long period of time, seal the stopper with wax and store in a dark place. If you wish to avoid the alcohol when administering a tincture internally, you may evaporate 98 to 99 percent of the alcohol from the solution by putting it into a little boiling water. Otherwise, simply add your tincture to a little cold or warm water or to fruit juice.

The average recommended dosage for tinctures made from berries, leaves, flowers, barks, root barks, rhizomes, and seeds varies from herb to herb, so consult a herbal practitioner for guidance.

Dosage for Everyday and Long-Term Use

Adults:	1 teaspoon of tincture that has been diluted in 5 teaspoons of water (or fruit juice), two to three times daily, for a total intake of approximately 3 teaspoons per day
Children aged 7 to 12:	half of adult dose
Children aged 3 to 7:	one-quarter of adult dose
Children under 3:	2 to 5 drops twice a day

Dosage varies from individual to individual and depending on whether or not a single herb or a formula is being used.

Commercially produced tinctures of a professional standard can be used. Some are of a very high quality, but always choose those that use organic or wild-crafted herbs. Some combine tinctures with infusions and decoctions for extra benefit.

HERBAL SYRUPS

A herbal syrup is basically a maceration, an infusion, a decoction, or occasionally a tincture to which maple syrup, vegetable glycerin, or honey has been added. These substances are added mainly to preserve the solution, but they also give the liquid a thicker and stickier consistency, making it much more palatable to children. I prefer to use maple syrup and have done so successfully in my clinic for several years. Most children can be induced to take any herbal tincture by adding 25 to 50 percent maple syrup.

Syrups were traditionally made by reducing a decoction down to less than its original amount and then adding sugar or runny honey. If you slowly simmer a decoction down to half its original quantity, you will have what used to be referred to as a three-power decoction. If you simmer a three-power decoction down to half this amount again, you will have a six-power decoction. By adding maple syrup to this, you get a three- or six-power syrup. Try to find organic maple syrup (instead of sugar).

Dosage Guide

Follow the dosage guidelines given for tinctures.

Onion and garlic syrup: This syrup can be used to prevent and ward off colds, chills, and fevers and to generally empower the immune system. Chop organic garlic and onions, or put them into the food processor or blender. If you use fresh organic garlic and onions, you can use the whole plant. Cover with vegetable glycerin and a pint of honey, if it is of very good quality — that is to say, the bees should not have been fed on sugar during the winter, and the honey should not have been heat-treated. Some rain forest honeys are good for this, or maple syrup. Add one tablespoon of lemon juice. Alternatively, you can puree the onions, garlic, and syrup together, which is quicker but requires more syrup.

Elder flower and elderberry compote syrup: Just as fruit compotes are made throughout the summer in Europe, you can make herbal compotes, adding herbs as they come into flower or fruit. Use vegetable glycerin, runny honey or maple syrup, and lemon juice if desired, instead of the brandy and sugar used in conventional recipes for fruit compotes.

Begin with elder flowers, which appear in June; their white, flat petticoats should be picked just as they burst out of their buds. Pull the white flowers off the green stalks and put them into a wide-necked jar. You can add more every day or so, but each time cover the flowers with the vegetable glycerin or maple syrup. For a combined mix, a good ratio is roughly a pint of vegetable glycerin to a cup of maple syrup to a tablespoon of fresh lemon juice. A cheaper version uses only vegetable glycerin with a tablespoon of freshly squeezed lemon juice added to every pint of glycerin.

Stand this mix outside to catch all available sunshine, but if the weather is relentlessly cold and gray, keep it in a warm, but not hot, place indoors.

As time goes by, the flowers will compact and the upper part of the jar will contain only syrup. Add more flowers and fill the gap, but never let the flowers rise above the syrup; this often proves difficult! Shake daily, preferably more than once, to keep them down, because if the flowers don't remain in the syrup, they will oxidize, turn brown, and ferment. After at least two weeks, you can strain the syrup off from the flowers, discard the flowers, and then add fresh ones to increase the strength.

In Britain and Canada in September and October, the wine-red elderberries of *Sambucus nigra* appear (a variety which is safe and healthy to eat and which is made into cough syrups due to its highly antiviral compounds); collect these when fully ripe but not moldy in any way and add them to the strained syrup, this time pureeing the whole lot in order to crush the berries. The resulting syrup is thick and full-bodied. Shake daily. You can likewise place it in any dwindling autumn sunshine, and strain and add more berries if you wish. The resulting brew, which is ready to consume by mid to late October, is so tasty that everyone who samples it will let you know immediately that they feel a little shivery—so make plenty!

HERBAL CAPSULES

There are two types of empty gelatin capsules—those of vegetable origin (preferred by vegans) and those of animal origin. To use, mix powdered herbs together (if using a formula) and fill the capsules by putting the powder in a saucer and scooping powder into both ends. Then push the two ends together; one will overlap the other. You can buy little machines to do this for you or purchase ready-made capsules. Capsules are ideal for use in bowel remedies, where the chemical constituents need to reach the colon. Otherwise tinctures, teas, decoctions, or freeze-dried herbs are preferred because they will be fresher or reach the bloodstream more quickly. For people who cannot take large quantities of fersh garlic, it can be chopped and put into capsules; but use them immediately, otherwise the garlic will dissolve the gelatin. Capsules can also be useful for those who are unable to take hot cayenne pepper on a teaspoon.

Dosage Guide

Adults:	2 capsules two to four times a day
Children aged 7 to 12:	1 capsule two to four times a day
Children aged 3 to 7:	1 capsule twice a day
Children under 3:	capsules often not advised

OINTMENTS

Ointments are used for their protective and emollient effect, liquefying when applied. They are generally made from a mixture of herbs, oils (preferably virgin olive oil), essential oils, and beeswax. The herbs absorb the oils, and the wax gives firmness to the ointment.

To make an ointment, pour olive oil over the chosen powdered herbs. A good standard is 1 cup olive oil for 12 ounces dried herbs. Place in a closed container (stainless steel, earthenware, unchipped enamel, or glass) and either put into the oven and leave there at low heat (100°F) for an hour, or stand in the sun or some other warm spot for a week. Periodically, take a fork and stir the mixture. Leave for a further week to macerate (if using the oven method, heat up again before continuing). Strain by passing the mixture through a piece of muslin lining a large plastic or stainless steel colander; alternatively use a jelly bag and hang overnight. Finally, melt 1.75 ounces beeswax in a double boiler or sauce pan with a very thick base using a very low temperature, and add the herbal olive oil. Have glass jars at the ready and put a little of the liquid into one to check that it is the correct consistency for use: solid but not hard, that is, still spreadable. Do not forget to label your ointments. See "Other Items" in chapter 11 for formulas.

Dosage Guide

Apply two to three times daily, or more frequently if necessary.

COMPRESSES

A compress is basically a herbal infusion or decoction applied directly to the skin using a piece of cloth, gauze, or towel, always one made of natural fibers like cotton. Compresses can be made with any liquid at any temperature, but a hot herbal tea or decoction is commonly used. Other possible ways to make a compress are by using various vegetable oils, apple cider vinegar, and essential oils.

To make a herbal tea compress, first prepare an infusion or decoction in the usual way. Then dip a piece of cloth into the solution, the size of the cloth being proportional to the area of the body you want to cover. Wring out excess liquid, and apply the cloth to the affected area. You may wish to keep the fluid hot and keep dipping the cloth back into it every few minutes as it cools. Placing a heavy towel, plastic wrap, or hot water bottle over the compress will help it retain its heat longer. Replace when the heat has ceased.

A good way to increase circulation in any area of the body is to alternate the hot compress with a cold one. Place a wet, ice-cold cloth on the area for a few minutes, and then follow with a similar application of a hot compress.

You may decide at some point to leave the compress on for a long period of time. In this case, you will want to cover it with plastic wrap and then extra towels, and definitely a hot water bottle. Leave on for up to two hours. Using different temperatures encourages circulation in the affected area and will relieve congestion. While the hot compress pulls impurities from the body, the cold compress temporarily constricts the blood flow and circulation to the area. This can soothe discomfort caused by too much exposure to heat and will reduce unwanted swelling and pain. A mixture of the two will increase circulation threefold.

POULTICES

A poultice differs from a compress in that, instead of the infusion or decoction being applied to the body, the herb or herb oil itself is applied. This can be done very simply by just "bruising" a herb leaf (crushing it slightly) and applying it to the skin; plantain leaves, mullein flowers, and comfrey leaf poultices are good examples and are ideal for sprains. Another common method is to mix dried, cut, or powdered herbs together and add water, apple cider vinegar, or another appropriate liquid such as olive oil to form a paste, which is then applied to the skin. I have found that also adding some mucilaginous herb powder, such as slippery elm bark, to the mixture creates a consistency that will adhere more effectively. With a non-oil-based poultice, a little oil applied over the area to be treated will make the poultice feel more comfortable.

When using a poultice on a hole in the body, or on a deep wound, you will first need to clean the area with a solution of essential oil and water—for example, one drop lavender essential oil and one drop tea tree essential oil in a cup of water—before applying the poultice. Then you will need to add some anti-infection herbs to the poultice, such as turmeric rhizome, myrrh resin, or thyme leaf. There is another rule for treating a wound: Once the poultice has dried, it may seem that some of it has disappeared or been absorbed into the body. Don't clean the remaining poultice off—add a new poultice over the old one and keep "feeding" the area. Once a poultice has dried onto a wound, I consider it a part of the body, just like a scab—it will come off when it's time, or it will grow into and become the flesh itself. There are, however, some types of poultice, especially drawing ones, that need to be changed frequently because they will have absorbed toxins that need to be removed from the body.

Poultices can be used to treat itching skin and other skin irritations and to draw out the poisons of stings and bites. They can also be used to heat an area (for example, a mustard plaster) and for glandular infections or congestion. A poultice can also be applied between two layers of gauze or light cotton if you don't want the actual herb to touch the skin for some reason.

As a poultice dries, it becomes taut and draws out impurities. You can add drawing herbs or even refined clay, which increases this "pulling" power. This type of poultice is ideal for tumors and cancers; herbs like pokeweed root may be used to assist in the treatment of breast cancer, while the addition of powdered charcoal will help purify the blood.

Vegetable poultices have also been used widely over the years, made from potatoes, onions, carrots, beets, garlic, cucumbers, aloe vera, and a wide variety of greens. Cayenne, ginger, mustard, and horseradish have all been popular for heating and stimulating poultices. Healing and soothing poultices made from comfrey leaf, slippery elm bark, marshmallow root, aloe leaf or gel, calendula flower, lobelia leaves and seed, and mullein flower have been used extensively. Seed and grain poultices have also been used over the years with very soothing effects, along with fruit poultices using bananas, figs, apples, papayas, and melons. Plantain leaf is a prime drawing herb used in poultices and is also a blood cleanser. Every kitchen contains an onion, and this can be heated in the oven and placed over the affected area for pain relief.

CASTOR-OIL PACKS

Castor-oil packs are useful for easing pain and inflammation. They can also relieve congestion and draw out toxins. Construct a muslin or flannel pack to the appropriate size and soak it in warmed castor oil. The temperature on the body should be as hot as is bearable, because the heat will force the castor oil into the area. After placing on the body, hold in place and cover with plastic wrap and a hot water bottle. The duration that the pack is left on will vary. Some packs are changed for new ones every hour or so in order to keep them hot. Some may be left on overnight, or just for thirty minutes. Another option is to apply a pack for thirty minutes every four hours.

GARLIC PASTE FOR FEET

This treatment is an excellent aid for any respiratory disorders. Peel eight cloves of garlic and puree with equal parts of olive oil, water, and slippery elm bark. Apply a generous amount of petroleum jelly to the soles of the feet (to prevent burning of the skin) followed by a layer of the garlic paste. Cover with fine muslin bandages and an old pair of baggy socks; you can even tie plastic bags over these. This paste should be checked every two hours to ensure that the garlic is not burning the soles of the feet.

SUPPOSITORIES AND PESSARIES

Suppositories and pessaries are herbal poultices that are used internally. The base is generally made with a mucilaginous herb like slippery elm inner bark powder and a lubricant such as coconut oil or cocoa butter. Other powdered herbs that treat the particular problem are added to the base. These are inserted into body openings (vagina, rectum, nasal cavities, ears, or mouth) in order to disperse their herbal constituents to internal areas. Suppositories and pessaries are made in the same way and are commonly used for rectal cleansing, vaginal infections, irritation, inflammation, and general problems in the reproductive area.

When making a suppository, you will need finely powdered and sieved herbs in order to make the result as smooth as possible. The size of the suppository will depend on the area that it will be inserted into.

Take a jar of coconut oil and place it in a bowl of hot water. In a short time the oil will melt. Mix the melted coconut oil with the finely powdered herbs until the mixture forms a pastrylike consistency. Form the herb mixture into the size and shape of suppository you desire.

Place the individual suppositories on a piece of waxed paper, or a stainless steel or glass plate, and refrigerate them. Refrigeration will make them hard. When you want to use one, take it out of the refrigerator, hold it between your fingers for just a few seconds (the coconut oil will begin to melt), and then insert. Use some olive oil to lubricate the area of insertion first. When the suppository is inside the body, the body temperature, which is always variable, will cause the coconut oil to melt and the herbs will be dispersed.

Vaginal pessaries: Use equal parts of the following in powder form: squaw vine leaf, slippery elm inner bark, yellow dock root, comfrey root, chickweed leaf and stem, barberry root bark, mullein leaf and flower, plus half a drop each of geranium essential oil and lavender essential oil in a cocoa butter base.

Candida pessaries: Use nine parts slippery elm bark, three parts barberry root, three parts *pau d'arco* inner bark, two parts black walnut hull, one part chamomile flower, one part lavender flower, and tea tree essential oil in a coconut oil base.

Start with a treatment of seven pessaries, using one every night, or one every third or fourth night. Insert into the vagina. If you wish, use a sanitary napkin to protect night clothing, bed linens, and so on; but the more air allowed to circulate around the affected area, the better. The coconut butter melts at body temperature overnight (or it may be longer, depending on the individual woman's basal temperature), leaving the herbs to be absorbed into the body. Any remaining herbs are easy to douche out every three or four days or can be expelled by doing pelvic floor exercises in a bath containing a few drops of lavender essential oil and five tablespoons of cider vinegar. On dressing in the morning, use a natural sponge to prevent leakage; you may even need the extra protection of a sanitary napkin.

Anal suppositories: Ideal for hemorrhoids. Use equal parts of black walnut hull, horse chestnut fruit, eucalyptus leaf, slippery elm bark, and yarrow leaves, plus a few drops of witch hazel essential oil in a base of cocoa butter.

DOUCHES

Douches are herbal liquids gently inserted into the vagina (using a douche bag), usually in the form of a herbal infusion or decoction using vegetable, nut, or seed oils, or aloe vera leaf gel.

An example of douche herbs would be a premade decoction of an equal amount of chamomile flower, *pau d'arco* inner bark, barberry root bark, and lavender flowers and leaves. This formula is capable of promoting resistance to a range of fungi and bacteria.

Douches can be used to wash out the residue of the pessaries or simply to cleanse the area.

ESSENTIAL OILS — THE COMPACT PHARMACY

Essential oils are extracted from flowers, grasses, fruits, leaves, roots, and trees. There are, at present, more than three hundred different types of essential oils available, which form an extremely efficient medical system. Many essential oils form the basis of modern pharmaceutical preparations.

The wonderful benefits of essential oils must be respected. Applied directly and undiluted to the skin, they will burn, except in the case of lavender. Some people, following advice in books, have put pure essential oils (particularly tea tree oil) onto cuts, skin abrasions, and skin problems. Tea tree burns are common because this essential oil has been advised for direct skin use. Some people can indeed tolerate it, but a patch test is advisable.

If an essential oil has been applied directly in undiluted form and is burning, treat with aloe vera gel, olive oil, wheat germ oil, or any thick vegetable oil you have at hand. Do not use water, as it will amplify the burning effect.

Methods of Use and Dosage for Essential Oils

Tissue and handkerchief: Put one drop on and sniff when required.

Inhaled as a vapor: Add two to three drops to a bowl of steaming-hot water and cover the head and bowl with a towel; keep your face a foot above the surface of the water and inhale the vapor.

Massage oil: Use approximately ¼ to ½ teaspoon essential oil to 1 cup base oil.

Baths: Add a maximum of eight drops.

Vegetable base oils: Nut or seed oils are best. If in doubt, use cold-pressed virgin olive oil.

HERBAL OILS

Place your chosen and preferably fresh herb in a blender with a little olive oil or fractionated coconut oil—both are nonrancid, safe, stable base oils in which the herbs can be macerated. The cutting of the herbs will release the essential oils into the base oil. The ratio is approximately 4 ounces dried material to 3 cups of oil, but if you use fresh material, use about 6 ounces. Place this maceration in the sunshine and allow to steep for two weeks. Shake regularly. If you wish, you can strengthen it by straining the liquid, discarding the residual herbs, and beginning the process again with a new batch of herbs.

For a warming body oil and rub, use a tablespoon of each of the following herbs: English mustard seed, hot chile powder, fresh ground ginger, and black pepper. Cover the ingredients with olive oil. Steep for a month and add essential oils of peppermint and camphor for extra heat.

Essential oils are being used increasingly today, and this demand has led, in some cases, to inferior quality. Toxins are sometimes not removed, and occasionally the best bits of the essential oils are removed. Testing for oil quality is expensive but vital, ensuring that they are safe and reliable. Making your own as described above is easy and ensures high quality with no adulteration.

SMUDGE STICKS

These provide a lovely way of "fumigating" an area. The fragrance will change the atmosphere and help clean it. Native Americans traditionally used wormwood or white sage. You can make your own version using a combination of English sage, thyme, eucalyptus, rosemary, and wormwood.

Hold the herbs together in a tight bundle, then bind the bundle even more tightly using thick, pure cotton thread. Dry the bundles thoroughly and quickly, otherwise they will become moldy and unusable. To use, light and allow flame to take hold, then blow out, and use when smoldering.

POWDERS AND TALCS

These can be very useful treatments for chicken pox, shingles, summer heat rashes, athlete's foot, or any itching disease, especially where there are pustules that are weeping. You can even use it on weeping eczema.

Use two teaspoons of arrowroot, cornstarch, or fine corn flour. Mix with one teaspoon of a combination of finely powdered black walnut hull, thyme leaf, barberry root bark, and dried lavender leaf and flower, or any of these herbs singly.

Vaginal dusting powder: This is suitable for moist discharges and infections. Use a combination of ¼ ounce fine white clay or bentonite clay,

½ ounce arrowroot powder, ½ ounce black walnut hull powder, ½ ounce barberry root bark powder or turmeric rhizome powder, ½ ounce neem powder (if available), and ¼ ounce lavender leaf and flower powder. Either apply to the area as a powder or mix the powder with aloe vera gel and insert into the vagina. Aloe will cool the area in hot weather; however, the powder will dry up and absorb discharge.

Book List

American Herbalism: Essays on Herbs and Herbalism by Members of the American Herbalist Guild, edited by Michael Tierra (Berkeley, California: Crossing Press, 1992)

Aromatherapy: An A–Z by Patricia Davis (Saffron Walden, Essex, UK: C. W. Daniel Company, 1988)

Aromatherapy Handbook by Danielle Ryman (Saffron Walden, Essex, UK: C. W. Daniel Company, 1984)

Common Sense Health and Healing by Dr. Richard Schulze (Santa Monica, California: Natural Healing Publications, 2002)

Making Tinctures by James Green (San Francisco, California: Wildlife and Green Publications, n.d.)

The School of Natural Healing by Dr. John Christopher (Springville, Utah: Christopher Publications, 1976)

❧ 4 ❧

Food and Nutrition

The body runs on the fuel it is provided with. When we were hunters and gatherers, this fuel came in the form of foods collected in the wild, encompassing a diverse range of health-giving chemistry, to include components far beyond vitamins and minerals. For instance, archaeologists have found evening primrose seed on ancient European sites, leading us to believe that prehistoric men and women knew the value of the oil collected from these tiny seeds.

Archaeologists and anthropologists are also able to tell us of the diseases of ancient peoples. There is evidence to suggest that cancer, osteoporosis, rheumatism, and arthritis were often exacerbated by their working and living conditions, but also partly because their dietary needs were not always met—just as with modern man. They did not, however, have high quantities of sugar literally eating away their vital calcium, magnesium, zinc, and mineral supplies, with processed junk food creating a plethora of bowel diseases, cancers, and other disorders. They had the stress of survival on a day-to-day basis, but the adrenaline they produced to deal with these situations was more readily burned off. I rather feel that their instincts and needs were completely intact and, therefore, that their hormones, glands, brain, and organs functioned with a more natural rhythm and balance. Until recently there were quite a number of peoples who ate well and with variety from the wild. Mountain peoples of Iran, for example, typically caught wild meat and ate dishes often containing thirty to forty species of wild plants and herbs. But now wild meat and lots of the wild plants and knowledge of what to collect and how to use them have dwindled. Modern-day people of the so-called progressive Western world also have become less instinctive and their health less stable.

At whatever age, it can be difficult to make sure that nutritional needs are met. In the past, people had to travel and explore the great outdoors in order to find necessary medicine; but what do we do now? So much of what society considers food today should actually be avoided. It is strange to think that, in the average supermarket, at least 70 percent of the food for sale should not be consumed. And in order to obtain what we require, we have to be prepared to spend a lot of time in the kitchen (a way of life that our grandparents accepted without question).

In the 1920s and 1930s, juicers, able to create a nonbulky and highly assimilable form of nutrition, became popular. The 1950s and 1960s saw the development of vitamin, mineral, and other supplements made from animal parts, sea and land vegetables, minerals, and other derivatives. More recently, "superfood" drinks have been created using primary plants like algae and lichens—that is, using nature's potent forces. Finally, at the beginning of the twenty-first century, people—not least, the leading supplement companies—are turning to combining supplements and herbs.

What should we choose? As a daily matter of course, I would suggest good food with liberal amounts of culinary and wild herbs, with superfood drinks to balance the effects of pollution and stress. For those chronic deficiencies picked up through tests or diagnosis, it is wise to choose supplements, superfoods, juices, or a combination of them all.

Food builds us physically as well as nurturing us on a more subtle, unseen vibrational level. Many great minds, not least those of botanists, archaeologists, and herbalists, have recognized that, in the prefarming era, health rested largely on humans' consumption of many different species of plants. This contrasts with the modern, genetically engineered and overproduced twenty or so species that are farmed today. It was this diverse array of plant chemistry that kept our systems honed and hardy and allowed our immune systems to act with force and spontaneity. It enabled our digestive systems to perform with vigor and digest almost anything. Since we stopped collecting and eating wild foods, which tend to be more bitter or sour (and altogether more rudimentary in their flavor), society has incurred a whole range of gut-based diseases that simply did not exist before. Many of our modern herbs were, originally, everyday foods, and it is the lack of everyday usage that has, in part, caused people to become physically weaker and more prone to an overall and ever-increasing degeneration of the body— not least through allergies. Therefore, we should get back to using our known culinary herbs in earnest. Herbs such as thyme, marjoram, coriander, mint, and garlic should be included in the diet at every opportunity, as should salads in the form of our garden "weeds"—dandelions, chickweed, young oak leaves, fat hen (also known as goosefoot or pigweed), and so on.

Being ill on an obviously physical level, like having a bloated stomach, arthritis, or a headache, might lead you to believe that somewhere along the line your diet may have been responsible. But very often it is easy to miss the more emotional and behavioral side effects of the wrong food input. Being poisoned, or else starved of the correct nutrition, can create anger, impatience, apathy, and a whole array of negative emotions, which you may simply regard as being "you." Strip away the coffee, tea, alcohol, sugar, and chocolate and replace them with more healthy foods (which balance stomach flora and kill off any opportunistic parasites), and you may be surprised at the person you meet! There are many herbs that greatly help this process of conquering "driven" addiction by altering the body's chemistry, balancing and overriding unwanted cravings.

The Options

When I think about food for myself and my family, when I talk about foods with patients, I hope to represent the plant that flowers cheerfully, sways in the wind, and has a good root system that grounds and stabilizes it. Food is there to be enjoyed and you need to be creative and flexible in order to do so. The basis of this should be a combination of intuition and knowledge about what promotes good body chemistry and happy, healthy beings.

Sometimes tremendous upheaval is needed in order to transform sickness into health. To many people it appears to be too hard to change long-established and often cherished patterns, tastes, and beliefs. Changes in food can be bewildering and challenging and many people cannot, or will not, attempt such changes. Getting outside help to devise what is right for your individual body type, body weight, health, and culture will further this often difficult process. For some, the love and joy of nourishing their own bodies and respecting their own beings is simple; others find it more difficult. Some find it easiest to make changes when they are well. There are, however, some cases in which people become so seriously ill that a drastic change of diet may be their only option. In these situations, making this choice may prove to be a lifesaver.

But remember, eating is a loving and highly social process. Don't become unbalanced and neurotic about the often sad state of our food-chain options. Do your best, enjoy what you have, and be grateful for what your purse affords.

Blood Types and Digestive Enzymes

Blood group tests are available, which some professionals believe can give you an indication of which foods suit your genetic makeup; more simply, you can just ask your doctor what blood type you are and then follow the general advice below.

Blood types can be broken down into group O, group A (which further differentiates into A1 and A2), group B, and group AB.

DIET FOR BLOOD GROUP O

Historically, the blood group O diet was apparently the first to evolve and is associated with hunter-gatherer societies. People who are Group O do well on diets that are high in proteins such as meat, poultry, and fish. Dairy products, corn, and most grains should be eliminated. Group O individuals are generally associated with higher levels of hydrochloric acid in the stomach, which helps to digest the higher amounts of proteins found with this type of diet. Fruits and vegetables should also be eaten in larger amounts to help balance the body's pH level.

DIET FOR BLOOD GROUP A

Historically, blood group A individuals have adapted well to an agrarian form of diet, which evolved later and consists primarily of fruits, vegetables, nuts, and grains. Generally, little or no meat should be allowed, and then only as a condiment. Milk and cheese should also be eliminated, especially in type A2 individuals. Grains and beans contain higher amounts of naturally occurring agglutinins (lectins), which make their assimilation by the body more difficult. Larger amounts of fruits and vegetables are recommended for group A individuals, who tend to secrete lower amounts of hydrochloric acid and thus metabolize calories and obtain energy at a slower rate. Raw fruits and vegetables are higher in natural enzymes, which promote digestion, absorption, and assimilation.

DIET FOR BLOOD GROUP B

Apparently, the blood group B diet evolved later than that of group O or A and is associated with nomadic and herding societies. People who are group B do well with diets that are high in fermented dairy products. These individuals do better on ovo-lacto vegetarian diets, which are higher in products that contain milk, cheese, and eggs. Natural agglutinins in such foods as chicken, sunflower, sesame, and buckwheat may cause problems for a group B person and should be used in moderation. Group B individuals are generally associated with lower levels of hydrochloric acid in the stomach and may need enzyme and hydrochloric acid assistance if higher amounts of proteins are ingested. Group B persons do well with a good balance of the different food groups allowed rather than emphasis on a particular food type.

DIET FOR BLOOD GROUP AB

Apparently, the blood group AB diet evolved last, and it is felt to be associated with modern diets. Because of the presence of both A and B antigens, group AB individuals are well adapted to vegetarian, grain, and seafood diets with small to moderate amounts of milk products. Natural agglutinins in such foods as red meat, chicken, potatoes, tomatoes, and many grains and beans may cause problems for a group AB person and should be used only in moderation. Group AB individuals are generally associated with lower levels of hydrochloric acid in the stomach and may need enzyme and hydrochloric acid supplementation if higher amounts of proteins are ingested. Group AB people do well with a good balance of the different food groups allowed rather than emphasis on a particular food type or group.

See *Eat Right for Your Type* by Peter D'Adamo with Caroline Whitney for further information on this subject.

Organic Foods

The word *organic* has become somewhat meaningless, thanks to the excess of acid rain and other environmental pollutants now prevailing. However natural a farmer or gardener tries to be, what drops from the sky does count! But the term *organic* still indicates that something has been grown in chemical-free ground, so organic products are still worth pursuing.

A friend of mine, who used to work in a mortuary, told me years ago that bodies are taking a lot longer to decompose because of the preservatives ingested with food while alive. The very thought horrified me; the idea of the "walking preserved" is a chilling one. The days of preserving foods and growing foods with the use of toxic substances are not, however, as recent as we might assume. In 1953, Professor Arnold Ehret talked about sulfur-dried foods, benzoid of soda, salicylic acid, and sulfuric acid, which were being used to preserve canned foods.

Consuming preservatives, pesticides, nitrates, and other substances used by farmers is dangerous to every cell in the human body. The major concern is, of course, for children. The Soil Association in Britain has drawn attention to the fact that a one-year-old could easily receive a maximum lifetime's dose of eight pesticides from just twenty commonly eaten fruits, vegetables, and grains. The association is trying to unite farmers, the Department of Agriculture, and the Drug Administration Agency in an attempt to utilize beneficial organisms and crop rotation instead of some pesticides. Nerve gases are still used by farmers. They are commonly known as organophosphates. These chemicals enter the food chain via vegetables, grains, and cattle feed, and are also transported by the wind. Many cases of motor neuron disease are now being reported among young children (and adults). Often these are farmers' children whom I, in turn, see in my clinic. Let us not forget household pesticides and those used in our gardens; these at least could be dispensed with.

The major sources of pesticide residues in the Western diet are meat, poultry, and dairy products. *Pesticide* is a generic term that includes insecticides, herbicides (weed killers), and fungicides, among other agents. One chemical commonly found in household, agricultural, and commercial-use pesticides is 2,4-D, a key ingredient found in Agent Orange, the defoliant put to widespread use during the Vietnam War. Frequent use of herbicides, particularly those containing 2,4-D, has been associated with twofold to eightfold increases in non-Hodgkin's lymphoma in studies conducted in several countries. Other agents, including triazine and organophosphate pesticides, have also been shown to increase cancer risks. As I have mentioned, pesticide use has increased thirty-three-fold since the 1940s, and there has been a tenfold increase in potency. Dr. Sheila Zahm of the U.S. National Cancer Institute has recommended that pregnant women avoid exposure to all pesticides, which is not easy if you live in an area surrounded by fields being sprayed throughout the year. The fetus is particularly susceptible to genetic damage, chromosomal aberrations, and carcinogenicity. Infants are also at higher risk.

The food most likely to cause cancer from herbicide residue is beef. The frightening thing is that extremely few slaughtered animals are actually tested for toxic chemical residues. In America the figure is as low as one in every quarter-million. Levels of DDT in nonvegetarian mothers' milk in America have been found to be as high as 99 parts per million, as opposed to levels of 8 parts per million in vegetarian mothers!

It is not surprising that staphylococcus infections are much more rampant and that resistance in humans is now really low. Penicillin used to be able to deal with them, combating them successfully and leaving only 13 percent resistant; now the figure is more like 91 percent resistant, the reason being that antibiotic-resistant strains of staphylococcus bacteria have developed on factory farms because of the routine feeding of antibiotics to livestock. At present, one can expect 80 percent of all farmed livestock and poultry to receive drugs regularly. Milk is also affected by residues of sulfa drugs — tetracycline and other antibiotics have been found. One hopes that the government will step in.

Doctors and health workers are aghast at the hijacking of antibiotics by the animal feed industry. They have been left with fewer resources with which to fight disease as our bodies acclimatize to antibiotics via the food chain, making their use less and less effective. Through the addition of hormones to increase speed of growth and size of animals, our fertility and hormonal balance are being thrown into chaos, producing disease and distortions.

All plant life has a vibration and a gift beyond its physical sustenance as food — both aspects are important. It has been shown that foods grown in loving, positive atmospheres produce more nourishment in nutritional and vibrational terms.

BUYING ORGANIC

Buy what is in season at an organic farmers' market or local health-food store. Organic fruits, vegetables, nuts, seeds, and grains have a very much longer shelf life than their pesticide-laden counterparts, so even if you need to buy in quantity at some distance, you can be sure that they will retain their vitality longer. Store them in a cool environment away from sunlight.

Organic farmers represented 1 percent of British agriculture in 1995, but in the same year they received only 0.01 percent of the $2 million in assistance for farming in Britain; so when I pay a little more for organic foods, I know I am helping to compensate for this lack of government assistance to growers. I am also keen to support those in other countries, including Spanish organic growers, who produce the lemons and avocados that British farmers are unable to produce.

If you cannot afford the extra that organic foods cost, then add garlic to your normal supplies; with its sulfur compounds and antioxidant chemistry, it will detoxify some of the harmful compounds. There are also fruit and vegetable wash concentrates that help remove chemicals, waxes, dust, atmospheric pollutants, and exhaust fumes. For those who are able to do so, growing your own using an allotment or your garden is cheap and fun. The herb milk thistle can also be useful, as it greatly assists the liver in its detoxifying role, which is essential for keeping pace with all the pollutants.

Culinary Herbs and Spices

Culinary herbs and spices are chosen for their flavors to delight the palate. To me they also represent fun, color, and health. They are masters at dancing with our taste buds. They are nature's aid to the relaxation of stomach muscles. They also encourage better production of balanced and sufficient gastric juices. They contain elements that help counteract toxic foods. Some contain antifungal, antibacterial, and antiviral ingredients, giving some help to harmonize food combinations that might otherwise fight it out and cause indigestion and gas; still others help the liver with its job of constantly negating and purifying. You can grow fresh herbs and spices and use dried or freshly imported ones.

The spice and herb section of any kitchen is one of the major medicine cupboards for any household. This section should be used for everyday eating and staying healthy. The whole kitchen should be full of live, healing, and tasty foods, but herbs and spices have a special gift. Remember that by adding these to all meals and rotating their use, you are bringing a diversity of healing chemistry into your diet, thus reducing the likelihood of disease in general.

Aniseed *(Pimpinella anisum)* is a sweet spice. It is excellent for breaking up mucus in the body and for the relief of cramping in the bowels, as well as colic and flatulence. It is also very calming, soothing the nervous system and alleviating sleeplessness.

Caraway *(Carum carvi)* is an excellent aid to digestion and relieves indigestion.

Cardamom *(Elettaria cardamomum)* is the king of spices; it warms the body and soothes indigestion and gas.

Cayenne *(Capsicum annuum)* is a medicinal and nutritional herb. It is the purest and best stimulant. It is an excellent food for the circulatory system, as it feeds the necessary elements into the cell structure of arteries, veins, and capillaries so that they regain elasticity. It also regulates blood pressure.

Used most beneficially raw, it rebuilds the tissue in the stomach and heals stomach and intestinal ulcers (the opposite is true of cooked chiles). It also produces natural warmth and, in stimulating the peristaltic motion of the intestines, aids in assimilation and elimination. Cayenne peppers have white seeds, which are the hottest part; they are good for colds and flu.

Cinnamon (*Cinnamomum zeylanicum*) is available as bark, shoots, and sticks. The bark is mainly sweet, but also slightly hot and bitter; the shoots have a very different taste and are not so sweet. Both are warming and tonic. Cinnamon and whole barley soup is good for all kidney problems, balancing water volume, general tone, and function and helping to cleanse the system. Cinnamon and cloves complement each other in cooking, warming and speeding digestion. Nausea, flatulence, and diarrhea can be helped with them.

Cloves (*Syzygium aromaticum*) are a stimulant and are effective for warming the body, increasing circulation, improving digestion, alleviating nausea and vomiting, and clearing phlegm. They are also capable of inhibiting viruses and fungi as well as parasitic eggs. Use sparingly, as the flavor is strong.

Coriander (*Coriandrum sativum*) is the queen of spices and an antiviral herb. As a seed it is a good thickening agent. It is stimulative, digestive, and considered universally useful and healing.

Cumin (*Cuminum cyminum*) is "cooler" than some spices, but it still warms and aids digestion. It is one of the best spices for the relief of flatulence. It is also a stimulant and antispasmodic, useful to the heart and uterus.

Fennel (*Foeniculum vulgare*) assists digestion and increases metabolic processes in general; it alleviates gas, bloating, and spasms and speeds up digestion. It dissolves and disperses mucus and fats. The lungs benefit from it when taken as a tea.

Fenugreek (*Trigonella foenum graecum*) is a useful healing spice; it is very nourishing and considered to be a tonic, as well as balancing blood sugar. It is a very useful thickening agent in foods. Three cups of fenugreek tea a day will help people gain weight. It will also calm an acidic or ulcerated stomach and increase milk flow for mothers with poor production, and it strongly supports the pancreas.

Garlic (*Allium sativum*) is the paragon of blood cleansers and, with its abundance of sulfur (eighty different sulfur compounds), it is capable of killing viruses, bacteria, and fungi. It can calm and feed the nervous system and help correct faulty digestion. The fresh juice is effective for cramps, spasms, and seizures. Combine it with ginger, French tarragon, or marjoram to prevent gas. Combined with onions it is very beneficial for colds and flu, but simmer rather than boil it, or it will lose much of its goodness. Those with high cholesterol will find that it is reduced by garlic. It is a major antioxidant, proven to help reduce the incidence of cancer and many other diseases. Garlic juice, diluted to 1 part in 125,000, inhibits the growth of most types of bacteria. In fact, the odor alone does so. Garlic is nature's own broad-spectrum antibiotic, but it works without killing off friendly bacteria, as drug antibiotics do. In addition, garlic is positive for your heart, as it lowers blood pressure and reduces clots and platelet aggregation. Garlic not only encourages white blood cell formation but also produces a bacterial agent that halts tumor growth. Garlic protects the body from toxic chemicals, harmful food additives, and rancid oils. It is also helpful in the treatment of AIDS, where lymphocyte clumping encourages the spread of HIV from cell to cell. Cooked and raw garlic should be a part of everyday life; a recommended dose is between one and three cloves daily. (However, 1 percent of the population cannot tolerate it.)

Those who shy away from garlic because of its smell should add freshly grated ginger to it; provided you wash regularly, keep generally healthy, and don't get constipated, the garlic odor will be minimized.

Ginger (*Zingiber officinale*) is one of the most versatile herbal stimulants. It is of great benefit to the intestines, circulation, and stomach. Use as a tea when you are feeling sick or headachy. It enhances the effect of all other herbs and spices. Make your own ginger honey (organic, cold-pressed) and use instead of marmalade. **Avoid use if you have very high blood pressure, or in cases of extreme inflammation, dry skin, or liver inflammation.**

Lemon (*Citrus limonia*) is not only delightful in flavor, but also one of nature's best kitchen healers. Gypsy lore says it is among the five foods that should always be in the kitchen. The fresh skins of whole organic ones can also be used. Lemon juice can be added to so much — including teas. Rich in vitamin C, a natural antioxidant, it encourages the immune system. Suck on an organic lemon if you have swollen glands. Lemon is so powerfully acidic that it is rapidly converted to alkaline in the gut, providing a powerful healing tool for detoxifying and healing.

Marjoram (*Origanum majorana*) is a powerful antiviral herb. It is also a stimulant, antispasmodic, antiseptic, and carminative, a combination of opposites that brings balance. It relaxes the lungs and digestion and expels mucus wherever it may be situated. It is helpful in many bowel disorders, easing, soothing, and healing. It can be used for cramps and nausea and adds a slightly lemony flavor to dishes.

Mustard (*Brassica hirta*, *B. nigra*, and other species) is a stimulant, alterative, and rubefacient that is excellent for the digestive system. The best mustards are those made from whole grains and mixed with apple cider vinegar rather than malt or white wine vinegar. Add it frequently to salad dressings and when cooking rice and other grains. Use the seeds whole on steamed cabbage, carrots, and parsnips to add crunch and spicy heat!

Nutmeg and **Mace** *(Myristica fragrans)* come from the same seed. Mace is the outer covering of the nutmeg. Nutmeg and lettuce soup is very good for depression and nervous disorders. Mace is an antiseptic and is delicious in sweet dishes. Sprinkle nutmeg and mace on cooked fruit, use with cinnamon in sweet dishes, or grate onto potatoes, cabbage, onions, or leeks. The effect is generally warming and soothing. Together they are supposed to be an aphrodisiac, but be aware that in large quantities they can be hallucinatory. Nutmeg encourages menstruation and can be abortive in large quantities — therefore avoid it during pregnancy.

Parsley *(Petroselinum crispum)* comes in many varieties, all of which are incredibly tasty and health-giving. Parsley has a very high vitamin and mineral content and is very rich in chlorophyll. I used it a lot when making my babies their first foods. Millet and parsley makes a good combination for protein, iron, calcium, vitamin C, chlorophyll, and many other nutrients. Try parsley in soups, stews, or salads, not just as a garnish, to which status it is usually relegated. It is a blood cleanser — the high iron content helps the blood. It also acts as a diuretic and digestive through increasing bile flow, so one could call it a digestive and a detoxifier. Do not make it into strong teas if you are pregnant or suffer from heavy periods, as the estrogen within it could be unsuitable.

Pepper *(Piper nigrum)*, specifically black pepper, is anticatarrhal, antimucus, antifungal, and antibacterial, as well as being a natural preservative. It should be freshly ground and added after the food has been cooked; cooking changes its chemistry, making it more aggressive to the stomach. White pepper produces acids and is almost a mature fruit when the skin is removed — use it only as a seed to flavor, and do not eat in large quantities. Green pepper, like black pepper, is an immature fruit. Those with liver problems should eat only small amounts of it.

Rosemary *(Rosmarinus officinalis)* is astringent, bitter, highly stimulating, and yet calming, which makes it useful for indigestion, colic, nausea, gas, nervousness, and fever. It is also high in calcium and is a natural antiseptic.

Sage *(Salvia officinalis)* is an antispasmodic, antiseptic, and astringent, and is helpful for slowing fluid secretions. Consequently, it is helpful in cases of excessive perspiration, night sweats, milk flow, and vaginal discharge. It has a slightly bitter taste, so limit its usage and certainly never consider it alone as a herbal tea. It requires careful dosage, but is invaluable if used correctly.

Thyme *(Thymus vulgaris)* is useful in cases of lack of appetite, chronic gastritis, and diarrhea. It is highly antiseptic and can activate and strengthen the immune system, and it warms and tones as it works. (However, excessive amounts can cause depression if drunk daily in teas.)

Turmeric *(Curcuma domestica)* is one of the most useful and versatile spices. Not only is it an excellent cleanser of the liver thanks to its bitterness, but it is also highly antiseptic and, as a blood purifier, is useful for eczema, pimples, and a variety of other skin complaints. It is helpful for all circulatory problems and for maintaining menstrual regularity; it also keeps all kinds of undesirable bacteria and infection at bay, including in the gut, where it is also soothing and anti-inflammatory. It is an antioxidant, but perhaps most useful of all, it is strongly antiviral.

Note: As you have probably realized, foods and spices in their different states—fresh, whole, and powdered—all have different flavors. Whole, unprocessed spices last the longest. If you are buying powdered ones, buy only small quantities at a time; alternatively, buy whole ones and grind your own in a coffee grinder. Perhaps the main quality of most culinary herbs and spices is that their essential oils all help with digestion, relaxing stomach muscles, speeding digestion, and killing off unwanted amounts of fungi, bacteria, and even parasites in some cases. They are generally tonic, feeding, and health-giving. Don't forget others not listed here, such as bay leaf, basil, and chives.

Digestion

This is the most important subject of this chapter and perhaps of the book, for without proper digestion, much ill health and many diseases can be created. The digestive system comprises the mouth, spleen, pancreas, stomach, liver, gallbladder, intestines, and colon. There is much work to be done by each of these; for instance, the mouth secretes digestive enzymes, and the entire digestive tract is populated by symbiotic bacteria whose job it is to break down the partially processed food and assist its decomposition by fermentation.

A few helpful tips on eating are

- Don't eat if you are angry or frightened; eating should essentially be a feeding, nurturing, and sensuous experience.
- If you are tired but hungry, choose easily digestible foods that need little chewing, like soup, broth, soft fruits, or vegetable and fruit juices.
- A relaxed state of mind means relaxed stomach muscles and an easy production of balanced gastric juices, resulting in proper assimilation and easy, natural elimination. A before-dinner joke is as important as an after-dinner one; laughter is the best relaxant I know. That, or simply take some deep breaths.

- Mothers with babies and young children often have enforced strange and disturbed eating routines, especially when nursing; therefore they need extra support and help at this time.

See also "The Digestive System" in chapter 9.

Flavors

Bitter flavors, which are first tasted in the mouth, help the immune system that lies within the gut; they aid production of white blood cells, generally empowering immune responses and helping to fight many diseases of the immune system, from candidiasis to AIDS. Bitter flavors help to burn up excess fats in the body, quickly providing the necessary energy. For the very underweight, few bitter foods should be consumed unless they are being used for a specific reason, like ridding the body of worms.

Bitters include gentian, artichoke, olives and olive oil, dandelion leaves, chicory, and nasturtium leaves. Bitters often come in the form of wild greens in spring, but they are still available in the summer. They are often combined with aromatics like fennel seed, cumin seed, and caraway seed to help cool, calm, and soothe the digestive tract. The Swedish bitters and liqueurs can be consumed to aid before- and after-dinner digestion.

We owe it to ourselves to eat bitters and sours. The taste helps to destress and calm the nervous system, balancing and grounding, preventing over-extensive output of nervous energy.

Sour heals and nurtures the liver and gallbladder by deep cleansing and cooling, making the digestive process largely passive, which in turn has a positive emotional effect. A cleansed and cooled liver and gallbladder readily release the positive emotions of joy and happiness. These are two important emotions for the well-being of the immune system in general. Sour foods include limes, lemons, sorrel, sauerkraut, pineapple, and apple cider vinegar. Pineapples are sour-sweet, and the bromelain in them is a prime digestive, scavenging for and helping to finish off half-digested foods.

You can pickle foods easily using apple cider vinegar. This type of vinegar helps regulate the balanced output of stomach acid, correcting overactive and underactive conditions. The sour flavor can really be exciting, and chiles, which couldn't ordinarily be eaten raw, can be when softened by the pickling process.

Salty foods heal and nurture the kidneys, adrenals, bladder, and thyroid. Salty flavor is in all sea vegetables, such as kelp, nori, wakame, and so on. Parsley and celery are considered salty and make an excellent "dried and sprinkled-on" substitute. Do not use too much salt, as the kidneys will suffer. The dangers of high salt intake are so well publicized that it is almost more important to say, these days, that a little good-quality salt should be consumed—some people need more than others.

"Spicy" really sums up two flavors, hot and pungent. Spicy foods support and nourish the lungs and colon, opening both and allowing them to operate with the ease they should. This category includes hot peppers, mustards, and horseradish. They generally aid circulation, encouraging the delivery of oxygen and nutrients and the expulsion of waste products and toxins.

Neutral tastes include, among others, rice, potatoes, sago, arrowroot, banana, yam, turnip, parsnip, and millet. They nurture and ground the body, feeding and toning. They are one of the most unifying of all flavors, providing harmony and balance.

Sweet flavor heals and nurtures the stomach, spleen, and pancreas, thus improving digestion, if used in a balanced way. Some positive sweeteners are real maple syrup, brown rice syrup, barley syrup, cold-pressed organic honey, date syrup, whole licorice, sweet herb *(Stevia)*, peppermint leaf, and certain culinary herbs.

Sugar inhibits the ability of white blood cells to destroy bacteria. Just two teaspoons is enough to diminish our immune-system response dramatically; it also consumes calcium, stripping the body of one of its most necessary minerals. If sugar is to be used, then real cane sugar is rich in essential minerals and vitamins and provides a better alternative than most. Blackstrap molasses is sweet and loaded with iron and calcium, which also makes it a good substitute for sugar. Try using a little licorice on occasion. Sweet herb *(Stevia)*, which is three hundred to five hundred times sweeter than sugar, does not feed yeasts, fungi, and other unwanted gastrointestinal microorganisms, and it helps improve digestion by stimulating the pancreas. Made as a tea and kept in the refrigerator, a small amount could be added to herbal teas. Both this and licorice are very useful for hypoglycemic people who need a sugar boost.

We all start life with a sweet tooth—breast milk is sweet and, as such, it nourishes and replenishes and is right for this vulnerable entry into life. With the constant availability of sugar reaching huge proportions over the past several decades, "sweet diseases" have increased and, in parallel to them, mental afflictions. It is not just our pancreas, teeth, and waistlines that are affected; our whole emotional state suffers. Artificial sweeteners are a further perversion of the problem—not only poisoning, but also increasing appetite in many cases! It is always advisable to read labels in order to see how the food you buy has been sweetened. Never use artificial sweeteners—proved to be carcinogenic, in the 1970s they were banned in Japan by the government. Look at health-store foods and see how many products have been sweetened by the inclusion of fruit concentrates. Even though this is far better than adding white sugar, it still represents work for the liver and other organs and systems.

Putrid fermented foods like miso, sauerkraut, and tofu support the immune system immensely and sustain the body. There is more on this subject later in the chapter.

Umami — the eighth taste — is used frequently in Japan to add "richness" to a meal. It is often provided by seaweeds, mostly kelp and kombu. These are rich in glutamates, isosinate, and nucleotides (the monosodium glutamate found in some Chinese cooking is the chemical and often side-effect-ridden version of this). Other foods containing *umami* naturally are Parmesan cheese, shiitake mushrooms, and naturally fermented soy sauce.

Oils (and Antioxidants)

The only oil that does not become rancid is olive oil. It is the only oil that benefits the heart, liver, and gallbladder (as well as cholesterol levels). It can also be heated and used for cooking at low temperatures without diminishing its character and life force. Used raw, it is excellent with salads. It is 80 percent monounsaturated and, as such, does not present the health hazards of saturated or polyunsaturated fats. For occasional variance, there are other oils that can be safely used such as walnut oil, safflower oil, grapeseed oil, sunflower oil, hempseed oil, and flaxseed oil.

Oils are attacked by oxygen almost within moments of harvesting and become rancid; more rancid, in fact, the older they become. This effect of oxygen exposure causes a chain reaction in our bodies producing free radicals, and it is these free radicals that attack, kill, or damage our cellular structure. Many, many plants help stop this destruction because they contain chemical components that act as antioxidants. The liver is particularly susceptible to free-radical damage because this is where fats accumulate and are processed. Foods containing high amounts of fats and oils should only be a minor part of the diet.

When you stir-fry with olive oil, keep the heat low and be sure to add water at any sign of drying out or overheating. Remember, fried foods are basically too rich and indigestible for our systems and cause fermentation and stagnation. There is some recent data linking free-radical damage to Creutzfeldt-Jakob disease. Scientists are also linking diseases like Alzheimer's and Parkinson's to free-radical damage.

Whole Grains

Grains have always existed in their wild state but have now been genetically altered to suit monocrop mass farming. These modifications have contributed to many of the allergy problems we see today, with wheat as the main culprit.

There are eight whole grains readily available: rye, oats, millet, rice, quinoa, corn, wheat, and barley. They are healthiest eaten in their whole state to retain maximum nutrient value and roughage. Using a slow cooker is an ideal way to preserve their life force and nourishment, thanks to its low temperature but lengthy heating. Alternatively, soak them in a saucepan overnight before cooking. Presoaking will enable grains to be cooked at a low temperature for a shorter period of time. For those who do not have the time, however, try using a rice cooker, which will cook the grains for you and then keep them warm for three hours if necessary. Whole grains can be eaten with at least one

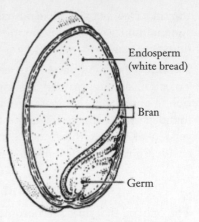

Endosperm (white bread)

Bran

Germ

The whole grain

main meal a day for a balanced diet. They are rich in fiber, and when fiber ferments in the large intestine, a chemical called butyrate is produced, which blocks the action of genes produced by cancer cells.

If you wish to eat raw grains, then growing organic wheat grass and sprouting barley, rye, and corn is wonderful (read *Light Eating for Survival* by Marcia Madhuri Acciardo for details).

Refined Carbohydrates

These are grains that have had their outer husks (roughage) removed, leaving just their inner section. Eating grains processed in this way tends to create body imbalances because the grains are themselves unbalanced. Refined carbohydrates have also very often been precooked. Mucus is a natural coating of mucous membranes and soft tissue, but consumption of refined carbohydrates creates too much of it. This excess mucus clogs and tires the whole body and exacerbates digestive problems, catarrh, asthma, and much more. Its sticky consistency invites infection. Sourdough rye and mixed-grain breads, Ryvita, rye bread, rice cakes, or sprouted seed bread are healthy alternatives to the average loaf!

Meat

Meat isn't what it used to be. Herbivores and poultry are now injected with antibiotics, fed on hormones and synthetic proteins, and were even, until recently, fed dead animals as a "recycling" policy, making them toxic to our bodies and especially to our livers. Beef contains high quantities of creatine, a member of the family of chemicals that includes caffeine and theine, which are heart and kidney stimulants. Pork is very high in fat (67.4 percent on average) and very low in protein (only 9.4 percent). All meat putrefies in the intestine and strips calcium from the body. If you wish to eat meat, then strive to find organic suppliers and avoid eating huge quantities, putting slivers rather than big chunks on your plate, more in keeping with our sedentary lives. Always cook meat with herbs like oregano and thyme to reduce parasites and microbes in general.

A four-ounce portion of red meat typically contains 100 mg of cholesterol, even after it has been skinned. The excessive fats found in meat raise cholesterol and uric acid levels in the tissues and interfere with the proper metabolism of carbohydrates. They encourage diabetes and dull the brain by causing clogging of capillaries, reducing the amount of available oxygen. Some cultures balance their meat consumption by mixing lean meat with grains, seeds, and vegetables. Meat, being a heavy protein, requires maximum digestive abilities and, if the body is too sick or undernourished to do this, toxicity and further sickness will result.

Genetically engineered meat may become more prevalent. These genetic creations are believed to be the future of meat, with extra meat and less fat being the goal; but some unpleasant side effects have been observed. I find it wholly frightening. It is not natural selection and runs contrary to principles of biodiversity.

If you want to move from meat eating to vegetarianism or veganism, take it very slowly over a period of a year or more to give your body time to adjust. It is also important to make sure you know where to gain adequate vegetable protein, which is vital for growing bodies. Organic meat is certainly an option, but ensure that the machinery used in the slaughterhouses has been thoroughly washed and sterilized to prevent the risk of cross-infection, which according to meat inspectors is prevalent.

Protein Needs

Levels of protein consumption currently far exceed official recommendations. Excessive animal, dairy, and egg protein can lead to many problems, from high cholesterol levels to excessive uric acid formation, cancers, calcium loss, and other ailments. We need amino acids (the basic component of all proteins) for growth, repair, and the production of hormones and enzymes. Yet an excess of amino acids forces the elimination of very important trace elements like zinc, calcium, magnesium, iron, and chromium, all of which are vital for emotional and physical well-being. The shedding of calcium, for instance, wears away the nervous system and depletes bone mass.

If you eat meat and fish, then consume no more than about one and a half pounds of flesh foods per week (approximately three to four ounces per day). For less active or nongrowing bodies, this amount could be reduced by about half. All meat dishes, particularly those containing red meats, increase the likelihood of uric acid forming in the body, causing arthritis, rheumatism, and bowel diseases. Poor digestion of even fresh foods can cause tremendous stagnation and create harmful bacteria and toxins. That being said, however, a balanced intake of protein in some form is essential. A totally vegetarian diet, without due care and attention being paid to alternative protein intake, is just as dangerous as an excess of animal protein. Lack of protein will produce visible symptoms like allergic sensitivity, bronchial and nasal congestion (lots of clear mucus), tiredness, and cold extremities, among others. These symptoms could continue for as long as one to two years after you change to a better diet.

The World Health Organization suggests that 4.5 percent of daily calories should be provided by protein. The U.S. Food and Nutrition Board suggests 6 percent. The approximate amount of protein needed for adults is two ounces daily; children require about three ounces daily.

VEGETABLE PROTEIN

Chlorella and blue-green algae are extremely rich in proteins (higher levels than meat), but spinach, broccoli, mushrooms, lettuce, and pumpkin are also good protein sources.

In order to obtain the twenty-two amino acids essential for complete protein formation and for adequate body function, use a combination of any grain and seed or legume. These are some ideas for grain and seed or legume combinations:

2 parts rice	plus	1 part broad beans
2 parts millet	plus	1 part sprouted alfalfa
2 parts corn on the cob	plus	1 part lentil stew
2 parts barley	plus	1 part runner beans
2 parts rice	plus	1 part sesame seeds

Dairy Products

Foods under this heading generally cause more concern and apprehension than any other. I see more sick people who have overindulged in dairy products than any other single food grouping. Milk and cheese are particularly damaging to children, and they can contribute to sinus problems, heart problems, allergies, colds, constipation, chronic fatigue, headaches, obesity, and dental deterioration. Many of us do not have sufficient natural lactase to break down the digestible lactose present in dairy products into assimilable sugars.

Dairy products often contain high levels of bacteria that can remain in these foods after cooking and even pass into unprotected food stored nearby. They do, of course, contain all the pesticides and herbicides the cattle have grazed on, unless they are organic.

Yogurt, though made from milk and therefore potentially just as harmful, does have the benefit of containing live cultures. Make it from organic goat's milk if you decide to eat yogurt.

Butter is almost free from mucus-forming substances and can be consumed, but use small amounts as it contains roughly 83 percent fat and 1 percent protein. But don't forget that it is basically rancid and has lots of free radicals. Avoid margarine completely.

Cheese is in a concentrated form and is often salted. Migraine headaches are frequently caused by cheese consumption, owing to the presence of the protein tyramine. Cheese causes excessive mucus production, which clogs up the intestines and other areas such as the lungs. This mucus forms a coating on the inner lining of the stomach that hardens, making an impermeable layer that prevents the absorption of nutrients. It can cause similar damage in the bowel, producing chronic constipation.

Milk and cheese have a history of causing allergies, such as hives and skin rashes. The reason is that they overstimulate certain stomach cells, producing a hydrochloric acid deficiency that results in proteins entering the bloodstream. In fact, milk neutralizes the hydrochloric acid necessary for food digestion, causing excessive mucus build up, which inhibits absorption of vital nutrients from all foods. In addition, 50 percent of the protein in cows' milk is indigestible anyway. The late Dr. Spock, the well-known child psychologist and nutritional expert, late in life advocated the withdrawal of milk from children's diet. In the book *Diet for a New America* by John Robbins (a member of a family that made a fortune from ice cream), milk, and other dairy products are cited as causing osteoporosis. Cows tend to graze on fields sprayed with pesticides. One pesticide that has been banned in Israel is lindane, an organochloride insecticide related to DDT. Fourteen other countries have banned lindane, with its use being restricted in still more. In Britain, however, lindane continues to contaminate our milk and put women at risk of breast cancer—the biggest killer of women between the ages of thirty-five and fifty-four in Britain. Search out organic milk perhaps.

Dairy products are generally consumed to add calcium and magnesium to the diet, but common foods and herbs are also sources of these nutrients. The recommended daily allowance of calcium is 800 mg to 1,200 mg, with sufficient sunshine or other sources of vitamin D to aid proper absorption of the calcium. The recommended daily allowance for magnesium is 350 mg to 450 mg.

Calcium-rich herbs and foods include valerian root, *pau d'arco* inner bark, kelp, wakame and hijiki seaweeds, nettle leaf, raw almonds (soak overnight and remove the outer skin before eating), dried figs, walnuts, raspberry leaf tea, boneset tea, fresh parsley, carrot juice, and sunflower seeds. Magnesium-rich foods include all of the above as well as Irish moss, oat straw, and turmeric.

All three recipes below are rich in calcium and magnesium:

- **Coconut Milk** — 1 cup grated coconut meat, 2 cups water, honey to taste if desired; blend and strain into a glass.
- **Almond Milk** — ½ cup almonds (remove the skins and presoak in the refrigerator), 4 cups water; blend and strain into a glass.
- **Cashew Milk** — 1 cup cashews, 3½ cups water; blend and strain into a glass.

Eggs

Eggs, like milk and cheese, are often alternatives to eating meat for vegetarians. Like milk and cheese, they are very mucus-forming, and cooked eggs deposit inorganic sulfur in the bowel. Therefore, if you wish to eat eggs, confine yourself to two free-range eggs a week. Eggs contain protein, but so do vegetables, grains, beans, nuts, and seeds in their correct combinations, while the B vitamins often missed when not eating meat can be obtained from vegetables, herbs, and yeasts.

Eggs are potential causes of diseases like arthritis, gallstones, and kidney stones, so if you suffer from any of these or have a tendency toward them, avoid eggs altogether. It is not advisable for women with gynecological problems such as menstrual difficulties or abnormalities of the womb or ovaries to eat eggs, as their consumption exacerbates this type of problem.

Eggs and flour are frequently the traditional binding elements in foods. Rice, corn, potato, and lentil flours can replace wheat flour. Other excellent binders include arrowroot and cornstarch. If a slightly spicy thickener is required, use ground coriander.

Fish

Fish now consume waste products that we liberally dump into the oceans year after year: drugs, radioactive materials, chemical waste, and heavy metals (particularly lead, cadmium, and mercury). Most of the fish in our rivers and lakes are equally poisoned in contaminated water. The notion of fish being a more digestible protein than meat (with almost no fat content) is becoming more irrelevant by the day. Trout and salmon, now "grown" in fish farms (fin to fin), live in water contaminated with antibiotics, antifungals, and other chemicals used to combat the diseases caused by unnatural overpopulation.

Chemical pollutants in the sea provide a nightmare scenario, but nitrate discharges into the sea are high and sewage discharges cause oxygen depletion, resulting in aggressive algal growth, which suffocates fish. Instead of using fish oils to decrease plaque buildups in the vascular system, use flaxseed oil or hempseed oil, which are richer in essential fatty acids like omega-3 and omega-6.

Drinking

What we drink is as important as what we eat. Drinking forms a large part of all our lives.

Coffee and tea both contain caffeine, a strong stimulant. Tea also contains theine, which is an additional stimulant, and tannin, which lines the stomach with an impermeable wall, making it difficult for assimilation and digestion to take place. Both drinks also contain theobromine—a harmful chemical that particularly exacerbates female gynecological disorders. Tea and coffee affect the adrenal glands, and long-term consumption can often lead to worn-out adrenals. The kidneys, too, are adversely affected. Coffee, in particular, will make the heart race, and palpitations and tachycardia are common. Yet these effects tend to go on constantly, so that most people do not notice the gradual degeneration of their bodies. Often, they are unable to remember what life was like before or imagine what it could be again. (When coming off tea, coffee, or alcohol, refer to "The Differences between Fasting and Detoxification" in chapter 6.)

Decaffeinated tea and coffee can provide a vital interim step for those wishing to come off the real thing. Springwater decaffeination is the safest process, and the labeling will indicate the process used.

Herbal teas are lovely made from fresh or dried (and preferably loose) herbs. Try them with the most natural sweeteners, such as pure honey or with lemon juice—or drink them just as they are. Herbal tea bags are very useful, but confine their usage to the office or for quick convenience on odd occasions. Tea made from fresh, loose herbs is fresher—no tea bag or dried herbal tea will come close to it for quality.

To dry your own herbs for teas, pick them as young as possible and preferably first thing in the morning. Dry in the air and away from direct heat or sunlight, covering with a brown paper bag to help preserve all their healing components. Store away from light.

Alcohol adversely affects the body, especially overloading the liver, but the purest alcohols are the best, such as 80-proof top-quality vodka or brandy or even good Champagne, which is double-fermented and organic. Anybody with liver, gallbladder, stomach, pancreas, or spleen problems should not drink alcohol at all.

Water cleanses and revitalizes the whole body. This is the best liquid to give you your daily needs. Its consumption tends to be overlooked, and its delicate taste underestimated. Often, it is just a question of having a bottle there when you need it—in the office or beside the bed. The habit grows on you. Well over half your body is made up of water, and you need it to constantly cleanse and regenerate all your cells and organs. Drinking a glass of water first thing in the morning helps clean out the body, especially helping to remove acids or foods left in the digestive tract overnight. If your airways are blocked or mucusy in the morning, add to your water some fresh lemon juice. It is best to drink water at least half an hour before a meal or half an hour after to keep your digestive juices from becoming diluted. Becoming excessively thirsty is a sign that you should seek professional help.

It's difficult to tell exactly what is filtered out by the local water company or by home water filters. Regularly found in tap water in the past was a chemical called nonylphenol, which mimics estrogen and causes disruption in the endocrine, nervous, and immune systems of both people and animals. There has been a 30 percent increase in prostate cancers over the past several decades, and many more male genital deformities are occurring. This has been coupled with a huge drop in male fertility.

Buying bottles of water can be useful for easy access to good-quality water. Compared to the rest of Europe, Britain buys the least bottled water—we are still committed to our tap water, it seems (according to 1998 statistics). Some people opt to use some kind of home water filter. This system generally relies on regular changing of filters and cleaning of equipment to ensure that the bacteria levels themselves do not become a hazard. Not all filters are capable of removing all the undesirable chemicals. Water distillers are yet another choice. They remove approximately 99 percent of impurities such as arsenic, barium, cadmium, nitrates, chlorine, and chloroform. They work by heating water placed inside the unit; as the temperature rises, light gases start to discharge through the ventilating system. When the water temperature reaches the boiling point, bacteria and viruses are killed, and the boiling water produces steam. As the steam rises into a stainless steel cooling coil, chemicals, salts, and other water contaminants are left behind. As the vapor is cooled, it recondenses as water. This water passes through an activated carbon filter in the spout, and the purified water is then collected in a storage container. Meanwhile, the contaminants are left behind in the stainless steel interior and can easily be cleaned away. They appear as a greeny, yellowy-gray sludge.

HOMEMADE BARLEY WATER

Barley water rejuvenates the kidneys. To make it, use half a cup of whole barley to five cups of water. Add one-quarter of a cinnamon stick and some grated ginger, and simmer for twenty minutes; then, after cooling, strain, add fresh lemon juice for extra flavor, and drink once a day.

Vegetables

Vegetables should be organic, and a proportion should be eaten raw. When cooking, use a steamer, as the vegetables retain their color, shape, texture, and flavor, not to mention all the vitamins and minerals. Try to eat a wide variety of vegetables to ensure a broader sweep of nutritional and medicinal needs.

SEEDS AND SPROUTING

Whole and sprouted seeds are a wonderful source of nutrition and can be used in cooking in a number of ways. Choose pumpkin (rich in copper, zinc, and phosphorus), alfalfa (rich in all vitamins, minerals, and trace elements, along with fiber), sunflower, or many others. If you combine sprouted sesame, sunflower, and pumpkin seeds, you can arrive at a total protein supplement. Sprouting is easy to do. If you have never tried it before, start with alfalfa seeds, because they sprout very quickly. Directions come with any sprouter box you buy from a health-food store.

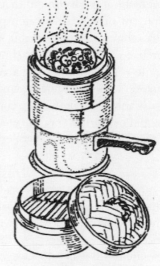

A bamboo steamer

GRASSES

Try growing organic wheat, rye, alfalfa, corn, millet, or barley in a tray with a little soil exposed to the sunlight. Once it has reached a height of one inch, cut it off and add to salads. It is incredibly rich in minerals, vitamins, and enzymes. It is also tasty, cheap, and versatile. For in-depth advice on this subject, read *Light Eating for Survival* by Marcia Madhuri Acciardo. Wheat grass is often dried commercially and can be found in good-quality organic nutritional drinks.

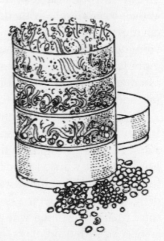

SEAWEED AND GREEN FOODS

Seaweeds are rich in minerals and trace elements, especially when harvested from the

A salad sprouter

least-polluted waters. Seaweeds are vital to a vegan diet and important to most others. It is in seaweed and algae that sunlight is most easily accessible to us. The plant structures are simple, and the sun's energy is readily released with minimal digestion. Seaweeds such as kelp, nori, dulse, and wakame are rich in iodine, calcium, and sodium, which are vital for the proper functioning of the thyroid. Spirulina algae, which are not quite the same as seaweed but are very similar, are rich in protein, chromium, manganese, niacin, riboflavin, thiamine, vitamin A, and zinc. Both can be sprinkled over food for a salty flavor and much-needed nourishment. Many green foods have a high chlorophyll content that is highly therapeutic. In fact, the chlorophyll content of any edible, nonsprayed weed will provide more nourishment than the average nonorganic store-bought vegetable. For instance, just four or five dandelion greens contain approximately 14,000 IU (International Units) of vitamin A, compared to only 33 IU in the same amount of supermarket iceberg lettuce. You need only a few dandelion leaves to gain a good daily intake of vitamin A, compared to the pounds of iceberg lettuce you would need to achieve the same result! Try drinking nettle tea daily, a cheap green tonic that can be collected or bought.

Organic Superfood

Nutritional superfood is made solely from dried organic plant substances that have a high nutritional value—rich in vitamins, minerals, amino acids, trace elements, antioxidants, and more—and can be assimilated in roughly fifteen minutes. These powdered supplements can be easily stirred into or blended with fruit juices, vegetables, or water. They nourish at a highly potent level, and relatively small amounts go a long way! They are targeted to give an all-round range of necessary nutrition and to provide bedrock care at the deepest level, giving the body true nourishment to which the varying chemistries found in medicinal plants can be added. They are ideal for young growing bodies, the elderly, the pregnant, or simply as a good beginning to the day for everyone. But they are vital where primary feeding is essential, especially in all forms of wasting diseases, including cancer and myalgic encephalomyelitis (chronic fatigue syndrome).

Superfood is good for convalescence of any kind, as it supports the body and involves minimal digestion. It is also excellent for toddlers, children, and teenagers, giving them the building blocks for healthy, vibrant growth. For teenagers worried about weight yet needing nutrition, this is the ideal food. For students, often away from home, taking superfood makes a good daily addition to cafeteria food. Anybody can use it as a quick meal substitute. Men and women who are prone to low blood sugar levels, perhaps associated with candidiasis, find it a good food that is capable of supplying a calorie-free snack between meals. It is ideal for supporting women premenstrually, helping to balance the liver, hormones, blood sugar levels, and mood swings.

Key ingredients in quality superfoods include spirulina, blue-green algae, chlorella, barley grass, alfalfa grass, wheat grass, purple dulse seaweed, and nonactive yeast flakes. Other highly beneficial foods include beets, spinach leaf, rose hips, orange peel, and lemon peel.

Spirulina and **blue-green algae** are indeed the most concentrated, nutritious foods on the planet. They are the highest natural source of complete protein known (75 percent).

Chlorella is second only to spirulina in food value. It is an extremely concentrated source of nutrition and complements spirulina well.

Barley grass, alfalfa grass, and **wheat grass** are wonderful healing grasses and are bulging with highly assimilable vitamins, minerals, enzymes, phytochemicals, and chlorophyll.

Purple dulse seaweed is an extremely rich source of assimilable minerals. It contains most of the minerals and trace minerals known.

HINTS AND TIPS FOR QUICK USE

For superfood to be used at breakfast, make up a batch the night before, leave in a plastic pitcher with a lid in the refrigerator, and shake before drinking in the morning, or leave some in a glass and simply stir. In wintry, cold weather, add in a knob of fresh gingerroot. In hot summer weather, chill some fruit juice before stirring in the superfood, or simply add ice cubes to the mixture. For a diabetic or low-calorie version, don't use fruit juice; instead add just the juice of two fresh lemons and springwater.

Fruits

According to some archaeologists, ethnobiologists, and zoologists, humans were originally designed to be fructivorous, that is to say, fruit-only feeders, as indicated by our eye placement and dexterous hands. Early humans lived in rain forests where fruit was readily available throughout the year. According to Dr. David Forman of the Imperial Cancer Research Fund's epidemiology unit at Oxford, fruit can substantially reduce the risk of stomach cancer. He says that a 30 to 50 percent lower risk of cancer can be achieved by eating one piece of fruit a day, and one-third of the annual deaths from cancer could be prevented this way. Fruit is not only tasty, but also full of fiber, minerals, and vitamins. Many fruits also contain large amounts of digestive enzymes, papaya and pineapple in particular (these are used by the supplement industry to enhance digestion). Proper digestion is essential for good health, so, on several levels, increased fruit consumption is a healthy move. When fiber ferments in the large intestine, a chemical called butyrate is produced, which blocks the action of genes produced by cancer cells.

If you feel cold in the winter, add paprika, powdered ginger, cinnamon, and other warming spices to fruit. Generally we eat more fruit in summer than in winter—a natural choice if we are not to feel too cold and watery—but fruit is vital at any time. It is best in season but can also be dried or canned for use out of season. Keep an unpeeled onion in your fruit bowl, and its sulfur content will keep the fruit fresher, keeping bacteria from spreading as quickly between the fruits and thus delaying decay.

Juices (Vegetable and Fruit)

Perhaps our greatest authority on the subject of juicing is N. W. Walker, author of *Fresh Vegetable and Fruit Juices*. He died relatively recently, aged almost 120 years, having helped many people. He said, "By juicing the vegetables and fruits one is keeping the vitamin, mineral and fluid content while discarding the fiber. This means that the goodness of the alkaline vegetables or fruit can be assimilated by the body in about 15 minutes instead of hours."

Who would chew through ten raw carrots, five sticks of raw celery, and two raw beets at one sitting anyway? You couldn't. The juicing process also sets free a lot of the food value that can remain permanently locked up in those whole raw vegetables because their molecular structure is too complex. For instance, the vitamin A (beta-carotene) in carrots is not surrendered except in light steaming or juicing of the vegetable.

Juices are one of the best ways I know for bringing sick and depleted bodies back to health, and for the healthy to enjoy ever-increasing vitality. They are also important for growing children, especially for calcium intake. Live, organic fruit and vegetable juices supply us with organic vitamins, minerals, and antioxidants that are very easily assimilated by our bodies. It is preferable to have your own juicer and to use organic ripe fruits and vegetables—preferably locally grown and in season. However, other fruits are also highly recommended.

The majority of the vitamin and mineral content of a fruit or vegetable lies just beneath its outer layer. It is vital, therefore, to juice the skin as well if it is organic. Also include the white pith, which is rich in immunostimulative chemistry. It is very important to chew the juices. This sounds funny, but they are more than water, they are food, and should therefore be well mixed with saliva and chewed for quite a while before swallowing to allow the greatest assimilation.

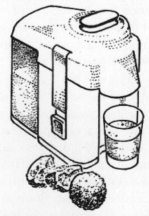

Cooking kills many enzymes, alters nutritional food values, and changes food from alkaline to acidic. However, fiber, as everyone   A fruit and vegetable juicer knows, is vitally important to one's diet for peristaltic movement and cleaning of the intestines, so sufficient whole raw food must be eaten as well.

Immunity through Fermented Food

Beneficial bacteria are vital for health; they inhabit the intestines, teeth, hair, appendix, and other places. They help digest food and create essential vitamins. Also, they play an important role in inhibiting the growth of disease-promoting pathogens and sustaining the correct amount of beneficial organisms. One's diet provides the balance of beneficial intestinal microorganisms that support the continued growth of "friendly" bacteria. Therefore fiber, as found in raw fruits and vegetables, is vitally important, along with sauerkraut, pickles (with apple cider vinegar), olives, yogurt, soy sauce or tamari, and sourdough bread, all of which add beneficial microorganisms. It has also been scientifically proved that these foods are natural antibiotics and anticarcinogens and are capable of breaking down and recycling toxins, much as the liver does.

Intestinal microflora (in the colon, lower small intestine, and stomach) are generally populous, forming a swarming and diverse environment containing many hundreds of beneficial species. It is their unique ability to change quickly with varying external environments and varying internal metabolic conditions that keeps us alive.

These rather intelligent microflora can help extract nutrition from everything we eat, while at the same time stimulating other aspects of our immune systems. They also inhibit the growth of pathogenic organisms by competing successfully for available nutrients in the intestines. If healthy, they will form a covering over all the intestinal inner linings. Having enough beneficial microflora helps digestion, primarily by cutting down on the amount of ammonia produced, which can cause gas, cramping, spasms, and more. Excessive production of hormones and steroids within the body can be balanced by having sufficient levels of beneficial microflora. Intestinal microflora also have the ability to keep the inner lining of every cell active, energized, and able to reproduce.

Eating fermented foods and having daily access to beneficial microorganisms is vital. The following options are all healthful possibilities.

Rejuvelac (homemade intestinal flora): Bowel flora are vital to enable the body to digest and assimilate foods. Rejuvelac contains B complex vitamins including B_{12}, along with vitamins K and E, lactic acid, and water-soluble minerals. Good rejuvelac has a somewhat lemony and sour odor and flavor. For variety, add your favorite herbs or seasonings. To make rejuvelac, use one cup of grain to two cups of water. Wheat is commonly used, but you can also try millet, rye, oats, brown rice, barley, or buckwheat. Always rinse the seeds first, and use the best-quality organically grown seeds. Soak the seeds for twenty-four hours, and keep covered in a warm place, between 60°F and 80°F. The rejuvelac is the water left after this process. Strain out the seeds and refrigerate the rejuvelac. Drink one or two cups daily, adding lemon for flavor. It can also be added to any cooking. To make another batch, add the same amount of water and repeat the process, using the same grains. They can be reused about five times.

Homemade sauerkraut: Generally, storebought varieties of sauerkraut contain malt vinegar or preservatives, so it is better to make your own. You will need a stone crock with a fitted lid, a glass jam jar with a plastic lid, or any large commercial glass jar—all are ideal for sauerkraut making. Use organic cabbage, and add green seaweeds like nori or wakame, along with herbs and seeds such as cumin, caraway, thyme, marjoram, juniper, ginger, turmeric, and coriander. Pour boiling water into the container to sterilize it, then empty it. Finely cut the cabbage. Add herbs and spices. Add some tamari to give a salty flavor and to ensure a good fermentation process. Put into a jar and cover the mix with whole cabbage leaves to within two to three inches of the top. Finally, put the lid on and weigh it down with a brick (or similar weight) to make sure no air enters.

Keep at a temperature between 70 and 80°F for three to four weeks. Open the sauerkraut every two to three days and remove any scum that may have been produced. When opening the lid, use a preboiled spoon and ensure you have clean hands. Use pH strips from the chemist to test the mixture. When the pH level has reached 3 to 7 and remained there for a week, it is ready. At that time, if you wish, you can add apple cider vinegar to it. This will ensure an almost indefinite shelf life. Keep it refrigerated. This is a successful recipe that I have used on numerous occasions.

Sourdough bread: Sourdough bread contains at least a hundred beneficial microorganisms. The resulting bread contains almost no gluten. Many sourdough breads use a starter made from flour and potato. Sourdough starters are easy to make, although you have to leave the mixture for a long time before it is ready to use.

Soy fermentations: Miso (a fermented paste made from soy, barley, and other grains) provides a tasty, salty, and very energizing food source. It can make a good and quick gravy, form the "body" behind soups, stews, and dahls, and be spread on bread or rice cakes.

Nutritional yeast: Nutritional yeast is a sprinkle-on nonactive-yeast product that can be used instead of grated cheese. Being nonactive, it can be eaten by those with candidiasis. It lends a nutty flavor to any dish. Its beneficial bacteria are *Saccharomyces cerevisiae*. It is also packed with B vitamins, protein, amino acids, enzymes, minerals, and trace elements.

Food Allergies

Allergy testing can be useful in order to highlight specific foods causing food allergies, but don't forget to look at the primary causes of food intolerances, which can often be sluggish digestive abilities, and make changes via balancing digestive enzymes that are not functioning correctly. Cleansing programs and herbs to support and stimulate enzyme production and general health of digestion-related organs, cleanses of major organs, and other natural regimes will help. Allergy treatments can initially be useful, but they can eventually exhaust the patient because they achieve their results through avoidance. A body that has become weak and poisoned can cope with only a few foods, but this does not mean that one will be so limited for the rest of one's life. A balance has to be struck in which a very broad range of foods comes to be tolerated as digestive strength is built up, giving greater diversity and, with it, good health. (Refer to sections on digestion throughout the book.)

Food Separation

One of the most noteworthy exponents of food separation has to be Dr. William Howard Hay who, more than sixty years ago, devised a "nature-cure" food approach based on separating out certain food combinations — a process he called "food combining." He ate many vegetables, fruits, nuts, and unrefined grains, and small quantities of meat and milk. He said that surplus acids are neutralized by the alkaline salts, namely sodium, potassium, calcium, and magnesium (all found in fruits and vegetables), and he suggested that acid wastes pile up in the body tissue when our alkaline reserves are grossly depleted, creating many problems. He suggested eating one totally alkaline meal a day. For some people, a closer look at food combinations can be very useful and, in some cases, vital. Perhaps one of the simplest ways to aid successful digestion is to separate foods completely, perhaps by eating fruits at breakfast, vegetables at lunch, and either protein or carbohydrates at dinner.

Cooked and Raw Foods

Cooking foods can be viewed on two levels. On the one hand, cooking destroys many vitamins, enzymes, minerals, nucleic acids, and chlorophyll. After a cooked meal, white blood cells increase in the stomach, thereby decreasing the body's immunity and leaving it more open to infection. In addition, cooked food is more likely to ferment or decompose in the intestines, resulting in toxicity. The stomach works at a temperature of 105°F, and food that is cooler or hotter can slow down the stomach's ability to function.

On the other hand, cooking adds certain energies into food, which creates a feeling of nourishment and warmth. Cooking is vital for foods that would ordinarily be indigestible or even toxic if left raw (including meat and some grains and beans). It is also useful for people with decreased stomach energy, which results in a lower metabolic rate and a reduced ability to digest their food. Anyone with a compromised spleen should take care that raw foods do not further weaken their spleen and pancreas. However, many people will thrive on raw food, which often makes the work of the pancreas easier. Eating only cooked food is unhealthy. Therefore it is suggested that a 70 to 80 percent raw-food diet is a good program to follow in the summer, or in hotter climates, while a 30 to 40 percent raw-food program is appropriate in the winter. Our bodies do not like feeling

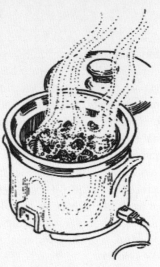

A plug-in slow cooker

damp, cold, and chilled, and hot food can balance those sensations.

Cooked food kills white blood cell activity, particularly in the stomach. Yet excessive raw foods will weaken some people by depleting spleen and pancreas function. Steaming is less aggressive than baking, and using a slow cooker, in which the temperature does not rise above 130°F, will ensure hot and wholesome food that is still very much alive. Sprouted barley seed and cooked barley create very different feelings inside us, and it is worth experimenting with each to see how you feel — grounded, tranquil, "high," stodgy, elated, or grounded. Climate, geography, and season will also influence your choice of food preparation.

Many foods become sweeter and more nurturing when cooked at low temperatures, including onion and turnip. I use a cooking pot that keeps an even low temperature for four to six hours, but you can also use low-temperature baking or steaming methods. You simply need to plan ahead a little. Food prepared using low temperatures has the comfort value of cooked food while retaining its nutritional value.

Kitchen Basics

This healing and deliciously tasty garlic and ginger cooking base can be added to a wide range of savory, cooked, or raw dishes. The potassium broth can be strained and drank as it is, or used in recipes that call for vegatable stock.

COOKING BASE

Use 4 cups virgin olive oil, ½ cup apple cider vinegar, 12 cloves chopped fresh garlic, and 2 tablespoons finely grated fresh ginger and blend. Use in all savory recipes. This will warm and revitalize circulation, additionally assisting immune capacity.

POTASSIUM BROTH

Using organic vegetables, fill a large pot with 25 percent potato peelings, 25 percent carrot and beet peelings, 25 percent chopped onions and garlic, and 25 percent celery and greens. Add minced fresh chiles (such as jalapeños) or crushed red pepper flakes to taste or cooler herbs like thyme and marjoram. Add enough springwater to cover the vegetables and simmer over a very low temperature for an hour. Strain. This will keep your body more alkaline and is useful for acidic conditions like arthritis or gout.

Book List

Avery Natural Therapy for Your Liver by Christopher Hobbs (Loveland, Colorado: Interweave Press, 1986, 2000)

Conscious Eating by Gabriel Cousins (Berkeley, California: North Atlantic Books, 2000)

Diet for a New America by John Robbins (Walpole, New Hampshire: Stillpoint, 1987)

Eat Right for Your Type by Peter D'Adamo with Caroline Whitney (London: Century, 1998)

Fresh Vegetable and Fruit Juices by N. W. Walker (Phoenix, Arizona: Norwalk Press, 1936)

Healing Liver and Gallbladder Disease Naturally by Dr. Richard Schulze (Santa Monica, California: Natural Healing Publications, 2003)

Healing with Whole Foods by Paul Pitchford (Berkeley, California: North Atlantic Books, 1993)

Healthy Digestion by David Hoffmann (Pownal, Vermont: Storey Books, 2000)

Light Eating for Survival by Marcia Madhuri Accairdo (Wethersfield, Connecticut: Omango Di Press, 1978)

The Nutrition Desk Reference by Robert Garrison and Elizabeth Somer (New Canaan, Connecticut: Keats, 1985)

Nutritional Herbology by Mark Pederson (Warsaw, Indiana: Wendell W. Whitman, 1994)

Prescription for Natural Healing by James and Phyllis Balch (New York: Avery, 1990)

Rejuvenation through Elimination by Dr. John Christopher (Springville, Utah: Christopher Publications, 1976)

School of Natural Healing by Dr. John Christopher (Springville, Utah: Christopher Publications, 1976)

Staying Healthy with Nutrition by Elson Haas (Berkeley, California: Celestial Arts, 1992)

Resources

For Juicers

Superior Health Products, 13549 Ventura Blvd., Sherman Oaks, CA 91423; tel: 818-986-9456; email: SuprHealth@aol.com; website: www.juicesforless.com

Discount Natural Foods, P.O. Box 16391, Hookset, NH 03106; tel: 888-392-9237

For Superfood

American Botanical Pharmacy, Glencoe Avenue, Marina del Rey, CA 90292; tel: 800-Herb-Doc

Herbs Hands Healing Ltd., Station Warehouse, Station Road, Pulham Market, Norfolk IP21 4XF, United Kingdom; tel: 011-44-0137-9608201; websites: www.super-food.co.uk and www.herbshandshealing.co.uk

For Water Filters

Ion & Light; tel: 415-346-6205; website: www.ionlight.com

The Soil Association, Bristol House, 40-56 Victoria Street, Bristol BSI 6BY, United Kingdom; tel: 011-44-0171-4901555

Friends of the Earth, 1025 Vermont Ave., NW, Suite 300, Washington, DC 20005; tel: 202-783-7400 or 877-843-8687; fax: 202-783-0444

For Food Dehydrators

Perfect Health, 4872 Casitas Pass Road, Ventura, California 93001; tel: 800-444-4584; email: sales@juicing.com

❧ 5 ❧

Natural Healing Methods

These various methods will support or radically promote the healing process.

Bodywork

SKIN BRUSHING

Skin brushing is a most effective technique for cleansing the lymphatic system by physically stimulating it. It also stimulates the bloodstream and is excellent for poor circulation. It gives you a refreshed, uplifted feeling on completion and makes you feel alive and energized. It takes no longer than five minutes, so don't skimp and try to do it in less—it can be done while running the bathwater. Use a skin brush made from natural vegetable bristles (nylon or animal bristles will be too rough and will damage the skin), with a long but detachable handle, so that you can reach your back if you are ordinarily unable to do so. Always keep it dry and strictly for this job, washing it in warm, soapy water every so often.

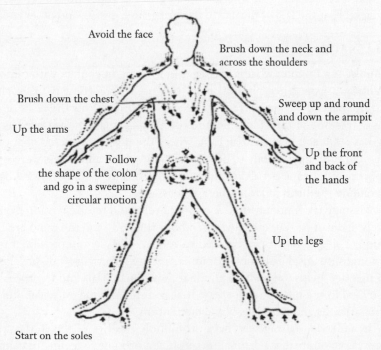

Avoid the face

Brush down the neck and across the shoulders

Brush down the chest

Up the arms

Sweep up and round and down the armpit

Up the front and back of the hands

Follow the shape of the colon and go in a sweeping circular motion

Up the legs

Start on the soles

Skin brushing

Do not touch the face. Make bold movements, passing only once over each part of the body in a sweeping motion:

- Start by brushing the soles of the feet.
- Work up each leg, over the buttocks, avoiding the genitals, and up to the middle of the back.
- Start at the fingertips and brush up the arms, through the armpits, across the shoulders, down the chest, and over the top of the back. Brush down the chest toward the colon.
- On reaching the area below the navel, use brush movements starting on the right-hand side, going up, across, and down, following the shape of the colon.
- Women should brush their breasts (it helps guard against lumps) but avoid the nipples, covering them with the fingertips. Basically, you work toward the heart and then bring all toxins toward the colon.

The face should never be skin brushed in this way, as this treatment is too harsh for it. Wet exfoliation, especially in grimy towns and cities, is a good alternative that should be done as part of your daily washing routine. Use a lotion containing oatmeal and abrasive particles like sand, adzuki beans, silica, or pumice. One treatment a day is quite enough for the face, preferably at the end of the day to remove grime, grease, and other residues.

MASSAGE

Think for a minute: what is massage? It is being in contact with our body. When we experience physical pain, our natural reaction is to touch the painful part of our body. This instinctive reaction forms the basis of massage. It is one of the oldest methods of healing: massage was used as long ago as 3000 B.C.E. in the Far East, where the positive benefits of applying oils and rubbing the body to prevent or relieve pain and illness were widely appreciated. In ancient civilizations, scented oils were almost always used — heralding the birth of aromatherapy massage.

Massage is commonly used as a tool to relax and release tension from the body and can be very effective when both the body and the mind are taken into consideration. It can be used to relieve many common ailments, including sinusitis, headaches, insomnia, and hyperactivity. The physical act of massage helps the body to eliminate waste materials and to process and use food in the most effective way. It also stimulates the muscular and nervous systems and improves blood circulation.

In addition, massage can have profoundly positive effects in those with depressive or anxious personalities, as it can promote a feeling of calmness and serenity. With this newfound calmness, people are often able to begin dealing with the underlying problems that initiated their anxiety or depression. Massage can be used in many other positive ways, including calming fretful babies and the rehabilitation of those with long-term incapacity problems (including those who are bedridden)—for example, lymph massage is often used in postoperative recovery from breast cancer.

Massage can be practiced in many ways. Just stroking your own or another person's body is a type of massage; this contact is incredibly important in order to gain some understanding and love for the human form. There are, however, four main categories of massage that are widely recognized: effleurage (stroking), friction (pressure), percussion (drumming), and petrissage (kneading). Most masseurs use a variety of these styles, depending on each individual case. Generally, they also use other personalized styles combined with other natural healing methods. This is often reflected in their choice of essential oils and carrier oils.

REFLEXOLOGY AND FOOT MASSAGE

Reflexology is a technique of diagnosis and treatment. It is believed to have partly originated in China approximately five thousand years ago. Dr. William Fitzgerald introduced reflexology into Western society. He identified ten zones (channels) in the human body, and these zones were considered to be the energy paths along which a person's "vital energy" flowed. The zones end at the hands and the feet. Therefore, when pain is experienced at one point in the body, it can be alleviated by applying pressure to the corresponding energy zone in the hands or feet. Today, in the main, practitioners tend to concentrate on the feet. There are many uses for reflexology, including pain relief. You can simply massage your own feet, which will go a long way toward relaxing, centering, and grounding you. You can use any oil that you like the smell of, massaging your feet when they are dry or simply rubbing them in the bath.

CHIROPRACTIC

The word *chiropractic* has its origins in two Greek words, *kheir*, meaning "hand," and *praktikos*, meaning "practical." Chiropractic is used for pain relief through manipulation and corrects many problems in the joints and muscles, especially the spine. Spinal disorder can cause widespread problems throughout the body, especially the hips, legs, and arms, and can also be the root cause of sciatica, a slipped disk, and other back problems. Furthermore, it can be responsible for conditions that on the surface have no relation to the spine, including catarrh, asthma, and constipation. Chiropractors use their hands in a skillful manner in order to perform different manipulative techniques. The process extends the joints to their fullest and then, with a short push, extends them further; which in turn relaxes the muscles around the joint and gives optimal movement and freedom to an area that was previously restricted in some way. This procedure may sound painful, but it should not be.

SLANT BOARD TREATMENT

A slant board treatment can help the spine, circulation, reproductive system, and more. It is really pleasant to use.

- Put a strong piece of wood, long enough to accommodate your height, on the floor with one end raised by six inches or a little more. (As you continue, you will increase the height, aiming at a height of two feet eventually.)
- Lie with your head toward the floor, feet on the raised end of the board. This will take the weight off your feet and relieve congestion in the hips, bowel, stomach, and lower back, as well as bringing blood to the head.
- Lie in this position for one minute at first, and slowly build up to fifteen minutes.
- When dismounting, do so slowly to avoid any light-headedness.

Do not use the slant board if you are pregnant or have high blood pressure, stomach ulcers, or heavy menstruation. There are also other times when it isn't advisable, so ask your practitioner.

You can buy slant boards or "tip-ups" from the Perfect Health Company (see the resource list at the end of this chapter). Alternatively, you can buy boots that hook over a bar, from which you hang upside down like a bat. You can also practice shoulder stands and headstands, which will have a similar effect.

Breathing

Correct breathing can really transform your whole life. It is the basis of all meditation, sports, singing, and other techniques. Insufficient, strangled, shallow breathing, gained through a life weighted down with illness, stress, or fear, will make your quality of life and emotional outlook much worse. You can learn breathing by joining a yoga class or by practicing easy counting techniques.

BELLY BREATHING

Do this exercise while lying down in a warm place or sitting comfortably in an upright chair, or else stand at ease with your shoulders relaxed.

- Gently become aware of your breath.
- Gently breathe into your belly or tummy by pushing it out like a balloon and breathing in through your nose. Count one.
- Breathe out by deflating your tummy and exhaling through your mouth. Relax your jaw and let go. Do this for a count of two.
- Repeat for two minutes initially, slowly building up to twenty minutes. You can also build up your inhalation time to a count of six, and your exhalation time to a count of twelve.
- Sometimes you may feel a little tired or even dizzy after breathing so deeply, so take your time and breathe normally for a few minutes before attempting to move around again.

Exercise and Movement

Some type of exercise is vital. Whether your preference is for football, swimming, tennis, whatever, it doesn't matter — just do it!

BAREFOOT WALKING

Walking barefoot on grass, sand, leaves, or pebbles has a grounding effect on the body. It helps to discharge static electricity from the body, calming the nervous system. Those who have tried this when they have been feeling particularly nervous, excitable, or tired have found that they feel calmed, rejuvenated, grounded, or, indeed, lightened; it has a very balancing effect.

DANCING

Dancing seems to come more naturally to women who, from a young age, like to move with grace and rhythm. However, I'm not sexist and believe dancing is a lovely meditation and joy for all.

POWER WALKING

Power walking (that is, walking very fast for sustained periods) is not as jerky for the body as jogging but is more balanced than running and easily sustained. Alongside yoga, it is one of the powerful ways of exercising and moving the lymph system.

YOGA

Yoga is a gentle, relaxing way to move the body safely and without strain. It will provide the body with much needed oxygen through its breathing strategies and additionally will massage and "exercise" internal organs.

Hydrotherapy

Water treatment, or hydrotherapy, is a very useful and natural way of improving circulation around the body. It complements exercise and massage but can also act as a substitute for people who are not able to exercise or cannot obtain massage. Very cold or very hot water or steam forces the blood to circulate more effectively, which brings nutrients and oxygen into and out of organs, easing congestion and stagnation.

HOT AND COLD SHOWERS

Try a cold shower after a hot shower or bath, adjusting the water slowly in order to acclimatize yourself. Direct the jet onto the area you wish to treat; this will encourage circulation and thus facilitate healing. If you do not have a shower unit, a cheap shower hose that fits over the taps will be adequate. A jug also works if nothing else is available, but the jet from a shower is far better. After the initial shock and gasp caused by the cold water, you will get accustomed to it. Start with thirty seconds under each temperature and build up to seven minutes; always finish with cold water.

SWIMMING

Swim whenever you can, in unpolluted sea- or freshwater where possible. When using swimming pools, be careful of the chlorination as the gas given off by chlorine is very toxic and will greatly affect those with allergies or a weakened immune system. Otherwise, wash the chlorine off afterward with thorough showering, using lavender or other essential oils to aid the process. Do a smell test afterward. If you can still smell chlorine on your skin or hair, then return to the shower!

SAUNAS

Saunas encourage perspiration, effectively opening the pores of the skin and driving water, toxins, and unwanted debris from the body via profuse sweating. They should not be used by the weak or frail; the very young, elderly, or pregnant; or people with certain heart conditions or high or low blood pressure. Frequent showering is vital during sauna sessions; concentrate the water stream over the top of the head as the skull heats up tremendously, which can cause nausea or dizziness.

SITZ BATHS

Sitz baths can be hot or cold baths in which the water line reaches the hips, womb, and ovaries but stays below the kidneys (so as not to chill them if the water is cold). The navel acts a good guide level. They encourage circulation of blood and oxygen to the womb and other associated areas and are very useful for aiding fertility and relieving endometriosis, PID (pelvic inflammatory disease), hip problems, sciatica, congestion, and so on.

Once you are in the water, swing both legs over the side of the bath. Alternatively, lower yourself into the water buttocks first, keeping your legs over the side of the bath. Whether you have the water hot or cold will depend on the particular problem you are aiming to treat. Sitz baths focus on encouraging circulation, increasing oxygen flow, and relieving any congestion or stagnation there might be in the lower abdominal area.

With cold sitz baths, it may be difficult to stay in the water for any length of time. Shout or scream, as this will relieve the shock and numbing effect of the cold water. Wear a sweater and socks if the bathroom itself is cold. Begin by staying in the water for one minute, and progress to five minutes as you get used to it. It is very important that you warm up quickly after a cold sitz bath. Placing a hot water bottle over the area, going for a run, or sitting near a fire are all good methods.

FOOT AND HAND BATHS

Water of varying temperatures may be used as a medium to carry herbs to all areas of the body by soaking the hands and feet. If the person feels hot, as is often the case with skin diseases, then cold water is used. Hot water would be appropriate with other conditions, such as flu. Herb decoctions or teas, essential oils, mustard, Epsom salts, or cider vinegar can be added. Soak your hands or feet in the solution for at least twenty minutes in order to absorb the plant extracts via the skin for topical or internal healing. You can use two bowls at once, each containing different herbs or varying water temperatures. One may be hot and the other cold—you can alternate between them. The famous French herbalist Maurice Messegue used this healing technique very successfully, and reading his book *Of People and Plants* will enlighten you about a whole system of healing for every known disorder.

Book List

Herbal Home Health by Christopher Hobbs (Springville, Utah: Christopher Publications, 1976)

Dr. Jensen's Nature Has a Remedy: Healthy Secrets from Around the World by Dr. Bernard Jenson (Los Angeles, California: Keats, 2001)

Resources

For Skin Brushes and Slant Boards

Perfect Health Company, 4872 Casitas Pass Road, Ventura, California 93001; tel: 800-444-4584; email: sales@juicing.com

⊰ 6 ⊱

Cleansing and Detoxification

You would not own a car and assume that simply by giving it oil, water, and gas it would keep functioning efficiently. You would realize that, at some time, it would need a complete oil change and a service. Interestingly, however, many people do not take similar steps to ensure that their bodies get the correct fuel and care. Yet they expect them to run efficiently. Detoxifying is like home servicing an engine, a self-help program to keep your body functioning well. A new breed of people are emerging who are prepared to give it a try and finding the results worthwhile.

Decreased immunity because of an increase in toxicity is evidently the key health issue of our time and will continue to be for the foreseeable future. But detoxifying and cleansing programs can help redress this problem. Cleansing the body of toxins by excreting, transforming, or neutralizing them frees the body. Every organ and system can sigh with relief as burdens are lifted, excess toxic baggage is towed away, and the effort of digestion is reduced to a minimum while nourishment is still provided.

What exactly are these toxins? They can be excessive mucus, abundant free radicals, fungal and other microbial infestations, parasites, and worms—in fact, anything that blocks tissues and suffocates cells, causing stagnation and the diseases that often arise out of an immunally or digestively compromised body. Free-radical damage is a common factor in chronic disease. Free radicals are irritants that cause tissue to inflame, blocking normal, free-flowing function at every level. Whatever the toxicity, and whatever its cause, the effects can manifest themselves in many ways. Cancer, diabetes, diverticulitis, obesity, fatigue, immune-system weakness, sexual disorders, swollen joints, headaches, candidiasis, and depression are just a few examples.

Good health relies entirely on a correctly functioning gastrointestinal tract that assimilates nutrients from food and swiftly removes toxic substances. Because this system creates harmony and balance, it stands to reason that appropriate foods or the lack of them can be the major mechanisms through which the body is healed or remains sick. Exercise, massage, hydrotherapy, and herbs have a supportive role in healing and should be used alongside healing food programs and other supportive therapies, such as acupuncture, radionics, and kinesiology. Exercise will always speed up the detoxification process because it helps to remove toxins by increasing circulation. Massage and skin brushing work similarly by stimulating the skin and are very valuable aids to health. Simple hydrotherapy should include alternating hot and cold showers, sitz baths, and saunas. It encourages circulation, promoting the movement of toxins and the delivery of nourishment to all cells, organs, and systems. For more on these therapies, see chapter 5.

General examples of herbs that may be chosen for various detoxification purposes include the following:

Blood cleansers: burdock root, red clover flower, plantain leaf, and lemon

Diuretics (water movers): corn silk, dandelion root and leaf, and celery seed

Laxatives (colon movers): barberry root bark, cascara sagrada bark, and Chinese rhubarb root

Liver supportives and cleansers: milk thistle seed, *Bupleurum* root, and dandelion root and leaf

Immune enhancers: echinacea root, arborvitae leaf, garlic clove, chamomile flower, olive leaf, and oregano leaf

Supportive and tonic herbs for the whole body: Siberian ginseng root, *Astragulus* root, *pau d'arco* inner bark, and *Schisandra* berries.

Food and Cleanses to Suit the Individual

Before you undertake a cleansing and detoxification program, there are several things that need to be taken into consideration in order to determine what kind of program is most suitable for you. In all cases, however, the body will require building and toning and then maintaining. Every program should include the use of water, juices, superfood, herbs, and specific foods.

Very often, only a selective grouping of foods should be eaten during this type of program. Foods should be specifically chosen to clean and detoxify the system that needs initial attention. It is important to remember that it is not the variety of food types that is important but, in this case, the quantity of the food type you are consuming. Often vegetables are chosen for these programs because they clean out the bloodstream, lymph system, kidneys, and colon while putting as little strain as possible on the digestive system and pancreas.

Ayurveda and other traditional healing systems look at body types and then advise on the duration of, and methods used for, a detoxification or fasting program that is appropriate to the individual. For instance, thin people with hypermetabolic constitutions burn up material quickly, and then the metabolism slows down. As this pattern decreases the likelihood of excessive detoxification, this type of person should be given a shorter program. People who have a slower metabolism and greater body weight can cleanse and fast more frequently and with increased intensity. People who are of medium height with red tones to the skin and hair and who maintain good levels of body warmth will find fasting and detoxifying programs an easy and productive process. If you wish to clarify your body type, consult an Ayurvedic practitioner. You can also simply start a cleanse and then stop if you are too overwhelmed physically and emotionally, returning to it at a later date.

For many relatively healthy people it is simply pleasant and rejuvenating to perform a cleanse at the onset of each season. Choose cleanses to fit the weather and your mood. The consumption of lots of juiced root vegetables, raw chiles, and ginger, accompanied by plenty of potassium broth (see under "Kitchen Basics" in chapter 4) and warming herbal teas, should be used in autumn and winter, while for the spring and summer, watery vegetables and fruits like melon and cucumber, along with an abundance of green salads, would be ideal.

For those wishing to cleanse only twice a year, the first cleanse should take place in spring. This is traditionally the best time of year to cleanse. It helps you to replenish your energy and shrug off the excesses of winter. Spring itself gives us the fresh ingredients for cleansing, such as spring greens (the sour varieties), dandelion leaves, young nettles, and new hawthorn shoots. Such plants can be used to thin the blood before the onset of summer heat. There are striking similarities between spring and autumn; for example, the damp nights and the golden days that give us green grass of such piercing vernal freshness. During the transitional season of autumn; you will again be able to find young dandelion leaves shooting up everywhere, and the nettles that have been cut down all summer will also begin to produce green, tender growth. Therefore autumn is a good time of year to cleanse the liver in preparation for the work it will have to do throughout the winter months, when the body and immune system are called on to endure the cold and the possible increase of infections.

Excessive fasting can slow down the metabolism and break down muscle, possibly leading to subsequent undesired weight gain.

The Differences between Fasting and Detoxification

Fasting involves total abstinence from food, with only water being drunk. This is a very good way of healing the body because only pure fluids, which do not require much processing, are entering the system, thereby giving the body a complete rest. But fasting should only be considered if you have a lot of experience with cleansing programs. Detoxification through cleansing involves more than water and can, in many ways, be more effective. It is certainly a more appropriate choice for the majority of people.

Those who are pregnant or breast-feeding should choose only a modi-fied, lighter, and shorter cleansing program using juices, raw foods, and herbs that are acceptable and complementary to pregnancy, along with gen-tle hydrotherapy. All should be professionally supervised and should not, under any circumstances, include enemas or colonics. Other people who should avoid fasting programs include those with a sluggish metabolism and congested organs, those already weak and depleted (as fasting can lower the body's resistance even further), those who are malnourished, those with low blood sugar levels, diabetics, and those contemplating strenuous tasks for their bodies in the near future.

Excessive use of laxatives, colonics, enemas, fasting, and cleansing programs can cause nutritional losses resulting in protein, vitamin, mineral, fat, fiber, and trace-element deficiencies. Remember, you are aiming to achieve equilibrium in your body, not trauma.

Healing Crisis

The phenomenon called *healing crisis* almost always accompanies these cleansing methods, causing your body to feel as if it is in both a physical and an emotional crisis. However, if you do not experience a healing crisis, it does not mean that the cleanse has failed. Your body is simply eliminating toxins in a different way. The whole process is a natural one whereby the body is healing itself by expelling excess toxins. Nevertheless, you may ini-tially feel as though your illness is becoming worse because of the unpleas-ant symptoms you are experiencing; in some cases it may remind you of the worst periods of any chronic illness or acute disorder you have experienced.

Many things can happen during a healing crisis, from headaches to aching limbs or rashes. Whatever form the reaction takes, it is a sign that toxins and stagnant materials that were previously poisoning the body are leaving it. The liver and colon are important areas to clean out and can release huge amounts of toxins accumulated over many years. The bowel can easily con-gest under the new regime being introduced unless careful advice and herbal help are given, so gentle laxatives are usually needed to accompany cleans-ing. Constipation at this stage works directly against what you are trying to achieve, and making sure the bowel is moving freely will speed up the general detoxification process. **The crisis stage may last three to four days but should never exceed seven days. This is an important guideline to fol-low, as ongoing symptoms would indicate that something else is amiss.**

A healing crisis can be slowed down if it is too dreadful by eating cooked food and reducing the number of days taken for the cleanse. Do not feel that you have failed if you do this; accept that your particular body needs to adjust more slowly and that you need to allow it to detoxify in smaller, less strenuous stages.

In the wrong hands and with certain diseases, a healing crisis could become a real crisis, resulting in excessive loss of weight from an already underweight and sick body. There is much to consider, physically, genetically, and emotionally before embarking on a cleanse, just as there is when choosing the right food program. It is vital to look not only at your body type and constitution but also at what your body is doing at the time. Under skilled professional supervision, weight can be allowed to drop in certain situations, but in these circumstances, daily massage with feeding oils and other natural healing therapies should be used as backup in order to maintain and support the body.

A one-day cleanse can provide a gentle start, allowing you slowly to progress to three days, five days, or longer at later dates, as you become more experienced and your body has fewer toxins to expel. Drinking water mixed with lemon juice will flush toxins through more quickly and, within a few days, the worst will usually be over. For the fit and able, extra exercise will help alleviate headaches and body aches by increasing circulation, thus moving and expelling the toxins more rapidly. For those who are sick and weak and find exercise almost impossible or very debilitating, cold showers are a perfect substitute. Alternatively, try a little yoga — deep breathing helps the lymph system work more efficiently. The fit and able must do all of these.

Speed of Elimination

It is important to keep in mind that fast elimination is not necessarily the best elimination. Excessive toxins forced through an organ can result in overload and crisis. A crucial rule to observe is cleanse a little, build a little.

The body's systems all have their own capacity, their own delicacy. A car engine doesn't run on jet fuel. Healing is the careful creative use of purifying elements. In a classic system, W. H. Cook (quoted in *The Textbook of Modern Herbology* by Terry Willard) described four groups:

Slow organs (e.g., liver) require slow remedies.

Rapid action organs (e.g., kidneys) require active remedies.

Sudden conditions require prompt and strong herbal remedies.

Slowly appearing conditions require slow, steady herbs.

Intuitive Fasting and Cleansing

An intuitive cleansing program or fast follows no specific rules. You comply with your body when it says, "I'm not hungry; I don't want to eat, even though it's mealtime." An intuitive fast can be for a single meal or for a day, and it's up to you to find some way of making it comfortable for others around you. Do not make the mistake of letting them cook you a meal and then turning it down! As meals are important social occasions, only you can decide when skipping one is convenient. Never eat when you are excessively tired, angry, or upset or when you are feeling overworked or depressed. Always eat when you are feeling relaxed and balanced. Some fruit or vegetable juice or light soup can be taken when you are feeling not quite able to digest but are still in need of food.

One-Day or Three-Day Cleanses

A one-day cleanse can be a gentle introduction to general cleansing. One day is not usually sufficient to induce the effects of excessive toxin release; if you do feel uncomfortable in any way on the night of the cleanse, there is no need to worry, as you will feel fine after eating a meal the next day. Eating naturally prevents detoxification.

A short detoxification gives the body time to rest, shut down, and do some repair work. It is usually perfectly safe for anyone to try. Choose a time when you have to do little or no work, either on the day of the cleanse itself or the next. Weekends are usually ideal. Choose the same day or days each month. The mind has a chance to rest and relax as well as the body, and the detoxification makes eating afterward all the more pleasurable!

First, drink a glass of pure, organic prune juice or fresh plum juice followed by a glass of purified water with a little cayenne, apple cider vinegar, or lemon juice in it and add a teaspoon or more of olive oil in order to cleanse the toxins from the liver. It can all taste surprisingly pleasant. You can also drink blood-cleansing teas. Include herbs like nettle leaf, cleavers leaf, burdock root, and red clover flower. Drink lots of springwater or distilled water to encourage the process. (Diabetics will not be able to undertake these cleanses.)

The next day, make your first foods fruit, then vegetables, building up to grains and the heavier proteins toward the end of the day. If you felt good on this one day, you may want to go on for a further two days, making it a three-day cleanse.

A ONE-DAY LIVER CLEANSE

A liver cleanse is specifically aimed at cleansing this organ and is something that can be done at any time of the year. It simply involves swapping your normal breakfast for a liver drink for one morning (or for three consecutive mornings, as above). This cleanse can give one a really springlike lift, whatever the time of year. Everything associated with spring can be regenerated with this cleanse (after the possible healing crisis): renewed energy levels, a greater feeling of joy, the desire to sing like spring birds, and even the emergence of new creative ideas as sloth and slowness ebb away. If you are feeling sluggish or out of sorts, this method of cleansing is paramount. People with liver and gallbladder dysfunction will definitely benefit from it. According to iridologists, those people who have brown or yellowish eye colors will particularly find relief with this gentle flushing process. It can also help those people with a history of either prescribed or recreational drug-taking. Cleansing your liver should lead to an improved sense of well-being. It is especially effective in breaking down cholesterol in the bloodstream by preventing the formation of fatty deposits along the walls of the arteries. Herbal cleansing once or twice a year will significantly help those people with an above-normal cholesterol level.

Start by cutting out all coffee, tea, and alcohol for three days. This will prepare you for cleansing, and already the body will begin releasing toxins, so do drink plenty of water to help flush them through.

Four foods are essential to the treatment: olive oil, garlic, lemon juice, and ginger.

Virgin olive oil helps to oxygenate your body internally; in its unrefined, uncooked state it is a prime antioxidant. Olive oil is a monounsaturated fat, which means that it does not clog your arteries with fatty deposits. It also increases the body's levels of high-density lipoproteins (HDL) or "good cholesterol"; this allows the blood to absorb more cholesterol so that it may be eliminated by the liver. Therefore it is important to choose the best-quality oil, that is, organic, virgin (first-pressing) olive oil.

Garlic is rich in sulfur and will help the liver perform and clear out better, as well as aid in keeping cholesterol and other levels in check.

Lemon juice is a wonderful blood cleanser and helps clear out excess acids.

Ginger will help ease any nausea associated with the cleanse and help to warm the whole body. Leave it out if your liver feels hot or inflamed.

To carry out a gentle flush of the liver, you will need to make up a drink to be consumed each morning on an empty stomach. For one person you will need

> 1 cup organic apple juice
> Freshly squeezed juice of 2 or 3 lemons
> 1 cup spring water, distilled water, or filtered water
> 1 clove fresh garlic
> 1 tablespoon virgin olive oil
> ¼ inch fresh gingerroot

Lemon juice is a citrus acid that becomes alkaline in the stomach, thereby aiding the cleansing of the digestive tract; it will also emulsify the olive oil. Should you be unable to consume any citrus at the time, use a teaspoon of turmeric instead. The garlic is best crushed before it is put into the blender. Blend all the cleanse ingredients until they form a smooth liquid.

Transfer this into a glass and drink it slowly; you can drink some organic apple juice afterward if desired. Fifteen minutes later, drink a cup of hot peppermint tea (using fresh leaves from the garden if they are available) or dandelion coffee with cinnamon sticks, cardamom, grated ginger, a little licorice, or any other flavoring that you have readily available.

If you feel a little headachy, it is because you are flushing your system. It will help if you drink plenty of fluids, especially water, and take some exercise. If you are unable to exercise, try hot and cold showers or massage.

Some emotions may also come to the surface—sadness and anger are associated with the liver—but their opposite emotion, joy, often replaces these feelings once the cleanse is over.

This is a gentle liver cleanse, and it's important to realize that toxins have been slowly building up in the liver for years. Therefore small steps are probably better in the first instance.

A ONE-DAY KIDNEY FLUSH

Pick a day when you can relax and keep warm. Start the morning with the juice of one lemon or lime, one quart of springwater, and a pinch of cayenne. Drink it all and, fifteen minutes later, drink a cup of kidney tea containing dandelion leaf, parsley leaf, bearberry leaf, and corn silk. Also take a kidney tincture if you have some, including all or some of the following herbs: dandelion root, marshmallow root, *Rehmannia* root, *Astragalus* root, chickweed leaf, lobelia leaf, burdock root, corn silk, Siberian ginseng root, ginkgo leaf, parsley leaf, and bearberry leaf. These herbs help to release excess stored water in all the cells of the body, as well as cleansing and healing all around.

At lunchtime, drink diluted fresh raw vegetable juices if you have any, or simply eat a large raw salad of sprouted seeds, dandelion leaves, lettuce, grated beet, and grated carrot. Use olive oil, apple cider vinegar, and lemon juice, with a little cayenne and black pepper, for a salad dressing. Have a cup of barley water (see recipe in chapter 4) with your salad. Continue the day with more raw juices and raw foods (but in winter avoid raw food and especially fruit if you feel the cold). In total, you should drink three cups of barley water, three cups of kidney tea, and approximately one tablespoon of kidney tincture. Also drink plain water at times, aiming to drink three to four quarts of liquid in total.

Advanced Cleansing Programs

Before you begin advanced cleansing programs, you must be proficient in the shorter and less intensive cleanses. Five-day programs achieve cleansing at a very deep level and will make a huge difference in your well-being. Get plenty of help, support, and advice prior to, during, and after the cleanse. Make sure all the ingredients for the cleansing program have been obtained and prepared before you begin.

A THREE-STAGE HERBAL COLON CLEANSE

Do not attempt when pregnant or breast-feeding. Do not attempt if taking prescription medication. Do not attempt this cleanse if you have any fragile bowel conditions, such as irritable bowel syndrome, spastic colon, or Crohn's disease.

Read through the section on the colon in chapter 9 for vital further information.

Cleansing the colon is a good initial step, because efficient waste disposal is essential in order to prevent the accumulation of debris and disease. Many modern bowels are accustomed to highly processed food and drink. The stress of our diet can cause a variety of disorders to arise, from a wide range of bowel complaints to less-obvious problems in other parts of the body like skin disorders, general allergies, and so on. A common problem today is poor stomach activity with depleted digestive juices, which contributes to making the colon less competent and more prone to underactivity or overactivity. Cleansing the colon is a good initial step toward increased health and well-being.

You can buy many different herbal colon cleansing programs from health-food stores. They all basically serve the same function. However, be careful to choose ones that have not been bulked out with a lot of psyllium husks. The program below is one that I choose to use with my patients and have found to be most successful over many years.

The herbalists Dr. Richard Schulze and the late Dr. John Christopher have designed between them three formulas used sequentially for thorough colon cleansing. The cleanse can last between two and three weeks or, if taken at a gentler pace, between two and three months. This cleanse should be directed and supervised throughout by a practitioner after initial checks for individual suitability. If the program is not appropriate for any reason, such as work commitments or children, it can be modified and used on a two-day basis, just like the short liver and kidney cleanses. Use the capsules and powders to suit individual requirements.

The cleanse *must* be accompanied by a good diet without coffee, sugar, wheat, dairy products, and so on. Mucus-forming foods must be avoided as they can cause excessive stickiness in the colon, slowing down passage of the feces and pasting old fecal matter to the walls of the colon. It is important to note that excessive mucus clogs up the whole body, not just the colon, so avoid animal products, eggs, cheese, and all wheat.

Useful additions while cleansing include

- Organic flaxseeds or psyllium husks (the fluffy, soft seed tops of a large fleawort, *Plantago psyllium*, found growing in Asia). Both plants soothe, heal, and attract water into the bowel.

- It is vital to drink plenty of water—two quarts a day at least, but four quarts would be better. Some find tepid water (nonsparkling spring-water) easier to consume and more detoxifying.

- Good foods: oats, rice, seeds, fruit, vegetables, herbal teas.

Chamomile and cascara capsules: This is very strong formula, designed for the modern bowel. It can be used on a weekly or daily basis on its own but is also a vital part of a three-pronged approach to the cleanse. I've known patients on massive doses of very strong bowel drugs who were experiencing painful side effects like gas, while still having very irregular movements. They have found this formula excellent; it is strong but gentle and contains the following powders: cascara sagrada bark, garlic cloves, barberry root bark, aloe gel, cayenne pod, senna pod, gingerroot, and chamomile flower. (Available from The American Botanical Pharmacy.)

People who may need to use this are those who are constipated because of an inherited lazy colon or through fiber and water deprivation or those who use morphine and other opiate drugs for pain relief. But there can be many, many other reasons for constipation. The number of people with lifelong genetic and behavioral tendencies toward this condition is rising by the day as junk-food consumption increases. The herbs help to retrain and regulate bowel function, promoting natural peristalsis; they also facilitate water absorption in the bowel and encourage liver, gallbladder, stomach, and pancreatic function. These herbs also clear out some of the old pockets of stagnant fecal matter that may harbor viruses, parasites, fungi, and bacteria. Should the bowel be inflamed, bleeding, and with pockets, this formula can still be used but with the addition of individually chosen herbs like meadowsweet leaf and flower *(Filipendula, not Spiraea)*, marshmallow root, and slippery elm inner bark. At first the formula may not quite suit the individual, but minor changes can be made until it does, such as using stool protectors and softeners.

Barberry capsules: Once constipation has given way to regular bowel movements, the bowel is ready to be cleansed in a different way. This formula is based on Master Herbalist Dr. Christopher's formula and is designed more for daily maintenance. Dr. Christopher originally had a dysfunctional and chronically constipated bowel. He wanted to design and use a herbal formula, containing no laxatives, that would maintain, strengthen, and gradually improve his bowel after he had cleansed and removed most, if not all, of the old fecal matter with strong herbs and healing clays. Combine this formula separately with psyllium husks, flaxseeds, and plenty of water on a daily basis.

The herbs he used, which now have more than fifty years' use, included

- Cascara sagrada bark—used in correct quantity, a gentle peristaltic tonic
- Barberry root bark—a liver and bowel herb
- Cayenne pod—to help circulation and peristalsis
- Fennel seed—alleviates gas and toxicity
- Garlic clove—protects against fungi, viruses, and other microbials
- Gingerroot—warming and circulating
- Licorice root—digestive and tonic
- Lobelia leaf—antispasmodic, relaxing
- Red raspberry leaf—stops bleeding, "feeds" the bowel, provides protective mucilage
- Chinese rhubarb root—gentle, tonic, and laxative
- Turmeric root—assists the immune system and liver
- Wild yam root—a prime digestive (alleviates gas) and liver herb
- Chamomile flower—soothing, antimicrobial, reestablishes bowel flora

Mix these together and place in capsules (see chapter 3). Many people use this formula on a daily basis, aside from taking it during a bowel cleanse, and it is quite safe to do so.

Clay and flaxseed powder: The third herbal formula (by Richard Schulze) is designed to draw and detoxify within the bowel. It is based on Russian and Native American herbal use of clays and herb powders and is used alongside the preceding two formulas but on a more limited basis.

The formula is made with the following powdered herbs: psyllium husks, bentonite clay, apple fruit pectin, flaxseed, slippery elm inner bark, sycamore charcoal, marshmallow root, and fennel seed.

This formula draws out poisons, toxins, and heavy metals (like lead and mercury), and even removes radioactive materials such as strontium 90. It removes more than two thousand known chemical and pharmaceutical drug residues. Another of its incredible abilities is that of softening hardened fecal matter so that it comes away from the colon wall easily and painlessly. At the same time, it soothes and heals the stomach, intestines, and colon itself.

Bentonite clay is able to absorb forty times its own weight and gently eases out old fecal matter, stale bile, and other unwanted residues. The clay is derived from volcanic ash and contains montmorillonite, which is a molecule five hundred times smaller than those that make up water (composed of hydrogen and oxygen), making it a far superior cleanser to water. These tiny molecules are capable of getting into the incredibly small nooks that water simply can't enter, which is vital for a thorough cleanse. Most toxic material is positively charged, while bentonite clay carries a negative charge. Therefore, toxins are immediately neutralized.

The pectin in apples removes radioactive substances from the body and generally detoxifies. Flaxseed and slippery elm inner bark lubricate, nourish, and cleanse. Marshmallow root similarly soothes, and its calcium and magnesium feed the nervous system. Slippery elm and marshmallow share an ability to promote tissue regeneration—useful in a bowel condition in which certain areas have worn very thin or old deoxygenated flesh is being exposed for the first time in years after being cleaned. Fennel seed is rich in phenols, which act in an antibiotic capacity. Charcoal cleans the bloodstream supplying the bowel. Psyllium husks provide gentle, healing fiber.

This formula can be taken half a teaspoon at a time (once or twice daily), mixed into juice, not just as part of a particular cleanse but by way of gently and consistently cleansing.

Please note: Because bentonite clay is so strong, any drugs prescribed by a doctor and upon which you rely, for instance for the thyroid or blood pressure, may become less effective. You may be able to increase your dose temporarily, but you must consult your doctor first. Otherwise you need to "negate" the shortfall. Also, you should not rely on any hormone-based contraception while using this remedy. Consideration must also be given to any drugs taken, as these will have a bearing on the outcome of the cleanse. How other organs and systems are functioning is also important. Some sort of healing crisis is to be expected, and for this a support network of friends or relatives can be of great help.

Stage 1

If you are constipated, then this is the preparation phase. Begin with one chamomile and cascara capsule just after supper. The following day you should notice an increase in your peristaltic bowel action and in the amount of fecal matter that you eliminate, the consistency of which should be softer. If you do not notice any difference in your bowel behavior or the difference wasn't dramatic enough, the dosage should be increased to two capsules the following night. You can continue to increase your dosage every evening by one capsule until you notice a satisfactory increase. Then continue at the same level for a couple of days before progressing to stage 2. It has taken most of us years to create a sluggish bowel, so be patient and allow time to get the dosage right.

Note: If you already have regular bowel movements (one to two daily with ease), then start with barberry capsules and build up in the same way.

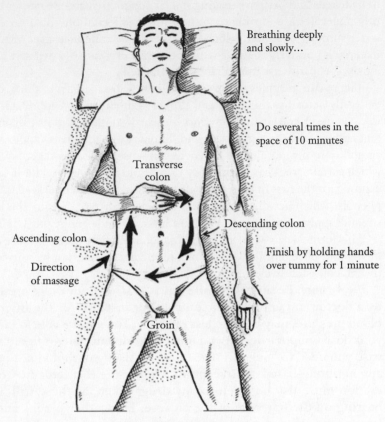

Breathing deeply and slowly...

Do several times in the space of 10 minutes

Transverse colon

Descending colon

Ascending colon

Finish by holding hands over tummy for 1 minute

Direction of massage

Groin

Abdominal massage

(Suggested dose: two barberry capsules and one chamomile and cascara capsule nightly.) You should be in regular contact with your herbal practitioner during this cleanse, and contact him or her immediately if you experience any pain.

Stage 2

Introduce clay and flaxseed powder into the program. Take ½ to 1 teaspoon of clay and flaxseed powder one to five times daily, according to your individual needs.

- Take the first dose one hour after a light breakfast of fruit or vegetable juice and springwater (with lemon juice, if desired). Drink immediately after mixing.

- Repeat midmorning, lunchtime, midafternoon, and before supper as required.

While taking the powder, increase the amount of chamomile and cascara capsules by one or two nightly to ease through the bulk created by the swelling powder. If you find that five teaspoons of powder a day is too taxing to your body (for instance, if you get headaches or bloating), you can slow the cleanse down. Reduce the amount of clay and flaxseed powder to a level that you find comfortable, such as two or three teaspoons a day, although even one or a half teaspoon a day will be beneficial. With lower doses like one teaspoon a day, some people sprinkle the powder into drinks or onto food, making a very easy way to perform the cleanse.

If you start to experience uncomfortable physical or emotional reactions and symptoms, then you are very likely experiencing a detoxifying reaction, which can last a few days. Please contact your herbal practitioner if this is the case, or simply apply a few practical self-help procedures:

- Drink plenty of water; increase the amount to help flush through the toxins.
- Try performing an enema—enemas quickly rid the body of toxins and can help reduce uncomfortable feelings (see below in this chapter).
- Rest, relax, and sleep as much as possible. The body is working hard, and rest will help its ability to keep going.
- If you feel very overwhelmed physically, then it can help to take some immune-boosting herbs (such as echinacea), which can help reduce the level of inflammation and generalized microbial reaction within the body.
- Use a castor-oil pack over the lower abdomen (see chapter 3).
- Take a relaxing bath with two tablespoons of Epsom salts.

Clay and flaxseed powder can be used for five to seven days if taking four to five teaspoons daily. This phase can be extended if taking a smaller dose, or the cleanse can be repeated in a few months.

Stage 3

Once you have finished the clay and flaxseed powder, use the more toning barberry capsules. These will help to regularize the colon again after the onslaught of the cleanse, which really forces peristalsis. For those normally constipated, it may be necessary to stay on these capsules for some time; it is better to use them regularly as needed rather than to slip back into old patterns.

This colon cleanse can be repeated twice a year. For those with long-term problems, however, several cleanses will very likely be needed. The feedback indicating its effectiveness may come in the form of a healing crisis, as toxic material is released from the body, causing a few unpleasant days of physical and emotional disturbance. The look of your bowel movements and how you feel are sure signs of having been through a healing crisis, especially if you suddenly feel much better. Often the brain clears and you feel emotionally positive and have a lot more energy. Each cleanse will leave you feeling more energized and generally stronger, more balanced both physically and mentally, and less prone to allergies.

During the colon cleanse, a professionally administered colonic will be of great use. A colonic is a gravitationally fed enema that is pumped into the bowel, using many gallons of water, to "sweep" the bowel clean. Water and herbs chosen for the individual are gently coaxed around the entire large intestine. It rarely hurts, except perhaps if an air pocket develops, and then some extra wild yam tuber in the water will expel the gas within moments. People's needs vary according to their bowel problems, so the number of colonics required will vary; a good therapist will use lots of herbs in the water. An individual with many old pockets will obviously need more sessions than someone who has a lesser problem. Colonics are particularly useful for people with old pockets full of putrefied and decaying fecal matter of many years' standing. Those with candida or parasitic infestations will also find colonics useful, and a good colonic therapist will be able to tell you how infested you are.

One-Bag or Four-Bag Enema

Enemas are useful for cleansing the bowel during and after the three-stage colon cleanse and for the majority of people unable to obtain a colonic. You can do a one-bag enema or a four-bag or "high" enema: the four-bag enema treats the entire length of the colon, from the anus to the ascending colon and ileocecal valve, whereas a one-bag enema may well only fully reach the descending colon. The enema ensures that all traces of clay and toxins are removed from the body. A herbal practitioner can select the herbal tincture mixture that best suits your needs. You will need an enema bag for this procedure.

1. Using your specifically chosen herbal tinctures, mix 4 teaspoons of tincture with one and a quarter cups of cider vinegar and two and a half cups warm springwater.

2. Ideally, make up four quarts of mixture and keep three quarts warm in flasks while you use the first.

3. The first quart goes into the enema bag. It is advisable to use a pint of coldish water initially for a few seconds; this contracts the bowel and makes it easier to "hold" the subsequent warm herb solution. The bag is hung on a bathroom door hook or some convenient place high up so that, using gravitational force, it can feed into the bowel.

4. The bathroom should be warm, with towels placed on the floor. Lie down on your back. Using Vaseline or a lubricating ointment, grease your anus and the end of the tube. Insert the tube into your anus. Then turn slowly onto your left side and get comfortable as the liquid slowly goes in. Stay on your left side and gently massage your abdomen, easing all the fluid in. Relax and breathe, so as to keep the fluid in as long as possible. Finally, let it go into the toilet.

5. If you are doing a high enema, repeat with another quart of fluid. Lay on your left side as before and then turn onto your back, encouraging the fluid to go into the transverse colon. Massage, breathe, and finally let go.

6. Continue with the third quart, but this time, after starting on your left side, move onto your back and then onto your right side; massage, breathe and finally let go.

7. When using the last bag, repeat all the movements of steps 1 through 6 in the same order, then stand up and massage the area over the ileocecal valve (the spot on the right-hand side of your bowel, where worms and fecal matter often collect). There is sometimes quite a strong and forceful reaction to massage of this area, so do stay in close proximity to the toilet! Finally, let it go; you have finished. Well done.

DOS (AND DON'TS) OF ENEMAS

- Do use during and after sickness.
- Do use during and after cleanses.
- Do use drops of lobelia leaf tincture on the tongue to relax you before and during the enema, and add a little to each enema bag.
- Afterward, thoroughly chew foods and juices to reestablish good digestion.
- Take some type of acidophilus to reestablish intestinal flora.
- Don't get addicted to the washed-out sensation or feeling thinner. You do lose several pounds of weight for a few hours, but this is due only to reduced water levels in the bowel, which will soon rebalance.

Intestinal Flora and Parasites

Maintaining healthy intestinal flora is vitally important in colon function as it aids many essential processes. Sufficient amounts are needed of these beneficial bacteria, which require fibrous foods to multiply. Antibiotics kill them, and it takes between six and twelve weeks to reinstate them to normal levels. Take daily probiotics to help cope with the release of unfriendly flora and to rebuild friendly intestinal flora. Many companies sell probiotics either by mail order or in health-food stores. Also drink chamomile flower tea or tincture; eat plenty of garlic and oregano, as they have natural probiotic action and kill off various antibiotic-resistant strains of bacteria. Soil organisms are also now being sold to help repopulate the gut, and these will also kill parasites, which is a bonus as parasites very frequently hide in dirty bowels. There are many herbs to assist parasite removal. This is just one formula — two parts wormwood leaf and one part black walnut hull, with cloves to remove the parasites' eggs (for adults, 3 capsules 3 times daily for 2 weeks). The use of cloves for parasitic eggs was originally researched by Hulda Clark.

Parasitic diseases and general systemic parasitic invasion of the body are more prevalent than many people believe. They range from microscopic organisms to threadworms to the well-known tapeworm. One in six people is believed to be host to some kind of parasite or another, and far from being a problem of "other countries," it is prevalent in the West. They can infest a weakened, sickly body, unable to fight their introduction, or conversely they can be introduced into a relatively healthy body and cause a slow or rapid decline, which shows baffling symptoms yet causes sometimes disastrous results.

These parasites do not kill directly, but they can cause a range of uncomfortable and debilitating symptoms according to the type of parasite. Some lodge in and "coat" the inside of the small intestine, preventing the absorption of nutrients from food. Others directly attack components of the immune system and can lower resistance drastically and even dangerously. Amebiasis and giardiasis (infestation with amoebas and *Giardia lamblia*) are two conditions now fully recognized as causing long-term illness. A book to help understand this complex and far-reaching subject is *Parasites: An Epidemic in Disguise*, written and compiled by Stanley Weinberger.

Specific herbs are very powerful and best used with other specific programs, such as bowel cleanses, liver cleanses, and immune support. Apart from the aforementioned wormwood leaf and black walnut hull, there are other very powerful herbs: *Artemisia annua*, well-known for malaria prevention and treatment as well as being a profound antiparasitic; and olive leaf, another wonderful and competent antiparasitic.

Liver Cleanses

A FIVE-DAY CLEANSING AND DETOXIFICATION PROGRAM

This program involves three days of a purifying food program (using raw foods) with a two days of juice fast in the middle. It should be undertaken only after the successful completion of the one-day version described earlier in the chapter.

Drink at least four quarts of liquid per day during the cleanse (if you weigh more than 140 pounds, increase this quantity by approximately one pint per extra 15 pounds). As you drink, keep a note of how much liquid you're consuming so that you consume enough before bedtime.

Day One

Breakfast: On rising, drink at least a pint and preferably a quart of spring-water. This is a great way to start your day. The water rinses your digestive tract and flushes out any leftover food or acids.

Within one hour, prepare a liver and gallbladder flush: Mix in a blender one cup of citrus juice singly or as a combination (for instance, mix the juices of one lemon and one lime and enough orange, grapefruit, or tangerine juice to make a cup) or apple juice. Then add the juice of two freshly squeezed lemons and a cup of springwater. Add one or more cloves of garlic, one or more tablespoons of organic cold-pressed virgin olive oil, and a ½-inch piece of fresh gingerroot. This mixture sounds rather strange but, in fact, it tastes like an exotic salad dressing and sits easily in the stomach. If you need to split up the juice and the water and the olive oil and garlic, then do so, but consume all within a few moments of each other. You may also mix in the herbs mentioned below.

You can add 1 teaspoon of a liver formula to this drink or dose it separately. This formula or one similar would be appropriate: six parts each of milk thistle seed, *Bupleurum* leaf, and wild yam root; four parts each of artichoke leaf, barberry root bark, *dong quai* root, gentian root, rosemary leaf, dandelion root, and turmeric rhizome; two parts each of agrimony leaf, burdock root, gingerroot, and lobelia leaf; and one part of mugwort leaf.

Fifteen minutes after taking this drink, consume two cups of tea made from a variety of general cleansing and specific liver herbs, such as plantain leaf, licorice root, carob pod, cinnamon stick, star anise, damiana leaf, mullein flower, and fennel seed.

If you are hungry before lunchtime you may have fruit, diluted fruit juices, or fruit smoothies (banana, apples, grapes, cinnamon, cardamom, vanilla extract, and rose water or lemon juice pureed in the blender). Stop all fruit or fruit juices at least an hour before lunch: it is best, while on this program, not to mix fruit and vegetables together.

Lunch: a salad incorporating a dressing of olive oil, raw apple cider vinegar, lemon juice, and any herbs and raw spices of your choice. Organic mushrooms, olives, dandelion leaves in season, parsley, chicory, and watercress are very beneficial and tasty. Drink potassium broth (see under "Kitchen Basics" in chapter 4).

Afternoon snacks: raw vegetables, diluted vegetable juices, sprouts, potassium broth, herb teas. All vegetable food must be stopped by 4:00 P.M.

Dinner (5:00 P.M. or later): diluted fruit juices, whole fruits, fruit salads, and herb teas.

Day Two

Repeat the program for day one.

Day Three

This is the first day to fast. Repeat the day one procedure up to and including lunch, then begin fasting, taking no solid food after 1:00 P.M. Continue to take diluted vegetable juices, potassium broth, and herb teas.

Day Four

This is the only complete day of fasting. Start with your water, morning drink, and herbal tea. Take diluted fruit juices and herb tea until noon, then diluted vegetable juices, potassium broth, and herb tea at midday and in the afternoon, and diluted fruit juices and herb tea again in the evening.

Day Five

This is the day to break your fast. Continue the fast until 1:00 P.M., and then you can have some fresh fruit. Chew it very slowly, and mix each mouthful with plenty of saliva. Remember, breaking your fast is a very important part of this program. Chew your food well and eat until satisfied, not full. You can always eat more later on if you are still hungry. After 4:00 P.M. you may have a vegetable salad, and fruit again in the evening.

Afterward

On the day after, start the same way as you did on day one, and then ease your way back into a good diet over a few days. This schedule can be done on a week-on, week-off basis until you feel that any deep-seated imbalances have really changed.

Things to Do Every Day

- Skin brushing, bathing, or showering with lavender essential oil.
- Hot and cold showers.
- Thirty minutes minimum of vigorous cardiovascular exercise to get your blood moving, preferably in fresh air.
- Twenty minutes of belly breathing exercises twice daily, preferably once in the morning and again in the afternoon.
- Take one teaspoon three times daily of a detoxification tincture containing red clover flower, plantain leaf, wild yam tuber, sarsaparilla root, bearberry leaf, gingerroot, licorice root, and myrrh resin.

- It is vitally important that you seek advice on bowel cleansing during this program.

Kidney Cleanses

A FIVE-DAY CLEANSING AND DETOXIFICATION PROGRAM

A kidney cleanse can be done at any time of year, but if a liver cleanse is also contemplated, do the kidney cleanse first. Very cold, damp weather is not an ideal condition in which to clear the kidneys, but as long as you keep warm and well wrapped up, it can be done during any season. Emotionally, you may feel weepy, vulnerable, and watery. Those who have felt this way have also felt that past issues were somehow accessed and flushed away.

You must consume at least four and a half quarts of liquid a day, plus three cups of barley water (see recipe in chapter 4). Keep vegetables and fruit separate on this program.

On waking, drink at least a pint of distilled water. This flushes the digestive tract.

Prepare a morning drink in a bottle: For the kidney and bladder flush, use the juice of two lemons or one lemon and one lime, one quart of springwater, and a pinch of cayenne pepper. You can, if you wish, add half a teaspoon of kidney herb tincture to the morning drink or take it separately. Herbs to choose would be similar to (or the same as) this formula: two parts each of dandelion root, marshmallow root, and *Rehmannia* root; and one part each of chickweed leaf, lobelia leaf, ginkgo leaf, *Astragalus* root, burdock root, Siberian ginseng root, parsley leaf, and bearberry leaf. A little maple syrup may be added to taste. Fifteen minutes after this drink, consume two cups of a tea made from dandelion leaf, parsley leaf, bearberry leaf, and corn silk. This really gets the kidneys awake and livened up.

If you are hungry, drink fresh fruit juices and fruit and herb teas until noon. Do not consume anything for one hour, then begin on vegetables or vegetable juices, using olive oil dressing with apple cider vinegar, spices, and herbs. Also have some potassium broth (see under "Kitchen Basics" in chapter 4); it aids the body in ridding itself of toxins. Eat only vegetables, salads, vegetable juice, and herb teas until 4:00 P.M. Eat nothing for one hour before switching back to fruit.

Supper: Eat fresh fruit and drink fruit juices and herb teas.

This program can be followed each day, but it is desirable to incorporate a day or two of fasting in the middle. For instance, on a five-day program, stop all solid food after lunch on the second day and stay with liquids only, including the potassium broth, until suppertime on the third or fourth day. Then take a little fruit and ease back into eating vegetables and fruit as before.

Every day, take thirty minutes of energetic exercise in the open air to get the cardiovascular system stimulated and cultivate positive thoughts. This is a time to nurture yourself and find out how to make the most of the food program—don't plan to do this program in a busy week.

On this program, the kidneys are stimulated and supported and, though it might seem that they are working overtime, they are relieved of coping with a heavy, exhausting diet with too much inorganic material and too little liquid. The adrenals also benefit. Distilled water, being "empty," can carry out of the body a much greater load of inorganic material that might otherwise collect in the kidneys, forming stones and irritation. Traditionally, the kidneys are the seat of energy in the body, and they are also associated with the emotion of fear. Purging this negative emotion is very important and has a radical effect on one's general outlook on life.

Weight Loss and Weight Gain with Cleanses

Weight is an essential issue for many people. There is no doubt that underweight and overweight conditions are, like any disease, partly due to inherited genetic patterns. Thyroid function, amino acid performance, metabolism in general, liver function, and the well-being of the stomach and pancreas all have great bearing on how well or badly we store or use our fat supplies.

We would all love to be just the right weight, but few of us are. Those who are underweight would love to be more formed, muscular, "filled-out," or simply warmer and having more energy; those who are overweight know only too well that it is unhealthy and slows us down. Obviously a whole-body tuning using cleanses and organic foods will help to compensate. Taking plenty of water helps remove excess toxins, which are always stored in fatty tissue. Eat less, but eat well.

Desired weight loss is aided by spirulina algae, kelp, evening primrose oil, chickweed leaf, dandelion root and leaf, and burdock root, whereas desired weight gain is aided by fenugreek seed tea or decoction, marshmallow root, and slippery elm inner bark.

Weight can plunge during cleanses in those with chronic diseases, and when switching to new food programs. This can be unavoidable, but olive oil massages will help "feed" the body. Slippery elm inner bark, fenugreek seed tea or decoction, and miso gruel will help to feed and nourish and keep undesirable weight loss at bay. Superfoods like algae or wheat or barley grasses will ensure proper nutrition while (or if) weight loss is occurring. Eventually the weight will creep back on and metabolism will be optimal, as all organs and systems find a greater harmony and well-being.

Young women heading toward anorexia, or indeed those already anorexic, may be unnecessarily force-fed stodgy food in an attempt to fatten them up when, in fact, good nutritious juices, broths, and superfoods would keep them feeling light and slim until more solid food is introduced, while herbs can help immensely.

TOXIC FAT STORES

Weight loss can also be achieved by bearing in mind your possible need for particular herbs for hormone balancing, relieving constipation, and treating a sluggish liver. Fat holds onto toxins even if you are not overweight. Fatty tissues attract toxic substances from gas, chlorobenzene, tap water, herbicides, and car exhaust residues. We also take in toxins from paints and lacquers. These can cause fatigue, headaches, tiredness, reproductive problems, immune deficiency problems, dizziness, eye discharge, and many other conditions.

TWENTY-FIRST-CENTURY REASONS TO CLEANSE

Toxic bioaccumulation isn't just a steady buildup in the fat stores of the bodies of overweight people. Most people have fatty tissue, especially women. All these toxins can be potential cancer promoters. There are at least fifty thousand environmentally harmful chemicals in use causing daily problems, and most of these are unlikely ever to be investigated. There are approximately fifty thousand pesticides alone used around homes, schools, and workplaces. Levels of car exhaust fumes are steadily increasing: approximately thirty thousand new cars are put on the road worldwide every twenty-four hours. This knowledge should give us a strong incentive to take regular care of our bodies by cleansing and detoxifying just to keep pace with all the poisons that flood our systems, no matter how careful we try to be.

Hints and Tips When Eliminating Certain Foods

	Coffee
Emotional effects	Coffee is a strong masker of flagging energies, and these will now be felt, sometimes making it hard to concentrate. You may feel sad, depressed, or angry as the liver starts to detoxify. You can also feel dizzy, anxious, or nervous. Irritability, insomnia, and depression can be other results.
Physical effects	The bowel will become more lazy because of a lack of morning peristaltic stimulation provided by the coffee. Headaches (throbbing, pressure), nausea (vomiting), and other such "liverish" side effects may be felt.

Tips and procedures to help the detoxification process

Reduce the daily number of cups and gradually decrease the strength of the coffee used. Decaffeinated coffee can be an intermediate crutch, but only briefly. For energy lows that come through lack of coffee's stimulating effects, take rosemary leaf tea and tincture of prickly ash berry and bark until the crisis is over. A few drops of lobelia leaf tincture will help balance and calm nerves, decreasing the overall need. Ensure that the bowels are moving daily and that the liver is supported via liver drinks once or twice a week. Drink plenty of water and herb teas—dandelion root, chamomile flower, and burdock root—in order to flush the body out. St John's wort flower can help some people with depression (and valerian root will aid sleep if needed). Dance or some other form of exercise will speed the release of toxins from the body. Saunas will help.

Tea

Emotional effects

Tea is a stimulant like coffee, but it doesn't kick the adrenal glands quite so hard, so in some ways it's a little gentler on the body and, of course, the emotions.

Physical effects

Lack of tea will slow down bowel function to a degree, and low energy will be a problem. Because tea contains a lot of tannin, you will gradually benefit from improved digestion and iron absorption.

Tips and procedures to help the detoxification process

The body won't feel as toxic as when coming off coffee. Please follow suggestions for coffee, as many of them will apply. Try green tea for a greater flavonoid- and antioxidant-rich alternative to help flagging energy. Finally, switch to herbal teas. Those that will be stimulative are rosemary leaf and flower, lavender flower, peppermint leaf, and prickly ash berry—alternate daily.

Alcohol

Emotional effects

(People with a recognized problem will need to attend AA or another similar program.)

Physical effects

You may feel vulnerable, craving, depressed, sad, angry, and low; anxious, paranoid, and irritable; fuzzy-headed and generally emotional or aggressive.

Tips and procedures to help the detoxification process

Common signs of alcohol withdrawal are shakiness and low blood sugar from a lack of alcohol sugars. The liver will be reflecting gastrointestinal difficulties, headaches, nausea (vomiting). You may get fevers, chills, and cramps, or hallucinations and seizures at worst.

Read the information on coffee—most of it will apply. Use St. John's wort to help with depression if it is appropriate. Milk thistle seed will help to protect the liver cells and encourage their regrowth. Support nutrition. Drink superfood because heavy drinkers are used to "empty" calories, and nutritional deficiency is probably present.

Wheat

Emotional effects

Irritability and muddleheadedness can emerge as the various allergies manifest from the wheat intolerance.

Physical effects

A relative feeling of relief predominates as the symptoms slowly subside.

Tips and procedures to help the detoxification process

Try sourdough and rye bread, rice, quinoa, sweet corn, and so on instead of pasta. Read the information on coffee for extra tips. Use herbs to help increase digestive powers, including gentian root and licorice root.

Sugar

Emotional effects

When sugar is eaten, an instant high will ensue. However, afterward the level of sugar in the blood drops, leaving you feeling vulnerable, weepy, angry, or chaotic, depending on the individual. Hyperactivity and poor concentration can also result.

Physical effects

You will probably have low energy. You might also suffer blackouts if weakness in the pancreas and spleen is critical.

Tips and procedures to help the detoxification process

Read the information on coffee, and use the applicable suggestions. Always keep blood sugar as balanced as possible; use licorice tincture or tea, or chew a licorice stick and sip sweet herb *(Stevia)* tea, which is three hundred to five hundred times sweeter than sugar. Chew on bitter foods to redirect taste and to "strengthen," such as dandelion leaf, dandelion coffee, olives, and chicory coffee. Support nutritionally to provide plenty of zinc, B vitamins, vitamin C, chromium, calcium, magnesium, and the amino acid L-glutamine.

Book List

Common Sense Health and Healing by Dr. Richard Schulze (Santa Monica, Califorinia: Natural Healing Publications, 2002)

The Cure for All Cancers by Hulda Clark (San Diego, California: New Century Press, 1993)

Healing Colon Disease Naturally by Dr. Richard Schulze (Santa Monica, California: Natural Healing Publications, 2003)

Parasites: An Epidemic in Disguise by Stanley Weinberger (Larkspur, California: Healing Within Products, 1993)

The Textbook of Modern Herbology by Terry Willard (Calgary, Alberta, Canada: Wild Rose College of Natural Healing, 1988)

Resources

American Botanical Pharmacy, 4114 Glencoe Avenue, Marina del Rey, California 90292; tel: 800-Herb-Doc.

Herbs Hands Healing Ltd., Station Warehouse, Station Road, Pulham Market, Norfolk IP21 4XF, United Kingdom; tel: 011-44-0137-9608201; web sites www.super-food.co.uk and www.herbshandshealing.co.uk

❧ 7 ❧

Immunity

I have heard many stories from history and traditional peoples about the use of plants, fire, air, and water to help the body defend itself physically—and also the reverse. Let's listen to a few.

Frenchwomen who packed lavender essential oil for the perfume trade in the seventeenth century didn't catch typhoid fever, and it soon became evident that lavender, just by handling it, could protect against the disease. The French are still known to use a great deal of lavender eau de cologne. Only twenty years ago, it was often used in place of a bath, with the name *lavender* stemming from the French word meaning "to wash."

When a small band of thieves was captured in France, staggering under the weight of gold, silver, and jewels they had plundered from the graves of the rich (many of whom were unlucky victims of a plague, which often killed off entire villages at a time), they were given a choice—they could escape the punishment of death if they told how they had avoided the plague while being continually in such close proximity to the very infectious dead. They disclosed all! The secret was simple: They collected a variety of wild thyme, marjoram, rosemary, and lavender, depending on their availability. They crushed the leaves and rubbed them over the entire body, releasing the pungent green, oily sap. A daily or twice-daily treatment had kept them free of the plague. What we now realize scientifically is that knowing it would work would also have increased their "happy hormone" output, thereby increasing the body's own abilities to defend itself.

Our family home, which was originally medieval, is a cottage in Norfolk; it had most of its south-facing windows blocked off during a very virulent plague. Knowing that the plague came from London to the south, the owners believed that a southerly breeze would surely blow the disease in through openings as you slept.

Europeans deliberately gave blankets exposed to smallpox to entire Native American tribes, with dire consequences. Much of the world still lives in fear that someone will eventually use smallpox as a lethal weapon.

Dirty water carries disease, especially whenever public waterworks break down—in war, earthquake, political upheaval, or famine. This problem still accounts for a large proportion of disease and death worldwide. Today the two major waterborne diseases are typhus and dysentery. The World Health Organization estimates that 2.1 million people are killed by these two diseases alone each year, most of the fatalities being children.

We often think we're steps ahead, only to find we're steps behind. A classic example was the law passed in the 1980s insisting that all chopping boards in catering kitchens must be made of plastic. Years later it was discovered that plastic chopping boards harbored unchallenged germs in tiny cutting grooves, whereas the natural essential oils, resins, and gums within wooden ones were natural and ongoing germ destroyers, constantly being released when chopped upon. It appears that wood is a living organism, rooted or unrooted.

Human beings, like other large species, evolve slowly. Microbes do not. They adapt and mutate incredibly quickly, and even if the world's wealthier countries eventually find some way to control them, they will still go on killing the inhabitants of poorer regions until those people finally become immune. The 1.7 billion people who were infected with tuberculosis bacillus in 1993, but who nevertheless didn't develop the disease, illustrate this process. Every year, 100 million people contract malaria. Two children die of it every minute, thanks to the collapse of a number of programs set up to eradicate it. The standard drugs being used are simply not as effective as they once were.

Many "old" diseases or diseases prevalent in the third-world countries have returned to and are spreading in the developed world — dengue fever, diphtheria, salmonellosis, pneumococcus, and listeriosis have all become more and more resistant to antibiotics. In fact, the U.S. National Institutes of Health has called it an epidemic of microbial resistance. Infectious diseases are still the world's leading cause of death, killing at least 17 million people each year. According to the World Health Organization, up to half the 5.72 billion people on earth are at risk of endemic disease.

Tuberculosis has made a big comeback, killing 3.1 million people a year with a more lethal strain of the disease that some say is potentially more dangerous than AIDS. The number of cases of hepatitis B has risen dramatically; in fact, viruses in general are on the increase, including viral meningitis, dengue fever, and so on. It is now thought that viruses that are able to hibernate for years may be the cause of many seemingly unrelated problems, from cancer to other chronic illnesses. Plants are able to disarm viruses and therefore we must learn more about them. Acute and chronic respiratory infections have risen to 4.4 million new cases a year. These alarming increases may be due to a combination of pollution and the overuse of antibiotics — sending out a clear message that we need to learn how to take care of ourselves.

American professor Paul Ewald has published a book called *Evolution of Infectious Diseases*, in which he strongly suggests that diseases long ascribed to genetic or environmental factors are actually caused by infectious diseases. He lists many: Alzheimer's, most forms of cancer, polycystic ovary disease, multiple sclerosis, Hashimoto's thyroiditis, cerebral palsy, lupus erythematosus, rheumatoid arthritis, a range of bowel diseases, and many heart and circulatory conditions. Of the latter conditions, he talks of the links between *Chlamydia pneumoniae*, and heart disease wherein live bacteria were found in arterial plaque fresh from operating tables. The same bacteria were found in a high ratio of Alzheimer's sufferers. He suggests that as time goes by there will be more and more examples of chronic diseases with an infectious etiology—*Helicobacter pylori* bacterium (the cause of stomach ulcers and disorders) being just one example.

The Layout of the Immune System

Immunity is not just a matter of balance, of germs versus our particular microflora and whether they can cope with invasion on a physical level. Looking at it in this way initially, however, can help us to understand the modern view of the immune system.

The *immune system* is the name given to particular cells and microbes in the blood, lymph, and some organs that defend the body against disease, harmful foreign microbes, and antigens that come into contact with them in the body, or indeed on the skin. The skin is our first line of defense—the armor of the body.

The immune system itself is a wonderful, subtle, and powerful system in which bone marrow, spleen, liver, thymus, tonsils, appendix, stomach, and adrenal glands have important roles to play. The system is intelligent and sensitive: for instance, chemicals issue from damaged cells in a form that allows them to pass through blood capillary walls and "eat" microbes by a process called *phagocytosis*. Their numbers increase according to the condition, as they are able to determine the severity of the situation. Certain cells can produce a chemical called *interferon*, which is useful because it limits the replication of a virus. Other cells secrete histamine, which causes blood vessels to dilate, which, in turn, helps the healing process. Still others increase their numbers during allergic responses, alleviating the condition by neutralizing histamine.

Different cells wander through the body seeking foreign bodies known as *antigens*. These cells enter the tissues to become *macrophages* (or "big eaters"), which can multiply as needed in affected organs. These *macrophages* are capable of isolating affected areas while they destroy antigens.

Cells have to be "educated" and activated as macrophages. Once they have been, their job is to find and destroy all invasive organisms, such as viruses and bacteria, that enter and endanger the body. They form what is commonly called the white bloodstream—the lymphatic system. This is a fine network that runs through the entire body, flowing in only one direction — toward the heart.

T cells are produced for fighting abnormal cell structures, for example cancer cells, cells invaded by virus, or transplanted tissue (as in heart transplants). They also fight pollen, fungi, bacteria, and some large-molecule drugs like penicillin. People in chronic disease situations like AIDS have too few T cells and are considered immune-deficient. In so-called autoimmune diseases, the T cells may act against themselves by mistake.

B cells, which come from the bone marrow, are activated by microbes and toxins. When they come into contact with a specific antigen, they secrete antibodies called immunoglobulins. Both B and T cells are capable of carrying out two jobs: one is to recognize antigens and remember previous encounters, while the other is to produce antibodies in response to them.

Current Immune Problems

One of the current worldwide — but mainly Western — immunity problems stems from the overuse of antibiotics in animal feeds. These drugs enter the human food chain and weaken our immune systems by killing valuable flora. Doctors now recognize this danger. The number of patients who contract food poisoning via contaminated meats and dairy products is constantly increasing. They cannot be treated with the available antibiotics because they have built up resistance via their food intake. Cases of food poisoning are rising by thousands each year. In fact, the U.K. Department of Health today regards salmonellosis as endemic, as it is now resistant to commonly used antibiotics. Pork, sausages, chicken, take-out restaurant food, and meat pastes are all in the higher-risk category. Intensive farming methods using antibiotics, steroids, and hormones are damaging both human and animal immune systems. It remains to be seen whether recent cleanup laws and revised procedures in abattoirs help to abate this trend.

Vaccination

I frequently get asked about vaccination, and I generally suggest that it is a good idea to read a lot about the entire immune system, and to research the ins and outs of individual vaccines and their short- and long-term side effects, before making a decision. After that, I would suggest a look at alternatives. These must include living an immunologically strong lifestyle and developing an ability to react well under potentially stressful and emotional conditions. In other words, you would be embarking on a lifestyle of responsibility. I have seen enough problems associated with vaccination to make me personally very wary and thus generally to avoid their use within my immediate family. I have had many children in my clinic suffering from lung complaints, digestive problems, bowel infestations, brain diseases, fungal and parasitic infestations, brain and speech breakdowns, and more. These conditions have been traced back particularly to the measles, mumps, and rubella (MMR) vaccination. It would seem that such a huge immunal assault on the very young often proves too much, and the body reacts adversely in a variety of ways.

Vaccination works because of the immune system's ability to recognize and respond, but it can tie up the body's B and T cell memory capacity to such an extent that the body's immune function ceases to be free to deal with any new challenges. *Natural coding*, whereby immunity is achieved through overcoming normal infections one by one in childhood, is more subtle: between 3 and 7 percent of memory capacity is tied up through natural coding, contrasting with 70 percent when a vaccine is used. (This gap was revealed in data collected by the Humanitarian Society in 1983.) Never allowing our immune system to self-educate, to recognize and remember for itself, is dangerous. Yet this is what may happen if antibiotics or vaccinations have been overused. Triple vaccines have been banned in some countries because of the increased danger of overstimulating a child's immune system. In Britain, however, it is still considered safe and acceptable. Although one brand of triple vaccine was withdrawn recently because of apparent links with meningitis, Britain still continues to use other types.

Instantaneous allergic reactions to vaccinations can be caused by excessive immune responses. This happens through the combining of antibodies with antigens to form allergies, which in turn stimulate cells to produce histamine. Excessive histamine can cause breathing difficulties and, indeed, bronchial spasm, which to a baby can be highly dangerous. Yet these immediate and worrying problems are minimal in comparison to the longer-term effects of vaccination and its overall strength.

If you decide to immunize your baby with the live polio vaccine, make sure you wash your hands carefully in essential oils after all diaper changes for three months afterward. Also, keep your baby out of contact with the following people because they are at high risk of contracting vaccine-induced polio: those receiving radiotherapy; those taking cytostatic drugs, systemic glucocorticoids like cortisone, potent corticosteroids for the skin, and adrenocorticotropic hormone (ACTH), or other immunosuppressive drugs; those with congenital immune-system deficiencies; and those with a history of paralytic disease.

If you or any other adults wish to be vaccinated, make sure you receive killed vaccines which have a higher safety record than live vaccines. Live vaccines are definitely considered riskier for adults. Also, take them separately (and spread the timing out), even if you have to pay more to do so. Multiple vaccines are cheaper, but they overburden the immune system incredibly.

Automatic Defenses

We have many automatic and natural defense systems for dealing with viruses, bacteria, fungi, and other foreign bodies. It is generally believed that viruses are different from bacteria in that bacteria operate outside cell walls while viruses choose a host cell in order to replicate themselves. Some can mutate—for instance, HIV dodges the immune memory system in order to survive. With all viruses there can be the added problem of secondary bacterial infection. Although modern drugs can deal with fungal or bacterial infections, they used to be unable to invade viruses or to penetrate the walls of cells inhabited by viruses. However, some are now able to overcome certain viruses' sophisticated defense systems. This development could lead to the production of entire families of antiviral drugs in the future, which could have a similar outcome to the story of modern antibiotics (see below). Should an antibiotic be given to a person with a virus, and should it enter the cell wall, aggressive side effects can take place; these may include severe nausea, dizziness, immune system imbalance, and emotional swings.

Antibiotics

Once reserved for life-threatening situations, antibiotics have now become abused substances, generally via the dairy and meat food chain. Repeated courses of antibiotics can disturb the immune system so much that they can become ineffective. Physicians have become much more aware of this problem, and avoid prescribing them where possible. Repeated use of antibiotics in children, toddlers, and babies can lead to severe conditions, which may include cases of unresolved tonsillitis (often resulting in surgery to remove the tonsils), chronic respiratory problems, skin disorders, middle ear infections, allergies, and hyperactivity. These are problems that, originating in childhood, may be reflected in a difficult and sickly transition into puberty, with deeper problems like myalgic encephalomyelitis (chronic fatigue syndrome), cancer, and other virulent immune disorders occurring in adulthood.

We now know, in terms of specific side effects, that prolonged use of neomycin can cause liver malfunction, tetracycline can stain children's teeth yellow, chloramphenicol can interfere with the production of red blood cells or cause potentially fatal underproduction of bone marrow. It is now generally understood that repeated use (in other words, three to four courses of broad-spectrum antibiotics in the course of several weeks or months) can so deplete a patient's immune system that chronic illness can set in very fast. This opinion is often reiterated by many enlightened doctors, nurses, and members of the public. It is now generally understood that once the "good" bacteria in the gut are gone—destroyed by antibiotics—yeasts and molds can quickly overpopulate the body, leaving it in a weakened state. What is less known is that, at that point, the body is vulnerable to a variety of other conditions ranging from digestive disorders, liver and gallbladder problems, and spleen and pancreas dysfunction to hormonal imbalance, thyroid insufficiencies, and bowel disorders.

We have created antibiotic-dependent cells in our bodies; we have coded our memory cells so that they are constantly looking for antibiotics. In other words, our cells have become drug-addicted. Thus, antibiotics that once worked now have little or no effect. In some parts of Africa and the Philippines, penicillin won't work at all. In other countries, where once one medium dose of penicillin would have worked to clear gonorrhea and staphylococcal infections, it now takes two huge doses of penicillin together with another antibiotic to deal with these conditions. *Staphylococcus aureus* is the most common type of bacteria that can infect humans. About a third of the population is colonized "harmlessly" by this bacterium, but it liberally passes to the vulnerable, especially in hospitals and care centers; and it has mutated into antibiotic-resistant forms.

Probiotics are organic substances for life as opposed to antibiotics (which kill germs, very often indiscriminately). Probiotics were originally called ecobiotics. Ecobiotics are substances that specifically treat intestinal flora and nowadays we call them probiotics—a term first used by Monica Bryant in 1986. Veterinarians have administered probiotic bacterial supplements for a long time to treat animals. It is only comparatively recently that these substances have been put to use with humans. What we now realize is that a balanced colony of beneficial bacteria will prevent intestinal toxicity and give good general protection from infection. The highest numbers of beneficial bacteria in the body are situated in the small and large intestines, perhaps as many as a trillion microorganisms. This volume of flora can easily weigh about four to five pounds! All bacteria have different actions, some living permanently in intestinal walls, others moving through the system, working as needed. This protective bacterial colony deals with invasive parasites, yeasts, and so on. Its other jobs include helping to break down bile in order to inhibit pathogenic organisms, assisting complete digestion, and helping to reduce toxic residues that encourage putrefactive bacteria. They assist in the making of B vitamins and important enzymes for digestion—particularly of lactose.

Where do probiotics come from? Some come from milk products, others from fermented vegetables and other sources. Ask your supplier for one that is suitable for you and appropriate for the problem at hand. Soil organisms are also being used very successfully to balance our own flora, reinstating the "peck of dirt" that used to be considered vital for our well-being, according to the old European saying.

How We Think and Feel *Is* the Immune System

The key to an effective immune system is the general well-being of our mind, body, and spirit. Being sick is not simply the result of one problem, it is a collection of many factors. Some diseases are regarded as being modern, such as depression caused by stress, pollution, and so on. We become frightened by these diseases and perhaps even feel guilty about them. These negative feelings are also factors in disease. Cancer is often talked about as a modern problem too, but archaeologists and scientists have told us that the skeletons of ancient peoples and animals have repeatedly shown signs of cancer, proving that this is an old, inherent problem affecting all living creatures.

In medical lectures on the immune system in top American hospitals, great emphasis is usually laid on a patient's state of mind as being the key to the health of the immune system. Medical experts have discovered through extensive research that the main, fundamental driver of the immune system is the hypothalamus, and that what dictates its performance is the way we think—that is, whether we are happy or sad, positive or negative. It is also important to look at the health and well-being of the adrenal glands, which support the hypothalamus. A stressed, overworked, unhappy life can lead to disease, whereas a positive attitude, happiness, and relaxation are vital in overcoming disease. In this modern era of gene testing, it is important to realize that we can all possess mutant genes with a potentiality toward cancer. Not only can we be responsible, in part, for whether they get switched on, we can also have the power to switch them off.

For those who are enlightened about positivity and who know about negativity and pain, the subject becomes something of a meditation itself. Maintaining genuinely good and positive feelings in any situation creates vibrations, and these vibrations create different auras and body chemistry. Kirlian photography and chromatography can reveal these normally invisible things. Body chemistry creates smells and fragrances that repel or attract and will affect you, other people, animals, insects, plants, stones—anything that has a vibration of its own. It is possible to hurt yourself with your own unhappy, angry, or depressed feelings because, by bringing this kind of emotional pain into your heart, you cause a kind of internal poisoning. If your childhood has been spent alongside parents or close relations who were often sad, angry, in pain, or depressed, this can affect your adult system. Your present immunity pattern may have something to do with early negative vibrations. Nevertheless, recognition that a parent or close friend was indeed emotionally disturbed can have a liberating effect. You can accept that this was the way it was in the past, and then move on.

We are beginning to explore such taboo subjects as sex, hopefully creating a society that is less sexually ignorant and more sexually loving, mature, and aware. Children treated with love and respect, who are accustomed to being listened to and responded to with freedom of knowledge about their bodies, their sexuality, life, and death, are more likely to grow up feeling relaxed in relationships and having the ability to recognize unhealthy vibrations in other people more quickly, rather than becoming victims who are unable to move on. People who have known and been surrounded by positive experiences as children will have that valuable asset, self-esteem. They will feel a balanced confidence and, being more whole, will be able to cry, laugh, grieve, feel, play, be silent, be noisy, and experience all the rainbow of emotions without becoming overly stuck in any one corner.

There are various ways to learn the art of maintaining genuinely good feelings most of the time, and this brings your lifestyle into the spotlight. Do you enjoy your job, your lover, your children, your neighbors? If not, then change one or another of them, or change yourself. Whichever initial approach you take, however, you'll need to spend time on yourself. Some form of meditation will have to become a part of you and your life. Without this, emotional or physical pain will be an unwanted companion. Understand that bad feelings hurt you, and bad feelings against someone vibrate most strongly back at you, so it is vital to transform this state. Counseling and voicing your problems can be very helpful, but to remain stuck in this mode for years merely becomes another excuse to avoid yourself. Meditation has the knack of allowing you to gain an understanding of yourself.

Physical pain is nagging, but is made worse by wishing to jump out of it. Exploring it and making peace with it can bring about a huge transformation. Of course, terror, fear, and anger usually hinder this transformation, but with time, guidance, and practice, it can become a reality.

Breath, Tranquillity, Laughter, Sounds, and Immunity

Like a contented baby who breathes with sublime bliss from its belly, we too can learn to breathe deeply again. Breath is the basis of any silent or moving meditation, just as it is the basis of dancing, singing, or laughing. Breathing from the belly is something we do in deep sleep. Most of us, during our waking hours, return to the more shallow breathing area of the rib cage, which utilizes only one-third of our lung capacity. Oxygen is so strongly connected to good health that it is helpful if we can learn to discipline ourselves to return to the more contented and balanced method of breathing, using the diaphragm and our entire lung capacity. Fear and anger are emotions that create controlled, frozen, or spurted breathing patterns high up in the chest. Outrage generally comes from the area of the gut, the belly. Laughter also comes from the belly and is always a strong, spontaneous medicine. At the age of three or so, a child's breathing moves from the belly more into the chest. This is a good age at which to remind children about belly breathing, teaching them to use it on occasion to calm grief, anger, fear, and other strong emotions. Adults, set in patterns developed and acquired during the course of life, often need more consistent practice. Breathing is a form of meditation on its own, and many old cultures still practice it. It is also the basis of all life: real, full life.

Perhaps the most attractive thing we are all capable of doing is laughing — whether at jokes, clowning about, funny movies, or slapstick humor. I make it my business to have these around me because I have always been attracted to laughter-making entertainment and find it vital for my own well-being in the work I do. Very often, after a day spent treating the pain and distress of others, laughter provides almost instantaneous medicine. I'm a great fan of comedy and have a growing collection of humorous videos so that I can get a quick laughter fix to balance all the other more serious things in life.

In the United States, where many progressive theories come from, music is being used directly for pain relief, relaxation, alleviation of psychiatric problems, and blood pressure reduction. In Britain's National Health Service, a hospital in Oxford is at present offering treatment using music for stroke patients, together with massage at mealtimes to help digestion and at nighttime to aid sleep.

Using Herbs for Our Immunity

Please refer to the section on "Immunity through Fermented Food" in chapter 4, which will give you further insight and a more comprehensive understanding of this subject.

Herbs that help the immune system can be used on a vibrational or a physical level, utilizing the chemistry of plants. Each plant has individual traits and diverse uses as a means for empowering the immune system. Some help to create interferon and T and B cells; some assist the absorption of oxygen, which keeps cells alive and healthy; still others act as antioxidants, preventing free-radical damage.

Sometimes it becomes difficult to know where the categorization of immune herbs begins and ends. There are many choices, so we will start with supporting the body both physically and emotionally by discussing adaptogenic herbs.

The category of **adaptogenic** herbs can help you to adapt more quickly to whatever is new in your surroundings, be it emotional, physical, or environmental. They can help to strengthen and change hereditary weaknesses. When the common cold virus came to Greenland from America, many Inuit died. The virus was so alien to them that their cells couldn't cope. Their adaptability was overwhelmed, for there were no immune-cell memories of the virus. The next generation fared better — something common to all disease throughout history. This is an extreme example of a situation in which adaptogenic herbs would be used.

In order to be classed as an adaptogen there are three qualifications the herb must possess: It must increase the body's immune function using a wide range of actions, rather than just one specific action. It must restore and maintain balance in all body systems at no expense or aggravation to them. And it should not produce side effects.

In general terms, adaptogens are described by herbalist Christopher Hobbs as working by supporting adrenal function, thus counteracting the debilitating effects of stress; increasing the concentration of enzymes that help produce energy in the body's cells; helping cells to eliminate the waste by-products of the metabolic process; and providing an anabolic effect that helps build muscle and tissue, helping the body use oxygen more efficiently and enhancing the regulation of biorhythms. Some famous adaptogens are Siberian ginseng root, *Schisandra* berry, *reishi* mushroom, and *Pfaffia* root.

The Russians have probably done the most research into adaptogens. They have concluded that there are also secondary adaptogens—herbs that are not quite as strong, but nevertheless very useful. These secondary adaptogens help to balance and normalize the immune system, nervous system, and hormone system. Those most recently studied include gotu kola, wild oats, *Astragalus*, and burdock.

Adaptogenic herbs can be used daily as food, in herbal teas, as tinctures, or in capsules. They are ideally suited to being combined with other plants as they mix well and remain balanced and supportive.

The beautiful **Siberian ginseng** or **eleuthero** (*Eleutherococcus senticosus*) is a herb of our time and, if used on a more widespread basis, could help balance major deleterious immune trends through its ability to fortify against environmental pollutants and radiation. It helps to regulate blood sugar levels and influences and nourishes the pituitary and adrenal systems. It protects the liver and helps eliminate drug residues from the body. Taken on a daily basis, Siberian ginseng increases our ability to resist infection; it has also been shown to suppress cancer cells by enhancing phagocytosis and the production of leukocytes. It is a good long-term tonic that should be used by those suffering from many conditions ranging from myalgic encephalomyelitis (chronic fatigue syndrome) to cancer and all the various autoimmune diseases, including multiple sclerosis. I use a mixture of this and milk thistle seed to treat and support those turning around from drug and alcohol addiction. Additionally, it increases endurance by improving the cells' ability to use phosphorus-containing molecules and by disposing of lactic acid and other unwanted and often-harbored by-products of metabolism. It is wonderful for stress, and one teaspoon of tincture before breakfast can really help the quality of one's day and of one's night of sleep. You can take up to three doses daily. It is a good idea to stop for two days in every ten and then repeat the cycle for up to nine months (or longer under supervision). Siberian ginseng also affects the adrenal cortex and will therefore have a slight hormonal effect—which could be estrogenic, but is more likely to be simply an endocrine tonic and balancer.

Although it is called a "ginseng," it is in no way related to true ginsengs (members of the genus *Panax*), either by its action or by its botanical structure. It got its name purely because it gives vitality. In order to avoid confusion, it may be wiser to refer to it by one of its other common names, *eleuthero*.

There are literally hundreds of herbs worldwide that stimulate the immune system and attack microbes: they include turmeric root, burdock root, plantain leaf, and oregano leaf, but of late echinacea root has been very popular. **Echinacea** *(Echinacea angustifolia)* is a well-known herb cultivated in Britain, America, and Europe. The only place it still grows in its natural habitat is North America. It is capable of rallying the top defenses of the immune army. Native American tribes have been aware of the benefits of this herb for many centuries. While white Americans grudgingly accepted its medicinal value toward the end of the eighteenth century, it has only comparatively recently reached Europe. It was used as a major immune-system stimulator by the indigenous peoples, who loved this pretty purple-pink-rayed flower with its attractive center. They sucked on the root, with its tingling, almost metallic taste, all day when they were sick.

The tingling is caused by the chemical isobutylamine. Many herbal scientists have said that the tingling is incidental to its healing properties, but professional practitioners have proved time and again that it is actually vitally important. *Echinacea angustifolia* is the preferred species, rather than the garden perennial *Echinacea purpurea*. The tingling and numbing of the tongue should be the deciding factor when buying the tincture or root. Alternatively, you could make your own.

As with all herbs, the quality of the tincture is of the utmost importance; some echinacea tinctures on the market are weak and ineffectual. Some people have told me that echinacea has made no difference to the way they felt; however, further investigation has revealed that they had bought poor-quality tincture. Tinctures are relatively easy to make if you have a quality benchmark to be guided by; otherwise you can buy them from reliable suppliers. You can also consume teas and decoctions or simply chew on the crude root.

Sioux, Cheyenne, Comanche, Pawnee, and other tribes all over America traditionally used echinacea in many ways, from stimulating energy or soothing toothache to treating deadly rattlesnake bites. Echinacea can be put directly onto bites, stings, and cuts, and enters the bloodstream that way. If the white blood count is very low and general immunity is severely depleted, echinacea cannot work fully unless vitality-building herbs and foods (and other immunity stimulants) are used alongside it to build up the bone marrow reserve. It was thought for a decade (the 1990s) that echinacea should never be used by people with autoimmune diseases; it was felt that it would only exacerbate the out-of-balance immune response, provoking it to "eat itself" and thus lower immune levels even more. These warnings were theoretical and as there is no convincing empirical evidence to support these ideas and as many autoimmune patients flourish on echinacea, the ban is lifted.

It was a hard battle to get echinacea accepted by the medical profession. They viewed it as a type of quack medicine; yet by 1914 it was scientifically proved to activate phagocytes. Recognized in Germany during the 1930s, it has been welcomed back in a new wave of interest there and is now being used more than ever. Germany is the largest producer and importer of echinacea in Europe, using the superior fresh tincture from wild organic plants from America. More recently Germans have been growing their own and making fresh tincture. They also produce hundreds of medicinal products with echinacea as one of the ingredients. Up-to-date scientific data shows that echinacea broadly acts by doubling or tripling the number of T cells in the body (although some tests have shown that it can increase available T cells tenfold, and some research has shown an increase by a factor of up to fifteen thousand). It also activates areas of the immune system that mobilize only for serious conditions (macrophage production); and it vastly increases the amounts of interferon, interleukin, immunoglobulin, and other important natural chemicals present in the blood. Echinacea actually boosts the number of immune-system fighter cells and then stimulates them into action by mimicking the function of the cell wall, which gives a signal to the body that an immune response is needed; a group of chemicals called *polysaccharides* is responsible for this stimulation. Short-term benefits include the treatment of colds. Echinacea also speeds up recovery from chronic immune depression illnesses.

The root of the endangered herb **goldenseal** *(Hydrastis canadensis)* is a wonderful immune herb, but it has been overused and often inappropriately used. Unfortunately, it has been wantonly overcollected and pillaged in the wild, though cultivated crops are now available. Dr. Christopher taught me its myriad uses for conditions ranging from eye problems to typhus, but if used for too long a period, the gut (and B_{12} production therein) and kidneys suffer. There is a useful substitute, **barberry** *(Berberis vulgaris)* root bark. Goldenseal and barberry contain two important chemical constituents, berberine and hydrastine, so can often be interchanged.

Barberry's tonic activity on the gallbladder and liver is supremely effective. Skin diseases are often alleviated, mainly thanks to this effectiveness on the liver. It makes an excellent tonic for the delicate, the weak, and children. American herbalist Christopher Hobbs reported that, when taken intravenously, barberry's antimicrobial effects are useful against a wide range of bacteria, fungi, and protozoa—*Salmonella typhi, Candida albicans, Neisseria meningitidis, Chlamydia,* and at least fifteen more microbes. In fact, its action is much stronger than that of many commonly used antibiotics. One of its fascinating qualities is that it releases compounds that trigger an immune response caused by increased blood supply to the spleen. It also activates macrophages and, in the laboratory, has been shown to inhibit tumor growth.

Garlic *(Allium sativum)* is the immune system's greatest friend. Fresh garlic, which is a stronger antifungal than nystatin, has been proved to destroy viral infections such as measles, mumps, chicken pox, herpes simplex 1 and 2, herpes zoster, viral hepatitis, scarlet fever, and rabies. It also defeats many types of bacterial illnesses including streptococcus, staphylococcus, typhoid fever, diphtheria, cholera, bacterial dysentery (travelers' diarrhea), tuberculosis, and tetanus. It should be used daily to keep immune levels balanced. See chapter 4 for further details.

The **apple** and **citrus** families: we have a beautiful fruit widely cultivated in Britian of which it is said, An apple a day keeps the doctor away. Apples should be organic and eaten whole—pips, core, flesh, and skin—or made into fresh apple juice. The apple is a sacred fruit and should be kept at the forefront of our fruit intake. It is a member of a particular category of plants that contain nitrilosides, which naturally occur, mostly in the seeds, in more than twelve hundred plants, among the best known of which are apple, apricot, cherry, flaxseed, peach, and plum. The Hunzas of Pakistan, who are noted for their consistanly long lives (age ninety and older), have been found to consume mineral-rich water and lots of organic fresh food, including apricot flesh and seeds, which are very rich in nitrilosides (B_{17}). Similarly used, the apple could give us equally long and healthy lives.

The beautiful family of plants known as citrus fruits are also important additions to our diet. In 1928, Hungarian scientist Albert Szent-Györgyi isolated vitamin C from citrus and other sources. He knew that in 1757 a British doctor had prevented scurvy aboard ships by using lime juice. Szent-Györgyi later isolated bioflavonoids, which he called vitamin P. He blended vitamins C and P and named it "citrin." We now know this compound to be a prime antioxidant. In nature, vitamin P occurs naturally in plants.

Fresh lemon juice on salads, in springwater, or added to herbal teas or cooked food is tasty and nutritious. It is able to cleanse the bloodstream and protect oxygen, and is also rich in vitamin C. I also use limes, always keeping a stock of fresh limes and lemons, plus their dried, powdered versions. Try this treatment for viral infections: Collect the white pith of twelve organic lemons and put into the blender along with a little peel and juice for taste. You can add some maple syrup if you like to counteract the sour flavor. Add enough spring water to loosen the mix, and puree to a light, fluffy, frothy "pudding." It tastes delicious and really helps if you are suffering from cold sores, candidiasis, flu, or colds. The vitamin C and the antioxidant qualities of the vitamin P in the raw white pith help heal the system. It makes an excellent one-day cleanse, combined with other herbs and teas that support the immune system.

Olive *(Olea europaea)* leaf is another very effective all-around herb, not least for being of great assistance to the immune system. It was used in 1927 to eradicate malaria in some areas. One of its chemical constituents, calcium enolate, seems to have particularly interested plant chemists who feel that it is largely responsible for fighting viruses and killing fungi, parasites, and bacteria. In the case of viruses, it is able to interfere with a number of key processes, thus inhibiting their spread, replication, and nutrition.

As I have said already, there are literally hundreds of immune herbs. Eucalyptus leaf, walnut husk, pine needle, *pau d'arco* inner bark, and elderberry are a small selection, capable of tackling a wide range of microbes, bacteria, and viruses. We could also add chamomile flowers, which can kill invasive bacteria, such as salmonella, that have evaded long-term use of strong antibiotics. But all herbs have their own special abilities and specific ways of disarming, which makes constant variety and the use of a number of immune herbs in any formula very useful in this twenty-first-century postantibiotic era.

Essential Oils

Essential oils are nature's antibiotics. About 1910 it was discovered through a scientific experiment that the volatile oils from various plants were as strong as, if not stronger than, phenol, a much-used chemical antiseptic. These oils include garlic, angelica, citrus lime fruit, lemon, and fennel. Lavender, oregano, and rosemary are not far behind. Eucalyptus and thyme are not as strong but are, nevertheless, potent antiseptics. Some Australian surgeons use diluted eucalyptus oil wherever a European surgeon would use a manufactured antiseptic—for instance, to swab out surgical cavities.

Recent research has shown that tea tree essential oil is supremely effective against the scourge of antibiotic-resistant bacteria, including *Staphylococcus aureus*. These bacteria are becoming more common in hospitals, where already vulnerable patients can easily pick up such opportunistic infections, and the usual treatments are ineffective. The resulting symptoms can range from debilitating to life-threatening. In tests, solutions between 0.2 and 2.0 percent of tea tree oil were added to cultures of these bacteria. The results indicated that as little as 0.25 to 0.5 percent killed the bacteria effectively. Vials containing no more than a teaspoon of tea tree oil, sold quite inexpensively in health-food stores, look like a cheap and effective godsend.

Pine tea, made from pine needles that are rich in essential oils, is a great antiviral aid. This is a traditional Native American remedy that has recently been discovered to be a prime antioxidant as well.

The use of essential oils can be part of keeping well and dealing with sickness. Oils can be added to the bath, used in the shower, put into shampoo and other hair treatments, added to toothpaste and mouth gargles, made into massage oils, added to foot and hand baths, and used as fragrances.

Use an essential oil supplier who tests the oils or has them tested using chromatography and other methods of analysis to ensure good-quality oils, devoid of toxins. Making your own oils at home is perhaps the most desirable of all. Collect the plants, flowers, leaves, or needles, blend them with olive oil, and leave in the sun, shaking daily, for two weeks. An easy antimicrobial oil would be made with equal parts of pine needles, ecualyptus leaves, and rosemary leaves.

Immune System Treatments

ASSISTING A FEVER WITH IMMUNE HERBS AND NATURAL HEALING METHODS

Fever is generally nature's way of getting rid of unwanted toxins, making it a healthy sign; the high temperature and consequent sweating burn and kill unwanted attackers. There are situations, however, in which it can be dangerous. Fevers in children and old people should be monitored, while in babies and those who are already chronically sick, good professional advice should be sought.

To help a fever in general, aim to keep your temperature up, but not too high—above 102°F but below 104°F. Make sure the fever is "wet" and not "dry." To keep the fever wet, drink hot real fruit juices such as apple juice with a stick of cinnamon and a pinch of pepper, or fresh lemon in hot water. Herb teas are ideal, too. Good ones for fever are yarrow leaf, red raspberry leaf, catnip leaf, peppermint leaf, elder flower, and boneset leaf. Drink as much as possible. Red raspberry leaf and boneset leaf not only help the sweating process but also provide calcium, which is lost in enormous amounts during sweating. Additionally, these herbs act to cleanse and clear the bloodstream and lymph system, which is a vital process. If you need a break from hot drinks, take sips of noncarbonated distilled, filtered, or mineral water, which must be at room temperature; you don't want to bring your temperature down.

Take five to ten drops of echinacea root tincture hourly along with five drops of barberry root bark tincture. If the bowels have not opened recently, have an enema, because constipation can push a fever up very high. An enema in certain fever situations can actually save a life, being the only thing that will bring a dangerously high temperature of 106°F or 107°F down a few degrees. Ensure that the bowels keep moving.

If your temperature is too high, get into a bath at a temperature of 98.6°F for approximately half an hour. If you feel low and exhausted, add one half-cup cider vinegar, two tablespoons Epsom salts, and five drops rosemary essential oil to your bath. Once you have dried off, use a skin brush, then go back to bed immediately and cover up well.

Use your thermometer frequently to keep gauging how you're doing. Once you've broken the fever, have another bath, this time finishing with a cold shower. Change all nightclothes, bed linen, and so on. Keep drinking the fluids you drank during the fever to maintain the detoxification process and to build up the lost calcium. This is a vital convalescent procedure. Also ensure that you consume appropriate liquid nutrients to maintain the healing process.

GENERAL IMMUNITY FORMULA

Immunity formulas vary according to an individual's needs or chosen direction of aid. Immune herbs will stimulate, disarm, and destroy fungi, viruses, and bacteria, while other herbs may be added to support different organs and systems, including the liver, lymph system, bowel, and circulatory system. A combination that includes red clover flower, *Pfaffia* root, echinacea root, chamomile flower, thyme leaf, pokeweed root, myrrh resin, barberry root bark, Chinese rhubarb root, cayenne pod, red raspberry leaf, arborvitae leaf, lobelia leaf, turmeric rhizome, pine needle, *pau d'arco* inner bark, burdock root, licorice root, and elder flower and berry would make a good formula. Using only one or two of these herbs would do equally well, however, and a selection would be best made with the help of a qualified herbalist using tinctures if possible.

Take approximately 1 teaspoon of your chosen herb formula selection three times daily for ten days and then, after a two- or four-day break, continue with 1 teaspoon three times daily for weeks, months, or longer in some cases. Addition of tonic support may be needed for deep-seated chronic conditions.

If the problem is very exhausting, supportive nutrition and nurturing herbs will be vital, as they will tone and build while giving gentle energy to the nervous, digestive, hormonal, and other systems. Such herbs might be slippery elm inner bark, Siberian ginseng root, dandelion root, burdock root, *Schisandra* berry, *Rehmannia* root, elecampane root, skullcap leaf, gentian root, nettle leaf, *Astragalus* root, saw palmetto berry, seaweed, red raspberry leaf, marshmallow root, fenugreek seed, lobelia leaf, and Chinese licorice root.

The Essiac formula is an old, yet still very effective, immunity formula that belonged originally to the Native Americans. It contains slippery elm inner bark, Chinese rhubarb root, burdock root, and sheep sorrel leaf. This formula takes into account some important basics—immune support, supportive tonic help, and bowel and liver detoxification. It is also highly regarded as a preventative and as a treatment for cancer.

SPECIFIC VIRUS FIGHTERS

Viruses are a problem for modern medicine, but many antiviral compounds are found in seaweed, fungi, and higher plants. Via a number of mechanisms, they are able to invade and disarm the viral cells. Clinical analysis needs to increase on this subject, but enough evidence exists that proves many plants' worthiness as potent antivirals. They include turmeric, lemon balm, olive, arborvitae, juniper, and oregano; there are hundreds more.

HOMEMADE IMMUNE SUPPORTER AND FIGHTER—"HOOCH"

This formula is a modern-day plague remedy, stimulating the blood while detoxifying. It benefits from being made on the new moon, then strained on the full moon, approximately fourteen days later.

- Fill a jar three-quarters full with equal parts of chopped fresh garlic, chopped fresh white onion (or the hottest type available), grated fresh gingerroot, chopped fresh horseradish if available, and chopped fresh chile peppers (the hottest available, such as African bird peppers). Other additions might be mustard seeds and black pepper.
- Top the jar with organic apple cider vinegar, cover, and shake vigorously.
- Let stand in a warm, dark place for two weeks.
- Filter the mixture through muslin or a fine sieve and keep the liquid. (You can leave some of the mixture unsieved and use it as a delicious hot relish with food.)
- Keep the liquid in the refrigerator.
- Dosage: one to two teaspoons two or more times daily. Gargle and then swallow.

Book List

The Book of Sound Therapy by Olivea Dewhurst-Maddock (London: Gaia Books, 1993)

Echinacea by Jill Rosemary Davies (Boston, Massachusetts: Element Books, 1999)

Herbal Antibiotics: Natural Alternatives for Treating Drug-Resistant Bacteria by Stephen Buhner (Dublin, Ireland: New Leaf, 2000)

Laughter, the Best Medicine by Robert Holden (London: Thorsons, 1993)

Olive Leaf Extract by Dr. Morten Walker (New York: Kensington Books, 1997)

Ginseng by Jill Rosemary Davies (Boston, Massachusetts: Element Books, 1999)

Tumeric and the Healing Curcuminoids by Muhammed Majeed, Vladimir Badnaer, and Frank Murray (New Canaan, Connecticut: Keats Publishing, Inc., 1996)

❧ 8 ❧

Life Stages

This chapter is a commentary on the natural development of the human body, with emphasis on those times when healthy growth and development may need extra care and attention—be it to ensure correct hormone balance or sufficient nourishment of certain organs and systems. All are aimed toward achieving a healthy and happy mind, spirit, and body.

Childhood

Children are the new generation and should therefore be given guidance, love, support, and appropriate protection to enable them to develop into healthy and balanced adults. Children do not belong to parents but have their own unique lives, yet parents are fully responsible for the unfolding and nurturing of their development—some task!

One of the best gifts children can be given is that of good health. Good nutrition is the basis of good health; it is the fuel that builds and sustains the physical body and also influences emotional development.

Calcium, vitamin C, and magnesium are essential for growing children; therefore consider food sources for all of these, like citrus fruit, walnuts, parsley, and sunflower seeds. Superfood is pleasant-tasting if made with fresh fruits and is full of essential nutrients. A daily cup of tea made from nettle leaf, dandelion root, chamomile flower, or hibiscus flower will also support children—in fact, any simple herb tea will be preferable to tea, coffee, artificial fruit juice mixes, and sodas.

If you choose to bring your child up as a vegetarian, you must ensure that you replace the nutrients that meat would have provided. Chapter 4 gives fuller information on all aspects of food and nutrition.

BABIES AND TODDLERS

When feeding babies and young toddlers, it is always best to use a variety of homemade meals. Some nutritious and easy recipes follow.

Breakfast

A good nutritional balance would consist of 50 percent ground organic millet flakes (or cooked whole millet) and 50 percent fresh alkaline fruit or vegetables—preferably organic, including apple, peach, banana, cauliflower, carrot, parsnip, and zucchini. With fruits, add powdered cinnamon, and with vegetables, add a pinch of powdered turmeric and a little finely chopped garlic. Soak the millet overnight and gently cook through over very low heat (sieve for very young babies). Add sieved or mashed fruit or vegetables and serve. If using vegetables, add finely chopped parsley for older babies, which will provide useful iron and calcium. This meal provides protein, iron, magnesium, calcium, B vitamins, and a range of other vitamins, minerals, and trace elements.

Rice and Seaweed Soother

1 cup cooked organic brown rice
¼ cup presoaked dried seaweed (any variety, such as purple dulse or bladder wrack—there are so many kinds, so always vary your choice)
½ cup steamed chopped carrot
1 teaspoon arrowroot
¼ teaspoon dried thyme leaves
½ clove garlic

Mix all the ingredients together in a blender. Add a little springwater if the mixture needs moistening. For extra protein, which is a vital body-building component for growing babies, add either 2 chlorella tablets or 2 teaspoons of superfood to the mixture while blending. Finally, stir in 1 to 2 teaspoons of virgin olive oil before serving. This meal supports good, easy digestion and provides a rich variety of vital food values.

Energy Meal

1 cup cooked quinoa
¼ cup freshly sprouted seeds, such as alfalfa or sunflower
1 teaspoon olive oil

Blend all the ingredients together. This recipe provides a good balance of protein, vitamins, minerals, and trace elements, with the bonus of the sprouts giving plenty of raw energy.

The White and Green Dish

1 cup mashed organic potato
½ cup mashed avocado
¼ cup chopped fresh parsley
½ teaspoon dried marjoram, or 1 teaspoon fresh marjoram leaves
¼ teaspoon fennel seeds, or 1 teaspoon fresh fennel fronds

Blend all the ingredients together. For very young babies, this dish is rich in protein and oils and contains a host of vital vitamins and minerals, while its herbs help digestion considerably.

Fruit Delight

> 1 cup apple puree
> ½ cup mashed prunes
> ½ cup vanilla bean, finely chopped
> ½ teaspoon powdered cinnamon

This recipe is excellent for digestion and slightly sluggish bowels. It is also easy to prepare. Add 1 teaspoon of uncooked arrowroot if more help is needed with digestion (and correspondingly a little water to loosen the mixture). Apple is a very healthy food.

Find a line of baby and toddler foods based on organic ingredients. Exposure to a variety of new foods will help babies and toddlers to develop a wider appreciation and encourage them to become more adventurous eaters as they grow up.

CHILDREN

When preparing food for children, make it appealing and fun. Occasionally, cover the table with many foods with different tastes — for example, sliced raw carrot, olives, olive oil, garlic, raw mushrooms, cauliflower, sunflower seeds, carob pods, and apple slices — then let them try each of them while you draw attention to the different flavors and colors. Children love to copy, so join in!

Children eat proportionally more food than adults. This is necessary because they are growing and, therefore, their metabolism is working at a much faster rate. They are also naturally more active than adults and use more calories, so it is always advisable to have nutritious snacks for them to eat, such as bananas, apples, or presoaked dried fruits. In the summer you can make your own fruit-juice ice pops.

Banana–Rice Milk Shake

This is a tasty and energizing drink that is ideal for children. To make, blend up to three bananas with ½ cup rice milk, soy milk, coconut milk, or almond milk; 5 bee pollen grains; and ¼ teaspoon powdered cinnamon.

What to Avoid

Children, like adults, will show clear reactions to certain food groups if they have allergies to them. They will also experience reactions if they are nutritionally deficient, including headaches, insomnia, lack of appetite, constipation, diarrhea, nausea, or catarrh. Candidiasis or a runny nose and general low health may indicate possible nutritional problems with reactions or allergies, stemming from inadequate digestion, malabsorption, or nutritional deficiency.

Avoid food colorings and additives in foods and limit the intake of sugar, especially hidden sugars like those in cakes, pastries, and chocolate. These can complicate and exacerbate conditions such as hyperactivity and attention deficit disorder.

Some 80 percent of children who have a combination of physical, intellectual, and emotional difficulties are simply afflicted by food-related allergies or childhood candidiasis. These cause a range of symptoms, including stomach, liver, and bowel disorders; chronic fatigue; eczema; aggression; and specific learning difficulties. Food allergy testing will help you identify foods that should be avoided, but a good rule of thumb is to avoid pesticide-laden vegetables, steroid- and hormone-fed meat, dairy products, and wheat products altogether. Some professionals believe that these difficulties may be due to the observed trend that children's blood grouping is changing. Many are now type A or AB, rather than the more common type O of their grandparents. This means that they have less hydrochloric acid in their stomachs, and this deficit, in turn, produces allergies if mishandled. Over time the digestive capacity of the child can be built up by using herbs like meadowsweet leaf and flower, gentian root, and slippery elm inner bark, with a range of foods that boost intestinal flora. Eventually the child should be able to process a wider range of foods with little or no reaction.

Immunization, the overuse of antibiotics, and an increase in junk food have radically altered the health of children, and there are now visible consequences of these changes. Children will especially benefit from flaxseed oil and other foods rich in essential fatty acids, which will support neurotransmitters, thus supporting the brain. (For more detailed information, refer to the section on the nervous system in chapter 9 and the dietary advice given in chapter 4.)

Zinc levels, so important for building up the immune system, are also often difficult to maintain in children because they use so much for growing. To help calm and soothe children on all levels, whether they are overworked at school or generally hyperactive, use the following formula: equal parts of lemon balm leaf, vervain leaf, lavender leaf or flower, dandelion root, chamomile flower, skullcap leaf, lobelia leaf, red clover flower, catmint leaf or flower, and Chinese licorice root.

GENERAL CHILDHOOD ILLNESS

Children can be quick to get sick but equally quick to recover, and essentially they have the potential for greater resilience and strength if every illness is treated correctly. Those who are supported with herbs, baths, massage, and good food, and left to fight out their illnesses without antibiotics and invasive, suppressive medicines, will build up better long-term defenses and consequently require less nursing in the long run. There is nothing better than parental care, home, and bed to deal with sickness; early, good support can keep the child out of both the doctor's office and the hospital. Having been involved in the parenting of four children, two from birth and two from the ages of nine and twelve, I know it takes effort, input, patience, and knowledge, but that the results are worth it.

First signs of illness can be anything from a lack of appetite to high or low facial color with shivering or fever. A child can be restless, loud, and angry or quiet, withdrawn, vulnerable, weepy, and in need of holding (or being near you). Be alert to behavior that seems odd for a particular child. Very often they complain of headaches or nausea or will simply need sleep at odd hours.

Knowing when to call in professional help is difficult, for we have fewer large family groups nowadays in which grandparents, aunts, and so on can help and advise: but seek help if you feel that you need it. **This list of warning signs may help you to know when to call for help: prolonged vomiting and diarrhea, convulsions, a temperature that fluctuates quickly between hot and cold, blurred vision, drowsiness, headache after a bang on the head, drifting in and out of consciousness during fever, turning pale or blue, shallow breathing, or eyes dull, sullen, or glazed can all be signs that you need prompt professional help. In fact, you will probably feel it when something is really wrong: you will know it by instinct—and trust your instinct.**

Giving lots of water but less food helps all illnesses. Children generally know what is best for them in these situations, much as animals do. But these gut instincts are becoming blurred as natural healing skills in the home diminish and nutrition loses its true value.

SOME CHILDHOOD CONDITIONS

Teething

When teething, your baby should have as much calcium and magnesium as possible. The teething pains will be greatly minimized if the new tooth can quickly break through by having adequate energy resources to do so.

To give your baby calcium, use what are called "tissue salts"; there is one specifically for teething, available from many pharmacies and health-food stores. Give nettle leaf tea (and occasional *pau d'arco* inner bark) with honey, if needed, in a bottle as a long-term measure. Short-term use of valerian root and honey tea (seek dose advice) will help the baby to sleep; it will also calm any fever and quickly supply large amounts of assimilable calcium, but it must be prescribed and dosed only by a qualified herbal practitioner.

When all the child's available energy is going in one direction, digestion can become upset. When this happens, provided they are no longer being breast-fed, give young children juices and superfood in a sippy cup. A little diarrhea is to be expected, but if there is constipation, use gentle laxative foods like prunes and olive oil. Children should also be encouraged to drink meadowsweet leaf tea three times daily before meals. A formula to aid poor digestion would be equal amounts of licorice root, cinnamon stick, and fennel seed taken as a tincture or tea (with honey).

Growing Pains

Growing pains can afflict toddlers, older children, and adolescents, especially if they have a poor diet. I have talked to many patients who remembered suffering weeks or months of aching limbs; their parents had told them that growing pains were a normal part of growing up.

What is actually happening is that the body is growing and stripping itself of the materials it requires for growth. Normal childhood growth can induce pains if the diet is not sufficiently balanced (see the section on calcium in chapter 4), but occasionally massive growth spurts take the body by surprise. If this occurs, extra calcium and magnesium must be given immediately by increasing the intake of herbs like boneset and nettle. Nettle leaf tea should be drunk daily; boneset tincture can also be given, but only for a few days at a time, until the pain has gone away and then for three to five days longer. Carrot juice, homemade or storebought, is also a good source of calcium. My children told me immediately whenever they got any aches; they were then given fresh carrot juice for a week, on top of their daily plant calcium and magnesium input.

Fever and muscle aches leach a large amount of nutrients from the body, not least calcium. If it is not replenished, what began as an acute and easily rectifiable ailment can become chronic, simply from the lack of calcium in the body. Drinking milk at this point is not recommended, as its neutralization of digestive foods would make an already hampered digestive system work at an even lower level. Get children to drink nettle leaf tea to increase levels of calcium and magnesium and use rice milk, soy milk, or other milk alternatives. Leg twitching during the night can indicate a need for calcium, magnesium, and iron in children, in which case nettle or red raspberry leaf will help, as they both contain large quantities of all these minerals.

Fever

When taking children's temperatures, remember that their higher rate of metabolism means that they can more safely sustain a higher temperature than an adult. Your first course of action should be to keep the child sponged down and ensure high fluid intake. If you are concerned about your child, call in professional help. Normal body temperature ranges between 96.8°F and 98.6°F. A fever is said to exist if a temperature is above 100°F. You must call for help if the child's temperature reaches 104°F. You can take rectal, armpit, or, in older children, oral temperatures. Rectal temperature readings are very reliable. Lay the young child or baby on your lap, tummy down, bottom up, and hold him or her down with one hand, allowing a small amount of movement. Lubricate the anus and slip the thermometer in as you hold the buttocks open. Insert at least one-third to half of the thermometer. Take a reading while it is still in place. Remove the thermometer and give the child a big cuddle. Refer to "Assisting a Fever" in chapter 7.

Childhood Convalescence

It is normal for a child to want to play the moment he or she feels better, but this stage must be handled carefully. If there has been a fever, much vital calcium, magnesium, and other vitamins and minerals will have been lost. These must be replenished rather than allowing the child to expend what little energy is left to the detriment of the body both in the short term and in the long term.

- Begin with fresh organic carrot juice and superfood—good sources of vitamins A and B complex, iron, calcium, and more. They are easy to digest.

- Feed the child rich broths and soups containing root vegetables and beans, whole grains, stewed apple puree, and other easily digestible foods. Additionally, blessed thistle tea will return digestive enzymes to normal, but also include a few slices of pineapple and half a papaya to assist.

- Move slowly back to normal eating patterns, without rushing this transition, even if the child is very hungry.

- Give nettle leaf or red raspberry leaf tea as they are both rich in calcium, magnesium, iron, and other nutrients.

- Massage the child frequently and use baths with essential oils.

- Keep the child stimulated with creative options that do not require excessive energy, but insist on rest periods.

The Hormone Arrival

Hormones prompt many of the next developmental stages in life. Adolescence is the period during which boys begin to become men and girls begin to become women. Girls start to menstruate, their bodies preparing for pregnancy, birth, and motherhood. Boys' bodies begin to change shape, their voices break, and they begin to grow facial hair. Hormones drive all these changes.

Plants contain many hormones, and their use has a full, rich history. There is still a vast amount of scientific research to be done on the world's hundreds of hormonal herbs, but it is known that the same herb can often affect men and women in varying ways in different situations. They mostly contain saponins, which have a steroidal effect on the body, acting as building blocks that can be converted by the body to the exact requirements that are needed. Sometimes these hormonal herbs increase or decrease the output of the pituitary gland or hypothalamus, while other times have a more broad-spectrum effect on the entire endocrine system.

What follows is a summary of the current knowledge regarding the three main male and female hormones, about which science is constantly discovering more enlightening revelations.

FUNCTIONS OF ESTROGEN, PROGESTERONE, AND TESTOSTERONE IN THE BODY

Estrogen

- guides the young female from fetus to babyhood to womanhood, partially explaining why girls behave like girls (such as playing nurturing games) and why eventually they grow breasts and develop higher voices and broader hips.
- helps in the growth of the endometrial tissue, which forms a "nest" for a fertilized egg. It is the fertility hormone.
- helps to relax blood vessel walls and aids circulation and tone in the genital tract. This relaxation causes cervical secretions that are inviting to the sperm.
- helps to retain bone calcium.
- needs to be balanced in order to prevent dramatic mood swings, painful cramping in menstruation, and more problems in later womanhood. A joyful woman has balanced estrogen.
- levels increase after menstruation and ovulation, then decrease premenstrually. Although this hormone is present throughout the whole cycle, premenstrually it can surge and decrease.
- produced excessively creates an imbalance in the production of a hormone called aldosterone, which in turn disturbs water balance in the body, resulting in swelling and tenderness of the breasts, stomach, and ankles. Excessive estrogen will lower progesterone levels and cause a chemical imbalance in the brain involving the hormones, adrenaline, serotonin, and dopamine. It will also cause poor metabolism of some vitamins, minerals, and fatty acids and will overstimulate the body, causing paranoia, anxiety, palpitations, hot and cold sweats, shaking, and lowered blood sugar.
- deficiency interferes with the successful breakdown of tryptophan and other mood-balancing and mood-enhancing chemicals in the brain.

Menopausal symptoms can reflect this problem but also others, including loss of bone density, lack of vaginal secretions, and many more.

- appears in great concentration, together with other steroid hormones, whenever the body is damaged by physical trauma, chemical action, or illness. This estrogen surge possibly serves as a stimulus or catalyst for cellular growth and body repair.
- encourages the development of female hormones in pubescent girls.

Progesterone

- is the precursor of the other sex hormones, estrogen and testosterone.
- is the predominant hormone in the second phase of the menstrual cycle, acting to maintain any fertilized eggs.
- mainly prepares for and supports pregnancy (in fact, the word *progesterone* is derived from Latin words meaning "supporting gestation"). Without it, spontaneous abortion can take place. It is vital for the survival of the embryo and fetus throughout gestation.
- protects against breast fibrocysts and endometrial and breast cancers.
- is a natural diuretic and can alleviate a premenstrual bloated feeling.
- helps use fat for energy: fat is built by estrogen, progesterone works to balance this production.
- is a natural antidepressant—lack of it will bring on apathy, sluggishness, and depression. But an excessive amount of progesterone may also cause depression, lack of concentration, and weepiness.
- helps thyroid action and resulting energy levels.
- normalizes blood clotting. If clots are seen during menstruation, progesterone herbs will help.
- helps normalize blood sugar levels; often premenstrual sugar cravings mean that there is too little progesterone available.
- normalizes zinc and copper levels, which are especially vital for the immune system.
- stimulates bone growth, which is vital for the development of children and to prevent osteoporosis in later life.
- is the precursor of cortisone synthesis by the adrenal cortex, which is essential for sustaining the balance of the adrenal glands. Cortisone in turn directly supports the thyroid.
- restores proper cell oxygen levels and therefore helps concentration and, in particular, mental agility.

- is vital during menopause just as much as estrogen for the balance of hormones.

Testosterone

- is produced primarily by the testes in the male body. The testes lie dormant throughout infancy and early childhood until the onset of puberty, at which time the male organs enlarge. If levels are low during the development of the fetus, the testes will not descend properly, if at all. The development of sperm may also be adversely affected.

- causes aggression—which, when channeled correctly, is a major human survival mechanism.

- promotes hair growth on the face, abdomen, pubis, chest, and armpits and increases laryngeal development, which lowers the adult male voice.

- increases the protein content of muscles, bones, and skin.

- encourages the development of male hormones in pubescent boys.

Adolescence

Every child is sensual to varying degrees, but the arrival of sex hormones adds a different dimension to these earlier feelings. If you look around, you will observe that girls are usually a few years ahead of boys in developmental terms as well as in their emotional moods and feelings, which are swayed by hormonal changes. Nevertheless, boys catch up and have their own particular problems to deal with. Girls can begin to menstruate as early as eight to ten years old, but it is more common around the age of twelve. With a stepdaughter, a stepson, and two girls of my own, I have watched these hormonal developments, and I'm happy to report that, with the use of good food, occasional herbs, and other balancing modalities, a lot of what parents refer to as "horrible hormone moods" can be partially (I do say partially!) alleviated and supported, making it easier for adolescents to step out of childhood and into adulthood.

It is essential to remember that adolescents themselves do not enjoy their own bodily fluctuations and emotional outbursts—or parental reactions to them. During adolescence, a great many new hormones are circulating in the system, dramatically affecting the whole energy of the body, along with moods and feelings. I feel that in cultures in which the passage of maturing into adulthood was traditionally celebrated, this recognition of the transition may have served to create for adolescents a greater understanding of the immense challenges that lay before them. To honor, respect, and take note of this phase publicly can only be beneficial, lending self-confidence, self-worth, and a sense of responsibility—all of which are very empowering, especially when the going gets tough. Unacknowledged puberty can be a chaotic and anxious time in which nature's blossoming is left denied, instead of enjoyed and celebrated. Young men and women need to know they are special at this time. Denial of this passage can lead to many problems, including anorexia, bulimia, and liver problems.

The liver plays an important role for menstruating young women and for those who are not yet menstruating but are cyclic. The liver produces many of the sex-related hormones itself as well as processing others that are produced elsewhere in the body. Occasionally, and particularly premenstrually when progesterone is high, the liver becomes congested with excess hormones. Unable for one reason or another to deal with them, the liver becomes sluggish. Toxins accumulate as a result of this incapacitation, and things can go from bad to worse. The liver is joyful if functioning properly and angry and depressed if overworked and underfunctioning, so at key hormone times, it can become quite an emotional time bomb. The liver can also work in harmony or at cross-purposes with the spleen, and both are worth looking at together on a regular and frequent basis.

The kidneys must also function well and, along with the adrenal glands, may need to be supported in times of stress, as weakness in these organs will adversely affect hormone production. In this case Siberian ginseng would help. A healthy bowel is also essential.

The endocrine or hormone system as a whole must be understood. Apart from the major hormones that have already been discussed, there are glands situated in key areas throughout the body that secrete very small amounts of other hormones. These glands include the adrenals, thyroid, pancreas, ovaries, and testes. Their healthy and balanced function is essential to adolescents, as they dictate to a large extent this delicate transition from childhood to adulthood. It is often observed that the endocrine system is very similar to the Ayurvedic system of chakras, so yoga exercises, deep breathing, and any other chakra-balancing exercises you may know of can help. Watching for the first showings of pubic and underarm hair and breast development will help mothers, fathers, daughters, and sons tune in to what is going on and be more alert to any uncomfortable mood swings that could be alleviated by foods, herbs, and exercise. (For young women who are already menstruating, read the section on menstruation for more ideas.)

Pau d'arco inner bark comes from a South American rain forest tree; it influences both the liver and the endocrine system. It can safely be taken over a period of time and is extremely rich in calcium, which is useful for growing bodies.

Wild yam root beneficially affects the liver, digestive system, adrenals, colon, and endocrine system. It is also a hormone precursor. It can be safely taken over a period of time by both sexes.

Siberian ginseng root and **Chinese licorice root** are major endocrine gland tonics and exhibit properties similar to adrenocortical hormone; they will therefore help exhausted teenagers. They will also generally detoxify and support the liver and bloodstream.

Dandelion root and **burdock** root make a great team as liver cleansers, and the burdock really helps to get rid of teenage acne; both are supreme endocrine tonics. Teas made of these two herbs are excellent with a little licorice to sweeten. The ratio should be three parts dandelion to one part burdock root.

Bladder wrack seaweed can be useful to the thyroid in underactive conditions and can really help with growth spurts or unexplained patches of tiredness.

Iron intake is vital, especially for girls, but adolescence generally increases the need for this mineral. Weekly or daily nettle tea will generally provide sufficient quantities for their needs.

All teenagers should avoid tea and coffee because they damage hormone production, clog the liver, and encourage problem skin. They also interrupt growth in children and adolescents, reducing the absorption of iron and calcium, both of which are vital for growing bodies. In addition, these much-used drinks can cause hyperactivity.

Herbalist James Green, author of *The Male Herbal*, is careful to point out that in many ways, boys and girls, men and women are all quite similar. He explains that the prostate can be interpreted as a male uterus and, although it manifests no cyclic menstruation, it is dependent on the endocrine system. Some would say it could also be considered the counterpart to the breasts in the female. He points out that it is a nourishing organ and says that testicles are ovarian tissue that has dropped down. When a male suffers a blow to the testicles, he says, much of the pain is felt in the vicinity of where the ovaries are located in a female's body. He goes on to draw similarities between vaginal and penile tissue and the hood found on both the clitoris and the penis; and he points out that the male scrotum and the female labia majora are made of homologous tissue.

Men produce ten times more testosterone than women. This gives men their more muscular features, just as estrogen produces the female curves. For the adolescent male, testosterone surges can be quite alarming and can be reflected in loud, reckless behavior, which is often difficult to handle for them as well as for those around them. Add to this a congested liver, and the result can indeed be explosive. Alcohol reduces testosterone levels and may result in stunted masculine development. Just as for women, the endocrine system is very important to male adolescent evolution. Similarly, acne can be a problem for male teenagers and confidence levels can swing, but with good food and herbs, these problems can be reduced. Good diet alleviates general growing pains and gives vital energy.

ACNE TREATMENT FOR BOTH SEXES

- Avoid sugar, coffee, tea, drugs, sodas, alcohol, tobacco, junk food, and food that is devoid of freshness and variety. Drink dandelion tea instead of coffee or tea. Drink plenty of water.
- Eat plenty of fresh fruit and raw olive oil.
- Evening primrose oil—containing mega gamma linoleic acid (GLA)—will help balance hormones.
- Use herbs for the liver and endocrine system: chaste tree *(Vitex agnus-castus)* berry is one suggestion for young women (check with a herbalist), and saw palmetto berry for young men. Use milk thistle seed (a liver herb) for both.
- Use a formula containing equal parts of sarsaparilla root, nettle leaf, barberry root bark, burdock root, cleavers leaf, and saw palmetto berry for young men and chaste tree berry for young women.
- Face wash: Mix together a few drops each of the following: witch hazel, tea tree essential oil, and sweet fennel essential oil, adding essential oil of geranium for women and essential oil of rosewood for men. Mix with a cup of water. Shake before use, as the oils will float on top of the water during storage. Dab affected areas with cotton balls two or three times a day. The oils will clean and unclog, giving antibiotic-like protection to the skin.

A MALE HERB

A wonderful male herb that helps to balance the body is saw palmetto. It safely and efficiently tones and strengthens the male reproductive system, enhancing the male sex hormones when required. It also helps relieve prostate enlargement, debilitation, and infection and benefits bladder efficiency and the nervous system. (It is also very useful to women in many situations.) Dosage: one teaspoon of saw palmetto tincture, three times daily.

A FEMALE HERB

For young women, even before menstruation has begun, there can be obvious cyclic patterns mirroring what will become full menstruation. For those already menstruating, pain and premenstrual mood swings can really be alarming. Hormone-balancing herbs may be overly strong for young women, and careful dosages are therefore required. A good choice is chaste tree berry in the majority of cases as it helps to regulate the female gynecological system. It is most frequently used for menstrual complaints in women (but also for involuntary ejaculation in men). It works by normalizing the secretions of the pituitary gland, hypothalamus, and ovaries, which then appropriately signal to balance the endocrine system.

Dosage: half a teaspoon of chaste tree tincture, three times daily (build up to one teaspoon, two times daily, over two to three months). Best taken in early morning to coincide with hypothalamic activity.

MENSTRUATION

Read the previous section on adolescence to remind yourself where and when this all begins. The effects of progesterone and estrogen need to be understood. But most of all, menstruation has to be seen as a natural occurrence whereby monthly weakness and vulnerability are clearly associated with the strength of women, especially their ability to procreate. Most women's views on menstruation are laid down in their early years, depending on the emotions surrounding it at the time. Mothers, family, and society create some part of this view. The rest is governed by the young woman's physical experiences, which may include discomfort and pain.

Women naturally feel more vulnerable both premenstrually and during menstruation. The physical pains associated with the premenstrual phase are often the most debilitating part of the menstrual cycle. The ability to help herself through these times using foods, diet, herbs, and other natural methods is a real gift to any woman. Understanding what can be done needs to become more widespread as it could change many negative feelings and beliefs surrounding menstruation and alleviate very real physical discomfort, which of course only dampens the joys of womanhood. Herbs really do excel when it comes to hormone regulation and should be used more frequently.

Menstruation should not be painful; the blood should flow with ease, with no clots (clots tend to suggest an estrogen excess), and should be brownish red rather than a bright red in color (the latter indicating poor assimilation and possibly an excess of sugar). If the flow is dark red and stringy, excessive unassimilable proteins, especially from meat and eggs, are likely to be the cause. The menses can last anywhere from a day or two to seven or more days, but between four and six is considered normal.

After menstruation has finished, you should feel uplifted as your hormonal balance changes again. Provided you have kept your iron and calcium levels up (blood loss lowers serum iron levels, and calcium is lost in womb activity) with seaweeds, nettle leaf, *pau d'arco* inner bark, yellow dock root, or red raspberry leaf tea, you should feel spirited, excited, and at peace. Menstruation can be an enjoyable time for a woman, especially if the bleeding is not too heavy or painful and the emotions are not excessively haywire. From the onset of premenstrual symptoms (up to ten days before the period) to one or two days into menstruation, tension, anxiety, tearfulness, depression, and even anger can build up, smolder, and erupt. Water retention can make you feel large and clumsy, while little upsets can become major issues. If you have these symptoms, you need help from herbs, exercise, and good diet. Some women can experience painful ovulation or even postmenstrual blues, but these can usually be helped and realigned so that symptoms are lessened or eradicated altogether.

Some Ideas to Keep a Healthily Menstruating Body

- If you have water retention problems, sprinkle plenty of celery seeds on your food. Drink dandelion root tea. Hormone imbalance often produces the situation in the first place, especially excessive estrogen with too little progesterone.

- Gamma linoleic acid (GLA) helps balance the female system. Take one capsule of black currant seed oil or evening primrose oil a day. GLA can also help aching eyes, fuzzy head, bloating, fatigue, and other premenstrual symptoms.

- If the adrenal glands and kidneys are not functioning correctly, they will need to be built up using Siberian ginseng root, among other herbs.

- Use relaxing essential oils for cleanliness and to avoid cystitis and vaginal infections. Organic lavender, geranium, and chamomile are wonderfully soothing and are in tune with your hormones—add one or two drops to your bathwater.

- Use plastic-free and chemical-free sanitary napkins. Try to avoid using any kind of tampon, but if you do, it should also be chemical- and plastic-free. Tampons of all descriptions keep stale blood where it shouldn't be, even if they are changed every four hours. (Some women even experience life-threatening toxicity from using tampons—known as toxic shock syndrome.) There is also considerable speculation that pelvic inflammatory disease and endometriosis can arise from tampon use over the years.

- Wear cotton or silk pants and avoid sweaty nylon pantyhose or other tight, airless clothing. Don't restrict your belly with tight skirts or trousers.

- Keep your circulatory system healthy; exercise and breathe deeply.

- Look after your nervous system and make sure magnesium and calcium levels are maintained (refer to chapter 4). Take care of your immune system: echinacea may be enough to boost it for a few days if you feel low.

- The contraceptive pill will upset normal menstruation. There are, however, some circumstances in which it is preferable to the risk of pregnancy. Consult your doctor, as some people are in higher-risk health categories and are therefore unable to use the pill. Ensure that you are fully briefed on the possible side effects of the type of oral contraception that your doctor prescribes.

- Don't plan exhausting work or social schedules around these times — stress disrupts the delicate balance of hormones. Think ahead and plan accordingly, giving yourself permission to take time off if you're able.

- The colors of menstrual blood are important. A good menstrual color is reddish-brown.

- Avoid tea, coffee, and alcohol. They are all known to disturb hormonal balance, increase sugar imbalances, and congest the liver. If you have sugar cravings, eat fruit or choose bitter and sour foods, which will offset the craving for sweetness.

- Avoid foods with a high fat content, such as dairy products and meat, as these affect prostaglandin levels in the body. Avoid all hormone-fed meat, dairy products, and eggs, as these will also disrupt your hormonal balance.

- Make up a tea that is especially good for premenstrual and menstrual symptoms, containing dandelion (for liver health and water balance) along with red raspberry and nettles, both of which are rich in iron and calcium.

- General hormone balancers include blessed thistle leaf and flower, chaste tree berry, sarsaparilla root, and red raspberry leaf.

- Liver health is important; therefore consider liver cleansing and supportive herbs.

- Bowel health is important (especially if you are generally constipated). Therefore bowel herbs and colon cleansing may be necessary — refer to "The Colon (Bowel) or Large Intestine" in chapter 9 and "A Three-Stage Herbal Colon Cleanse" in chapter 6.

- For menstrual cramps, use equal parts of cramp bark and black cohosh. Also ensure that you have sufficient calcium and magnesium intake.

Infertility

The current infertility figures for both men and women are very distressing. Findings show that 25 percent of infertility cases now relate to men, compared to 10 percent a few years ago. Much blame is laid on chemical pollution, including the widespread use of organophosphate pesticides, along with dioxins in meat and dairy products and PCBs (polychlorinated biphenyls). Nevertheless, good food and a few herbs can go a long way to redressing the problem.

For more detailed ideas on how to treat infertility, see the book list at the end of this chapter. Some hormone tests are helpful for both sexes, though they may not be able to pinpoint the exact problem in men. Be warned, however, of possible side effects of some hormonal treatments. Patients of mine have told of cysts and fibroids developing at the same time that they were taking drugs used to stimulate egg production. *The Lancet* has published studies of ovarian cell tumors occurring in women undergoing fertility treatment. The scientific director of an infertility clinic at Nottingham University estimates that one cycle of fertility drugs may be the equivalent of up to two years' natural egg production.

Men should take male hormonal tonics like saw palmetto berries, nettle root, damiana leaf, and squaw vine leaf. Adaptogenic herbs like Siberian ginseng root will feed the adrenal glands, which are the masters of all hormones. Women should use female hormone balancers like chaste tree berry, which helps by increasing luteinizing hormone levels and prolactin secretion and decreasing follicle-stimulating hormone secretion, as well as squaw vine leaf (and other aerial parts) and black cohosh root. All the men and women I have worked with in this situation have needed a total health review, personal programs of treatment, and adaptogenic herbs such as Siberian ginseng. A whole-body approach to natural healing is needed, involving proper diet, healthy function of the digestive system, the use of cleansing programs, exercise, and hydrotherapy.

- Nutritional support should focus on organic foods, thus avoiding synthetic hormones fed to animals and pesticides in plants, all of which can affect conception.
- Eat a generally wholesome diet, reducing dairy and wheat intake and increasing fruit and vegetables.
- Consume at least three quarts of water daily.
- Ensure that your bowel is working well and your liver is working efficiently, rather than laboring under hormone imbalances.
- Exercise will be important. Sitz baths will really help; see chapter 5.

Pregnancy

Creating magic in our bodies is part of the miracle of life. Pregnancy is a time of bliss, vulnerability, femininity, creativity, and change.

It is a time to build and tone the body, to balance feeding oneself and the baby within, with not overburdening the heart, circulatory system, and other organs with unwanted weight gain or any other condition. Before pregnancy is even entered into, it is wise to cleanse the colon, liver, and kidneys (see chapter 6), and to be consistently eating nutritious foods. This pattern should be established long before conception, if possible — even though pregnancy is not, of course, always planned!

Pregnancy is not the time to cleanse and detoxify the system heavily, though some minor cleansing work can be carried out with guidance and under supervision. Good food, herbs, and a well-functioning colon are vital. Once the placenta has grown (by the third month) and the fetus has its own line of nutrition and detoxification processes, you should attempt only very minor cleansing programs, guided by a professional. A suitable mini-cleanse could be aimed simply at decongesting the liver, which has a tendency to become overworked, overheated, and overcongested just by the pregnancy itself, with all the extra hormonal commitments it has to cope with. Likewise, the colon can become a bit sluggish, owing to hormonal changes and the extra bulk of the baby filling up available space in that area. The kidneys, the home of female nurturing, need to be able to perform the important role of helping to detoxify waste.

I strongly advise reading chapter 4, as the very best nutrition is vital while building another human being. Do not consume fish, meat, or dairy products raised on synthetic hormones, as these can complicate and unbalance the body's own carefully balanced hormones. Do not take stimulants like tea, coffee, and alcohol, and do not smoke: these will all disrupt, among other things, the baby's nervous system, sugar balances, and circulatory system. See "Anemia," in chapter 10, for information on iron and folic acid.

DAILY HERBS FOR PREGNANCY

You may need to take herbs to help the colon, but seek a practitioner's advice, as some colon herbs will be too forceful. Constipation is more likely to manifest or get worse during pregnancy and must be treated. Increase your water intake, drink fresh fruit juices, and eat flaxseed and psyllium husks.

Liver herbs are important — a simple daily choice is dandelion root, brewed as a "coffee," for liver and kidney function. Ten drops of milk thistle tincture is safe and a little stronger, useful for practitioner-indicated situations.

Many herbs are contraindicated in pregnancy, so seek professional advice on which ones to avoid. Nettles and chickweed are ideal choices to use. Any pregnant woman who feels she ought to rush to the vitamin and mineral counter at the pharmacy in order to do the best for the development of her baby should stop to consider that, if she has the time, her best source for these nutrients is essentially nature and her plants. The body finds natural sources easiest to assimilate, and these should come first, and the synthetic versions second.

Iron, calcium, and magnesium levels should be boosted by eating lots of seaweed or by taking kelp tablets and drinking three cups of strong nettle tea daily (for extra calcium sources, see chapter 4). Folic acid and iron are often given to women at the onset of pregnancy or after the first three months. You will find excellent folic acid and iron sources in chlorella and other algae. Folic acid in particular is vital in the first trimester as it is important for healthy bone formation in the fetus.

For calming and feeding the nerves, and for relaxing after a tiring day, drink weak chamomile tea each evening.

Pregnant women can use a range of safe hormone-balancing herbs during pregnancy to alleviate morning sickness, but only after consultation with a herbalist. There are many herbs that should be avoided in pregnancy, especially during the first three months. This is the time that the fetus is most vulnerable as, having no placenta, the baby is defenseless against anything toxic. Herbs that are rich in alkaloids, or those used to induce menstruation, are among those to avoid. They include barberry root bark, pokeweed root, blue and black cohosh root, nutmeg seed, yarrow leaf, angelica root, motherwort leaf, pennyroyal leaf, mistlotoe leaf, cramp bark, male fern, sage leaf, wormwood leaf, arborvitae leaf, coltsfoot leaf, and comfrey leaf. Echinacea, however, is a very useful herb to know about should you have an infection or virus while pregnant. As it is a complicated herb with many different dosages, seek guidance from a herbalist.

The same rule applies to using essential oils. However, making your own rose and lavender oils, by soaking rose petals and lavender flowers in a base almond oil and wheat germ oil for twenty-four hours in sunshine, would be safe and a lovely idea, producing a nourishing scented gift for your skin.

NATURAL HEALING

Take gentle, rhythmic exercise, but do not overdo it. Extensive running, swimming, and jogging should be reduced; aerobics could be replaced by yoga. Listen to what your body is telling you, and work in tune with it.

Breathing is very important, and practicing different breathing patterns will get you ready to use them to ease pain and steer labor when the time comes. Deep breathing in the belly during pregnancy provides extra oxygen for the fetus and is very calming for it.

Devote more time to relaxation, and be creative. Notice colors or delight-ful sounds, and cut out shocking or upsetting television programs, argu-ments, and stress. If stress does enter your life, talk to your baby in calming tones so as to form a close relationship. This helps to minimize trauma in-side the womb and, later, outside it.

Consult a practitioner for individual problems like protein in the urine (this often means that B vitamins are low—particularly choline), high blood pressure (in this case cayenne pod and hawthorn berry, leaf, and blossom should be used), or heartburn (this indicates that the liver is overburdened and needs help).

THREATENED MISCARRIAGE

If you have a history of miscarriage, you would be well advised to carry out a serious health, nutritional, and lifestyle check before getting pregnant again.

Vitamin A and folic acid are very important for physically strengthening the "hammock" of womb muscles designed to hold the baby. Consuming car-rot juice, chlorella, and Engevita yeast for B vitamins before and during the first trimester will provide these nutrients. Folic acid helps to form correct genetic blueprints, thus reducing the likelihood of spontaneous abortion caused by faulty combinations.

MISCARRIAGE

Should miscarriage occur, seek professional advice immediately.

Herbal douches, vaginal cleansing suppositories, herbs to rebalance the sudden change of hormones and help to support the nerves—including chaste tree berries, skullcap leaf, passionflower flower, and a little lobelia (Indian tobacco) leaf—will all help you come to terms with the physical and emotional traumas associated with miscarriage.

LABOR

Labor should, ideally, be a relaxed affair. Whether you give birth at home or in a hospital, you should take every possible means to feel as confident and at home. Special music, familiar pillows, and nice smells can all help.

There are herbs that can be used to help a birth along, should it become apparent that intervention, such as forceps or a cesarean section, may be needed. Yet it is important to let the body do its own thing as far as possi-ble, so herbs should be used no less reluctantly than any other interven-tionist methods.

Pennyroyal leaf can help stimulate contractions; squaw vine leaf and aer-ial parts and red raspberry leaf will generally support the labor; and cramp bark will relieve any contractions that are too sharp or painful. **However, these herbs should not be used in a self-help fashion ever.** Small amounts of chamomile tea may be drunk or sipped during labor to relax and help concentrate the breathing, though large amounts will relax the contractions too much. I prefer to keep things simple unless intervention, herbal or otherwise, is really necessary. One herb I would choose would be lobelia leaf tincture smeared on the lips, because it will provide relaxation and stimulation as required. **However, only a qualified herbal practitioner must ever prescribe all these herbs in this situation.**

AFTER THE BIRTH

Pains after birth can be treated with a combination of cramp bark and lobelia leaf. Nettle leaf tea will restore vitality, help mend torn or injured tissue, and provide iron to compensate for lost blood. Should there have been considerable hemorrhage, high and constant doses of nettle tea should be kept up. To stop the hemorrhage itself, take one teaspoon of yarrow tincture every half hour.

Equal parts of squaw vine leaf (a hormone balancer), fennel seed (a galactagogue—that is, it encourages the production of milk), nettle leaf (for calcium, magnesium, and iron), and marshmallow root (for calcium and as a galactagogue) will help balance you hormonally and provide a good supply of nutritious breast milk for your baby. British women breast-feed their babies less than any other European women. A breast-fed baby receives vital lifelong immunity factors as well as irreplaceable physical and emotional nourishment. Breast milk also helps form good brain cells. I have never seen herbs fail a mother who really wants to breast-feed. Fenugreek seed, fennel seed, marshmallow root, and motherwort leaf are classified as galactagogues and will all help provide an abundance of rich nutritious milk. Intake of plenty of water is important, but by drinking plenty of these herbs as teas, your fluid intake will be up anyway.

Breast-feeding should start at delivery—the clear colostrum that comes at birth and lasts for the first two days is vital immune-enhancing and nourishing food for the baby. Only stay in hospitals where you are encouraged to sleep all night with your baby and to feed the baby the colostrum. You should be allowed to feed as needed. If you feel very tired, look at the broader pick-me-up herbs such as Siberian ginseng root, which is the primary choice, but also *Pfaffia* root, *Schisandra* berry, *Rehmannia* root, *Astragalus* root, burdock root, red raspberry leaf, marshmallow root, fenugreek seed, licorice root, and damiana leaf if you feel particularly exhausted. You can also take evening primrose oil capsules. If you suspect that you may be anemic, it is important to treat the problem quickly.

NUTRITION AND NATURAL HEALING

Plenty of rest is important while recuperating from labor and the nine months of pregnancy. You have to have the energy to care for and feed this new bundle of joy. Being constantly woken up in the night to feed can be very draining if there are not occasional blocks of time when you know you don't have to keep an eye or ear open, but can sink, instead, into a completely undisturbed sleep. Good food is, of course, vital, and if you are looking for a good ready-prepared source, superfood will be ideal. It may be that you need to seek some extra professional help at this time to find out how best to meet the nutritional needs of the two of you. But as a general rule, look for calcium and iron sources to back up the nettle leaves and marshmallow root, do not forget to support your nervous system by using herbs like vervain leaf and oat straw, and take Siberian ginseng root and a little Chinese licorice root as they will support the adrenal glands.

Practice pelvic floor exercises. You should have learned these during pregnancy to make labor easier. They are also very useful throughout one's menstruating and lovemaking life. These exercises help maintain a healthy womb, along with bladder and rectal control. You can do them while sitting, standing, or lying down—my midwife said, "Do them while you're washing up!" Squeeze your "hammock" muscles as if you were trying to stop urination. Squeeze even harder, count to twelve slowly, then slowly relax again. Breathe evenly and naturally. Repeat the whole process ten times.

A lot of women rush around too soon after birth. This makes it very difficult for the uterus to return to its right size and correct position, and may also lay the foundations for prolapse later in life. It is important to rest for at least ten days in order to allow the repair process to take place. During this time, pelvic floor exercises are best done lying down. After six weeks, get the position of your uterus checked. If it is not in its correct position, a professional should be able to realign it.

POSTPARTUM DEPRESSION

Postpartum depression is a sad fact of life, especially in the West, but herbs can really help those women affected by it. Attention to the nervous system and adrenal glands is vital. However, all women need some kind of hormonal and nutritional rebalancing after birth. The squaw vine tuber and some or all of the milk-producing herbs will generally be sufficient for most mothers, and you could even add some chaste tree berry. An additional formula for postpartum depression is made up of equal parts of damiana leaf and St. John's wort flower (the latter must be used only at the directive of a professional). Under the influence of this illness, some women lose respect for their bodies by becoming violent or uncaring and can become a danger to themselves. Alternatively, they may become depressed and uninterested in their new baby. With the right herbs, this condition can be quickly rectified. There must be an extra intake of calcium, magnesium, and B vitamins (refer to chapter 4 for suggestions).

Menopause

This is the third cycle for women, after puberty and the time of childbearing. Its name means "moon pause"—the final long pause in the monthly moon cycles.

How graceful menopause is depends partly on how much we can express our pain and our physical changes, and partly on how we can view our new position in life emotionally. In my experience with women, the ones who suffer most are those with stress in their lives. A disturbing marriage, sick or elderly parents, and rowdy young adults still at home provide three of the most common stress patterns that can triple the incidence of hot flashes and other menopausal symptoms. The role of the caregiver leaves little time for personal care or reflection.

Not all women will suffer. In fact, it is estimated that as few as 10 percent go through a really difficult menopause, with vaginal dryness, hot flashes, night sweats, depression, and insomnia. The rest may encounter one or two of these symptoms without too much distress, while at least 20 percent will hardly notice any change at all. Statistically, in Britain, women go through menopause on average at the age of forty-seven. But some experience menopause much earlier. This can be due to illness, poor nutritional care, genetic tendencies (in other words, one's mother or grandmother did so), or extreme stress. Some women don't reach their menopause until they are in their mid fifties. On the whole, though, the recent trend has been for women to become menopausal earlier—mirroring the pattern of women menstruating earlier.

"In Germany 70 percent of physicians successfully prescribe herbal remedies for the menopause, instead of using hormone replacement drugs," reports Dr. M. Schmittmann. This trend to support menopause with herb use is an increasing one in Britain.

There are three stages of menopause: perimenopause (sometimes referred to as premenopause), menopause, and postmenopause. Medically speaking, *menopause* is defined as the last menstrual period, or the cessation of menstrual bleeding. The transition to menopause is known as *perimenopause* and may last as long as eight to fifteen years. *Postmenopause* is considered to start approximately one year after menopause has occurred.

Contrary to common belief, most women's estrogen levels remain relatively stable during perimenopause, or even may increase slightly. On the other hand, progesterone levels begin to fall. The result can be a condition called estrogen dominance. This causes a myriad of uncomfortable symptoms similar to premenstrual syndrome, only ten times more severe. Maintaining adequate progesterone is important for building up the uterine lining during menstruation, as well as for proper blood clotting, blood sugar regulation, healthy bone formation, and fat metabolism. Herbs are a real support during this time, particularly ones that increase progesterone levels, such as chaste tree berry. They initiate a progestogenic response in the body by having a dialogue with the pituitary gland and subsequently activating the ovaries. By regulating the hormones, any deficits or dominance are redressed, whether estrogenic or progestogenic. Proportional amounts of black cohosh and other estrogenic herbs can be additionally taken and the overall effect will be most welcome.

Hot flashes are the most common symptom of menopause transition, and changes in the blood's hormone levels are the main cause of naturally occurring menopause. The same herbs as above can continue or start to be taken with great success. When a woman has not experienced a period for one year, this means that the ovaries are not producing eggs and have greatly slowed down production of estrogen. Progesterone is no longer secreted, and the uterine lining does not develop. Since there is no endometrial lining to shed, there are no more periods.

During postmenopause, there is a slow, gradual decline in the sex hormone levels, eventually reaching a very low and stable level. If the adrenal glands are healthy, they will take over estrogen and progesterone production at a low rate. But exhausted adrenals exacerbate a different set of changes in the body, which tend to be more long-term. The adrenal glands are supposed to secrete a certain quota of hormones throughout the day, but tired and exhausted ones will not do so. Vaginal dryness and incontinence are two of most distressing symptoms of this problem, but the risk of heart disease, blood sugar disturbances, and osteoporosis are of course to be considered. Therefore, of great help to support the adrenal glands at this time are herbs like Siberian ginseng, licorice, and rosemary, which will directly feed and help replenish the adrenals. But very often, adrenal exhaustion can be largely avoided just by supplying the already mentioned hormone herb support.

Hot flashes and sweats are caused when the nerve centers are affected by blood flow, which triggers a hot, prickly feeling as the body searches for estrogen. During the perimenopausal stage, periods will become less frequent and scantier. Occasionally the opposite is true, sometimes resulting in flooding, as the body attempts to galvanize the ovaries into activity and overproduces estrogen in the short term. Caucasian Western women are eight times more likely to suffer calcium loss than other women worldwide; therefore care must be taken to obtain enough calcium and magnesium. (See "The Urinary System" in chapter 9 and the food and nutrition advice in chapter 4.) Other symptoms experienced can be as diverse as heart palpitations, depression, more frequent vaginal infections, chronic night sweats, nervousness and anxiety, irritability, anger, fatigue, insomnia, aching joints, headaches, weight gain, and mood swings.

NUTRITION

A good diet will go a long way toward stabilizing hot flashes and other symptoms. Cut out or considerably reduce the amount of coffee, tea, alcohol, sugar, and chocolate consumed, as well as foods with chemical and steroid additives.

Weight gain or loss is often associated with menopause. Thinner women will not be as able to produce estrogen as plumper women. Body fat helps to produce estrogen; therefore eat well and keep to a healthy weight.

Increase your intake of whole grains, including rice, millet, oats, barley, and quinoa. In addition, eat plenty of fresh vegetables and fruit. Lots of sprouted seeds, along with tofu and other soy products, will also help, as well as fennel, garlic, fenugreek, rosemary, sage, and bananas. All of these foods are rich in natural hormones. Take superfood daily. If you wish, you can also take one tablespoon of bee pollen daily.

HERBS

- Herbs to help general menopausal symptoms are very diverse, but here are just some: chaste tree berry, saw palmetto berry, vervain leaf, licorice root, *dong quai* root, *Astragalus* root, angelica root, yarrow leaf, sage leaf, lobelia leaf, hawthorn berry, dandelion root, black cohosh root, sarsaparilla root, hop strobilus, and wild yam root.

- Herbs to help hot flashes, sweating, and insomnia include many of the above, but low blood sugar can also produce these symptoms, so it would be worth testing blood glucose levels.

- Herbs to help calm the nervous system include valerian root, hop strobilus, wild lettuce leaf, oat straw, and pasqueflower.

- To promote sleep at night (beyond sleeplessness associated with hot flashes and sweating), use valerian root and passionflower.

- To help with depression, use St. John's wort flower.

- Herbs to help adrenal glands weakened by stress and hot flashes include Siberian ginseng root, wild yam root, and Chinese licorice root.

- Make sure your intake of calcium and magnesium is good and well-balanced.

- Liver health is important with regard to the balanced and even flow of hormones, and a liver cleanse is always helpful. Also drink dandelion root tea and put fresh dandelion leaves in salads. Consider milk thistle seed, artichoke leaf, and other liver herbs.

- If you already have a heart problem or high blood pressure, seek professional advice on treating the two problems together. Take hawthorn blossom, leaf, and berry and possibly motherwort leaf.

- Sometimes the immune system can become weakened with all this hormonal fluctuation; take echinacea root and Siberian ginseng root.

- For vaginal dryness caused by decreased estrogen, take *Pfaffia* root internally, as it stores sisterol, which produces enough estrogen to help the situation without producing an excess. It is also a very supportive herb that generally acts as an adaptogen and immune supporter. Diet and lifestyle adjustments will eventually balance enough to produce more lubrication. Meanwhile, make a mix of slippery elm powder with aloe vera gel, and teaspoon it into the vagina while lying on your back. Always use a lubricant when making love—macadamia oil is very good, or use olive oil. Other estrogenic herbs are hop strobilus, red clover flower, parsley leaf, and fennel seed.

- If there are any deep-seated problems, it is advisable to cleanse both your liver and your colon.

NATURAL HEALING

Take up new pursuits and do other creative things with your life—perhaps painting, gardening, or sewing. Indulge your life and your body. Soak in essential-oil baths and listen to music. Take up meditation and tune in with your new life phase. Enjoy your sexuality in its new maturity. Exercise: do keep moving as this is vital for healing all organs and for systems to work properly.

HORMONE REPLACEMENT THERAPY (HRT)

HRT can work for many women. But unlike herbal treatments that can eventually be stopped, HRT can only be leveled off to a maintenance dose that simply protects calcium stores and maintains hormone levels, once severe menopausal symptoms have been assisted at a higher dose. The onset of menopause has only been put off! All of the hormones used in HRT are synthetic and therefore do not have the natural "cutoff switches" available in herbal hormone precursors. Even the so-called natural versions like Premarin (made from urine collected from pregnant mares kept in confining pens) can cause blood clots. For those prone to liver disease, thrombosis, or heart disease, HRT carries the same risks as the contraceptive pill, and American research announced in summer 2002 has now confirmed all this.

Progesterone cream is another alternative that is available by prescription. It is made from soybeans. Read Marilyn Glenville's book *Natural*

Alternatives to HRT for a valuable insight into this product. For many reasons, she does not advocate its use, though I know other natural-healing therapists who do and who personally find it works well. I rely solely on herbs. A practitioner can help anyone who wants to come off HRT slowly, but the transition requires professional supervision to make it painless and easy. HRT side effects are numerous, and I have seen many women presenting many alarming symptoms without realizing that the HRT was to blame. They include weight gain, anger, aching joints, fluid retention, abdominal and leg cramps, migraine, loss of appetite, bingeing, and depression.

Old Age

According to many sources, including the World Health Organization, as time goes by we are going to have far more elderly people around who will not necessarily be in good or better health. Their prediction is that the number of cases of cancer and bowel diseases will dramatically increase.

As life expectancy extends, it is perhaps time to develop a good understanding of home self-healing methods. Anything that can ordinarily harm the body will simply continue to do so for longer, the older we get. So whether it is the bowel congesting or the liver stagnating, the answer lies in learning about and implementing natural healing routines designed to cleanse and rejuvenate the body's organs. This may, at first sight, appear to be a tough option for the elderly, who are sometimes more rigid or dogmatic in their approach to their lifestyles, as they justifiably relax into the evening of their lives. It certainly requires those noble elder qualities of wisdom, enlightenment, balance, and courage in order to make these changes.

Nutrition will have a different focus as digestion becomes less efficient and as shopping for food and cooking become more tiring. Additionally, older people tend to eat less as they require fewer calories and less protein to fuel their daily activities. For them, a combination of liquid foods balanced with fiber, good-quality fruit and vegetables, juices, superfood, and some good-quality and well-chosen supplements would be ideal, while also making sure that what little food is eaten is of excellent quality and taste. Every day, a salad should be eaten that includes some of the following ingredients: grated carrots, beets, cucumber, and ginger, added to dandelion leaves, lettuce, and sorrel. Vary the ingredients each day if possible. Now is the time to grow a few herbs like thyme, oregano, coriander, and garlic and to use them to flavor each meal.

Some older people find that memory and brain agility begin to fail them, just at a time when memories are more delightful to recall and they have all the time in the world for crosswords and conversation. Ginkgo (which is already used in copious amounts by the elderly) will really help, as will other brain restoratives such as Siberian ginseng root, rosemary leaf, gotu kola root, and prickly ash berry—refer to "Parkinson's and Alzheimer's Diseases" in chapter 10.

Brittle bones are an increasing problem as we grow older; some two hundred thousand hip fractures are reported each year in Britain and, likewise, cases of osteoporosis are increasing. Refer to "Osteoporosis" in chapter 10.

The immune system must be lovingly cared for so that colds, flu, and other respiratory disorders and diseases do not have a chance to become established. Include herbs like garlic clove, burdock root, and Siberian ginseng root daily in order to maintain your immune system. Use olive leaf or echinacea root, or both, if you should get an infection.

Take care of the liver and avoid accelerating tissue and cell degeneration through free-radical damage. Use olive oil wherever possible and consume lots of fresh fruit and vegetables to ensure that your body receives plenty of antioxidants.

Gentle but regular exercise is vital for this age group; in fact, this is the time to increase the amount that you do, especially if you have the time available. If you are infirm, hydrotherapy and massage will be essential treatments.

Book List

Herbal Healing for Women by Rosemary Gladstar (New York: Simon and Schuster, 1993)

Herbal Medicine for the Menopause by Andrew Chevallier (Rochester, UK: Amberwood Publishing, 2001)

The Male Herbal by James Green (Berkeley, California: Crossing Press, 1991)

Natural Alternatives to HRT by Marilyn Glenville (London: Kyle Cathie, 1997)

The Tao of Health, Sex and Longevity by Daniel Reid (London: Simon and Schuster, 1989)

The Women's Guide to Herbal Medicine by Carol Rogers (London: Hamish Hamilton, 1995)

Resources

Herbs Hands Healing Ltd., Station Warehouse, Station Road, Pulham Market, Norfolk IP21 4XF, United Kingdom; tel: 001-44-0137-9608201; website: www.super-food.co.uk and www.herbshandshealing.co.uk

American Botanical Pharmacy, 4114 Glencoe Avenue, Marina del Rey, CA 90292; tel: 800-Herb-Doc; website: www.800herbdoc.com

❧ 9 ❧
Body Systems

The Digestive System

The digestive system runs from the mouth through to the rectum. In many ways it is the focal point of the body. It is our earthy center. Whatever we eat, we must have the ability to absorb and make use of it. Most illnesses, from chronic diseases such as cancer to many modern allergies, arise out of gastrointestinal debility, with a range of causal factors that include bacterial, fungal, and viral overgrowth. One such condition is "leaky gut," in which the integrity of the stomach becomes thinned and leaky like a colander. One survey has shown that the high incidence of asthma among children—and, no

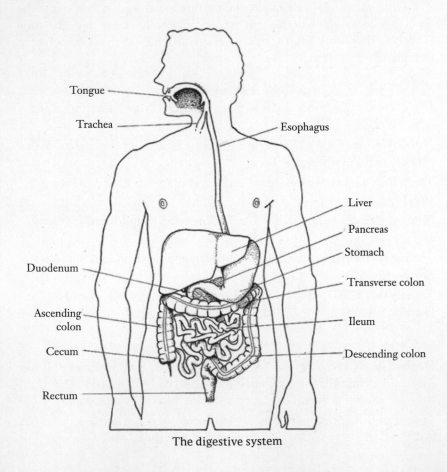

The digestive system

doubt, the whole spectrum of allergies—is caused by low hydrochloric acid levels, leading to low levels of vitamins B_{12} and B_6 and magnesium. Note also that if you are in blood group A or B, you may have a tendency toward low hydrochloric acid levels, resulting in poor digestive enzyme activity.

NUTRITION

Working out which foods suit you and can be processed efficiently by your body is a key factor in the upkeep of your digestive system and balanced health. As a general rule, you should avoid common food intolerances, vary and rotate foods, and increase fiber intake by eating whole grains, vegetables, and fruit. It may also be necessary to take probiotics occasionally. Pineapple, papaya, and apple cider vinegar will help digestion, while slippery elm inner bark will soothe and protect if necessary.

HERBS

Meadowsweet, a northern European herb that grows plentifully in Britain, is capable of stimulating the cells in the stomach to produce hydrochloric acid and pepsinogen. It is also capable of treating overacidity with tremendous results. There are many other herbs that can stimulate and support digestion in a variety of ways, not least the common culinary ones such as oregano, marjoram, fennel, coriander, basil, garlic, and ginger. Additionally, drink a tea of meadowsweet leaf, peppermint leaf, or chamomile flower after eating. It may even be necessary to avoid herbs that could be too harsh on the stomach for some, like *pau d'arco* inner bark. Your stomach will generally tell you if herbs don't suit you, but do consult a herbalist.

NATURAL HEALING

Good chewing is vital, and you can check on how good you are at it by looking at your stools. If you are able to recognize much of your food, then chew more! Even if you are desperately hungry, restrain yourself because your haste may easily backfire. In the short term it may produce gas, and in the long term, poor assimilation and ill health, not to mention a backed-up bowel, resulting in constipation or diarrhea. Take it slowly and chew.

Bad dental care and mouth problems can hamper your ability to chew well, so go regularly to the dentist, brush your teeth, and take care of your mouth. Mouthwashes containing salt, oak bark, fennel seed, and myrrh leaf are helpful for abscesses, receding gums, and infection. They can be especially effective alongside regular brushing.

Any natural healing technique that helps the process of digestion will be useful. Start with sound sleep and exercise accompanied by cleansing programs where necessary, especially of the colon and liver.

For more on the digestive system, see "The Pancreas," "The Liver and Gallbladder," "The Colon (Bowel) or Large Intestine," and "The Spleen," below in this chapter.

The Pancreas

The pancreas is mainly concerned with secreting digestive enzymes in order to break down protein, carbohydrates, and fats present in the duodenum. It neutralizes the acids issuing from the stomach. It is key to the overall balanced functioning of digestion in the body and therefore an extremely important organ for all the digestion-based diseases and disorders.

The health of the pancreas relies on an effectively functioning stomach, spleen, liver, and gallbladder, as well as the entire endocrine system. The pancreas produces two hormones required to control and balance the body's glucose and fatty acid levels. One of its jobs is to release insulin, which reduces glucose production in the liver. When the body's blood sugar levels rise, they affect the production of glucagons, which increases glucose production. The pancreas regulates blood sugar, so its health dictates the balance of sugar levels. Many people, especially women, have low blood sugar levels. In these cases, pancreatic health must be at the forefront of a support program.

NUTRITION

Refer to the section on digestive-system nutrition and to chapter 4, using the full spectrum of flavors from neutral to bitter. Eat seaweeds and garlic, both of which help to normalize blood sugar. Garlic does so by stimulating the pancreas to produce sufficient insulin. Poor pancreatic function often goes hand in hand with low or high blood sugar levels. Sweet herb *(Stevia)* helps to balance blood sugar and safely stimulates the pancreas while providing a sweet flavor (three hundred to five hundred times sweeter than sugar). Other supportive foods are fenugreek seed and leaf and sweet root vegetables like yams, while one of the best fruits is kiwi. Generally, eat little but often (six meals a day) to help support blood sugar levels. Be sure to eat some protein-rich foods in order to stabilize blood sugar levels. Liver health via food cleanses will, in turn, greatly assist pancreatic function. Excessive alcohol harms the pancreas and liver and can give rise to pancreatitis.

HERBS

Consume two or three garlic cloves a day, fenugreek seed and Chinese licorice root along with burdock root, Siberian ginseng root, *Schisandra* berry and *Astragalus* root. Add wild yam root because it helps normalize blood sugar levels. Liver and colon cleanses will be vital (pay particular attention to any colon congestion around the splenic flexure, which can press on the spleen and pancreas).

NATURAL HEALING

Take hot and cold showers, but if you feel fatigued or experience symptoms of low blood sugar such as light-headedness and dizziness, concentrate more on cold than hot.

The Liver and Gallbladder

The liver is the largest organ in the body and one of the most important for overall health. It is situated under the lower right rib cage. The liver is capable of complete self-renewal at a faster rate than the rest of the body. Given this ability to restore itself via good foods, rest, and herbs, the root meaning of its name, "live" or "life," is very apt. The liver makes and releases into the body an amazing amount of useful substances and sustains us in a myriad of vital ways. It also stores vitamins, minerals, and sugars. Deficiencies in any of these are due to a congested, poorly working, and underpar liver, and can contribute to a huge number of conditions, including low blood sugar levels, diabetes, menstrual problems, and other hormonal problems.

The raw material for all these chemical processes comes from food. Nutrition is the key to keeping the liver healthy; it absorbs food via the intestine and then releases it into the body at the necessary rate.

The liver is the body's main detoxification unit: using two specific processes, it detoxifies a range of internal and external toxins (of which there are more and more in our modern, polluted world). The end result of these detoxification processes is the excretion of toxins, via the bile if large and via the urine if small. Enzymes are vital to allow the phases of detoxification to be successful, and good nutrition plus herbs can greatly help. Additionally, the gallbladder and bile production need to be at optimum health in order for proper toxin elimination to take place.

The gallbladder is a small organ attached to the underside of the liver. It is here that bile is condensed and stored until it is required, once it has been received from the liver. The job of the gallbladder is to eject bile into the duodenum when food passes from the stomach into the intestine. Bile has many functions, and one of its uses is to help digest fats. It is also a natural laxative because it acts as the liver's own personal eliminatory channel.

The liver creates immune substances and also purifies and filters the blood by neutralizing poisons. During its many chemical reactions, it produces a great deal of heat that can warm the whole body. If the liver is pushed and overwhelmed with the work it needs to carry out, perhaps because of excessive hormonal demands or toxicity, it can become "overheated." This, in turn, will deleteriously affect other organs and systems. The liver also instigates some hormonal processes and inactivates others; it plays a major role in the premenstrual phase, menstruation, menopause, and other endocrine phases for women.

This cleansing, manufacturing, and storage center, through its influence on nutrient and energy supply as well as detoxification, has a direct link with the mind and its function. Emotionally, one can feel very depressed or even angry, sad, weepy, and at worst jealous if the liver is overextended by one's daily input. Fortunately, the liver is also very capable of making us feel happy, joyful, balanced, sprightly, and energized when it is functioning well. Such drastic differences are often plainly seen before and after a liver cleanse.

NUTRITION

When the liver is sick, avoid fatty foods except for extra virgin olive oil, which is very good for it. Increase your intake of antioxidants, as they protect the liver—foods like peppers, parsley, chlorella and other algae, fresh vegetable and fruit juices, garlic, carrots, greens, citrus fruit, and soaked or sprouted whole seeds, all eaten raw or gently steamed. Choline (a B vitamin) is vital for the balanced use of cholesterol by the body; soybean products are rich in this. Adults should keep their protein intake to an optimal one to two ounces a day, as Westerners eat far too much protein, which disrupts liver enzyme activity. Eat foods that contain sulfur—for instance, garlic, leeks, chives, and spring onions—as they decongest the liver. Keep your intake of refined sugar to a minimum. Eat lots of sour foods such as lemon juice, which is thought to initiate enzymatic releases that detoxify the liver. Avoid cooked spices and test to see whether raw ones are appropriate for you. Raw spices will have a more cooling effect on the liver than if cooked. However, if the liver is very heated and maybe even inflamed, then only use cooling culinary herbs for flavor, such as mint, thyme, and marjoram. Listen to your body and take note of its reactions. Eat steamed rice and vegetables and organic wheat. Avoid consuming coffee, tea, and alcohol—in fact anything that stimulates, including heating spices like chiles.

By keeping the gallbladder working properly, the liver can work less stressfully, thus relieving the bowel, the heart, and the kidneys. Raw juices make good liver and gallbladder cleansers; blend together 60 percent carrot juice, 30 percent beet juice, and 10 percent cucumber or apple juice and drink one to two cups a couple of times a week. Dr. Christopher always warned that those drinking large amounts of carrot juice can look as if they are suffering from carotene poisoning, developing an orange tint to their skin. However, he added reassuringly that this is just the liver clearing, when bile flows out in quantity, and that normal skin color will soon be restored. In my experience, before returning to normal many patients have had a hard job calming down anxious friends and relatives about their skin color, so before embarking on liver cleansing, it may be wise to give them due warning.

Grapes activate the liver to stimulate glycogenic and bile secretions. Ripe mango is invigorating and stimulates appetite. Rosemary is beneficial in cooking or salads, owing to its bitter flavor. Radishes and their green leaves can beneficially be taken daily for jaundice. Drink a glass of tomato juice mixed with cayenne pepper if you suffer from a sluggish liver (but avoid if your liver is hot and inflamed—see above). Turmeric—fresh or dried ground root added to food—is a prime Indian liver and gallbladder cleanser (avoid if gallstones are present). Globe artichokes contain cynarine, which promotes the flow of bile and stimulates liver cell regeneration.

Dizziness, eye problems, and a flushed face could suggest a deficiency of liver enzymes—eat more dark green vegetables and cabbage.

For a liver cleanse based on foods, see chapter 6.

HERBS

Many liver herbs are bitter or sour; these act as a digestive stimulant. Some common and wild liver herbs in Europe and the United States are dandelion leaf, sorrel leaf, angelica root, watercress, and wormwood leaf and, in the kitchen, turmeric and lemon. If the gallbladder is actually inflamed, then gentle herbs will be needed, like marshmallow root, dandelion root and leaf, gentian root, wild yam root, and chamomile flower.

All of the following herbs can be used to help the liver and gallbladder, either by stimulating bile flow, or by helping to protect, cool, and clear the liver: milk thistle seed, *Bupleurum* root, artichoke leaf, barberry root bark, *Schisandra* berry, wild yam root, burdock root, gingerroot, lobelia leaf, mugwort leaf, gentian root, dandelion root, olive leaf, turmeric rhizome, rosemary leaf, and peppermint leaf.

Chamomile flower tea, taken daily, helps digestion and liver function and replenishes bowel flora. It is ideal for calming children as well.

Herbs for the bowel, bloodstream, and lymph systems can also be of vital assistance to the liver: mullein flower, lobelia leaf, burdock root, and cascara sagrada aged bark.

Neck or breast lumps may point to a congested liver with insufficient blood and oxygen. Probably digestion is poor and in need of repair. Cleansing the liver and toning digestion will greatly help. Use dandelion root, milk thistle seed, and gentian root.

Weak tendons and ligaments and brittle nails can be a result of an over-stimulated sympathetic nervous system and overworked liver and gallbladder.

Eat lots of cabbage and broccoli and use burdock root, dandelion root, yellow dock root, barberry root bark, and *Bupleurum* root in teas or tinctures.

Skin disorders such as acne and psoriasis usually suggest that the liver and digestive system are in trouble. Milk thistle seed, dandelion root, barberry root bark, and burdock root will all help. Performing a liver cleanse will also be of great benefit (see chapter 6).

Digestive, spleen, and liver imbalances are often mirrored in blood sugar problems and indigestion—use wild yam root, Siberian ginseng root, *Astragalus* root, licorice root, burdock root, and dandelion root and leaf.

For the emotions of the liver—anger, sadness, emotional depression, and frustration—use milk thistle seed, lavender leaf, and dandelion root and leaf. Drink herb teas like mint, lavender, and chamomile.

NATURAL HEALING

Spring is when sap rises and trees and plants burst into new growth. Birds can also be heard joyfully singing their songs of love and wooing. In ancient Chinese medicine, the element of wood ruled the liver and gallbladder. Spring cleanses are therefore traditionally centered on liver cleansing (see chapter 6). Additionally, massage the liver area daily for one minute. Take daily hot and cold showers. Use castor-oil packs over the liver if it is swollen (see chapter 3). Release anger and anxiety constructively so that they do not get stuck in the liver and gallbladder; exercise will greatly help. Don't forget to drink plenty of water in order to flush out all extraneous toxins, hormones, and other unwanted congestive elements.

The Colon (Bowel) or Large Intestine

In 1995, nearly thirty-one thousand people in Britain were diagnosed with colon cancer, and twenty thousand are expected to die as a result. It is the third most common cancer, and could easily upgrade to second if our eating trends and accompanying lack of exercise continue. When combined with other colon diseases, it is already the second largest cause of death in Britain. When the colon starts to become clearer and cleaner, the symptoms of the disease begin to ebb away slowly, layer by layer. Remember, if you do not cleanse the colon, your other organs and systems will not be able to cleanse their wastes either, and an autointoxication situation can easily arise, causing extreme ill health.

Check whether close relatives, especially older members of your family, have bowel problems. This way you will be able to see if your own tendencies might be hereditary. As always, prevention is the key. The late Dr. Bernard Jensen, a well-known American herbalist, has written many books on the bowel; they are worth searching out, not least for their photographs of autopsies showing the variety of distorted colon shapes found in the deceased. These distortions were caused by old fecal matter piling up by the pound, creating pockets, narrowings, balloonings, and so forth.

In these balloons, old fecal matter slowly becomes part of the bowel wall itself, hardening and impacting, layer upon layer, encouraging viruses, bacteria, and fungi to take hold and thrive, with opportunistic parasites also setting up home—all draining the entire body of health and vigor. The ensuing strain on the colon walls also causes thinning and, where the wall has become too thin, fluid bowel matter can slowly seep into the rest of the body. It is not only toxins that can cause bowel problems. Beneficial microbes in the colon can become dangerously pathogenic if they escape from their regular environment.

Many common viruses and bacteria lurk in bowel pockets of both men and women. Candida is commonly found in the bowel pockets of women in particular, and can often stubbornly proliferate when parasites are present. Whenever ballooning of the bowel wall occurs, narrowing before or after the affected area results. These strictures then make it difficult for fecal matter to pass through. Very often the result is fecal matter being dumped into the existing balloon or pocket after attempts to negotiate the stricture have failed. What little fecal matter does get through is often very watery and thin, and this is the form in which diarrhea sometimes presents itself, especially if it comes after years of constipation.

HOW OFTEN SHOULD I HAVE A BOWEL MOVEMENT?

One needs a bowel movement roughly one to three times a day, depending on the daily food intake. Normally, you should eliminate four-fifths of your food intake over an eleven- to nineteen-hour period of time. Every eight hours there is a peristaltic urge triggered by the gallbladder. If a bowel movement is achieved on waking at 7:00 A.M., then the next one should be at approximately 3:00 P.M. Candida and other bowel flora imbalances can severely hamper peristalsis, much as liver and gallbladder dysfunction do. Many people find that having a meal triggers a bowel movement. The reason is that the filling of the stomach triggers the emptying of the colon. This idea to many people seems horrendous and ridiculous—they feel they don't want to give away that much! Nor do most of us check the amount of time that food takes to pass through. Try swallowing some sunflower seeds —the white seeds show up well against the other colors of the fecal matter and are a useful way to measure the amount of time food takes to pass through your system.

NUTRITION

Eat a diversity of food types according to your individual needs. One of the most important things to remember is that all foods must be completely digested in order to move successfully through the colon. Consuming plenty of water and fiber will help enormously.

HERBS

See chapter 6 for information on colon cleansing. Drinking aloe vera juice will soothe, heal, and help to repopulate bowel flora in all conditions. Liver and kidney cleansing may also be beneficial.

NATURAL HEALING

Try keeping a footstool in the bathroom. This is useful because we are really designed to squat when having a bowel movement—a position not encouraged by the design of most modern Western toilets. Using a footstool will help align your body in a more natural position.

As with all bodily functions, the spinal column provides nerve supply, and the lower vertebrae, if misaligned, will cause problems in the bowel. Therefore, consider a visit to an osteopath or chiropractor in order to make sure that your vertebrae aren't hindering the correct flow of impulses and fluids.

Massage will help, especially along the whole length of the intestine, where it will encourage and increase the intestine's vitality.

Self-massage can really help the bowel. Always use circular movements, starting on your right side at the bottom of the abdomen and moving up to just below your ribs, across to the other ribs, and down to your genitals. Use a soft, light touch until you get to know how deeply you can go. Eventually go as deeply as feels comfortable, stroking and kneading (like working bread dough). If you ever reach a painful spot, stop and hold your hand over the pain for a while till it ebbs away. For a relaxing oil, you could try diluted frankincense essential oil (one-half to one teaspoon in one cup of base oils). Other essential oils may be recommended for particular problems, but black pepper and camphor are two others for general use. You should also practice deep breathing exercises, and yoga will be of great benefit, as some of the postures deal directly with internal massage.

The Urinary System

The kidneys constantly regulate, distribute, sort, and filter matter. Without this ability, the body cannot survive for long—it will become poisoned. To do this job properly, large amounts of water are required in a body that is itself composed of 70 percent water, at least two quarts a day to prevent dehydration. The kidneys also maintain the pH balance within the bloodstream. With an adequate intake of fluids a more alkaline state will prevail, which is the base of all good health.

In addition, the kidneys have quite a number of hormonal functions. They help to process calcium and magnesium. In women, this is done in connection with estrogen. The kidneys also help produce an enzyme called *renin* that is vital for regulating blood pressure. Weak kidneys can sometimes be the root cause of blood pressure imbalances.

NUTRITION

Too little salt can be as harmful to the kidneys as too much is (excessive sodium causes the body to store too much water). Choose and use a variety of salts, from rock salt to sea salt. Consume two to four quarts of water daily, according to your size and body weight. Drinking water, any water, is vital. Tap water is the least advisable, but even that—with all its nitrates, chlorine, and so on—is better than no water. Better is bottled springwater or filtered water. *Your Body's Many Cries for Water* by F. Batmanghelidj is an excellent book on the subject (see also chapter 4). Keep the urinary system healthy via simple supportive and detoxification methods in order to deflect cystitis, water retention, and other problems.

Common foods and drinks such as tea, coffee, chocolate, and, to a lesser extent, peanuts, rhubarb, tomatoes, and spinach, contain oxalic acid, which creates more work for the kidneys. Some foods are strongly active on the kidneys and bladder, and eating them in season can help maintain, cleanse, and thus balance the kidneys and bladder, preventing stagnation, stone formation, and infection. Asparagus, for instance, is useful in late spring, but don't eat it if your kidneys are known to be, or suspected to be, inflamed. Also avoid asparagus if you already feel exhausted or tired, as the diuretic effect could increase these feelings. Parsley and nori seaweed in salads, soups, and stews provide a nice year-round addition, while blackberries, raspberries, cranberries, celery, watermelon, and watercress are good summer choices. Whole barley and sweet corn in soups and stews could be used in the autumn and winter months. If you have inflamed, weakened kidneys, make a soup of 70 percent zucchini and 30 percent potatoes. Carrots, lettuce, and cabbage are also very helpful. Oxalic acid–rich foods must be avoided by those who are prone to kidney problems, as they are known to help create kidney stones. Finally, drink barley water—refer to chapter 4 for the recipe.

HERBS

It is important to note that, because of the forceful nature of their action, some herbs are just as capable of exhausting the kidneys as are synthetic diuretics available by prescription. Therefore they should be used only for specific purposes and only for a short period of time. A prime example would be horsetail leaf. It is true that they don't leach potassium from the body because, like all plants except licorice root, they are rich in potassium and low in sodium (usually present in a ratio of three to one); if used for long periods, however, their potent diuretic action on the kidneys will cause weakening and draining.

The safest herb, which cannot harm the kidneys yet helps shed excess water in the body, is dandelion. As Dr. Christopher puts it, "it's the safest diuretic in the botanical kingdom." It also has the ability to aid the work of the liver. Others in combination include parsley root, marshmallow root, corn silk, and bearberry leaf.

NATURAL HEALING

Cold, damp, too little or too much water, wintry weather, and fear can negate the effectiveness and balance of the kidneys. Your environment and lifestyle and the climate in which you live can all make a difference, depending on your body structure. The kidneys and the urinary system work hardest or stagnate in extremes of weather, either hot or cold. So in winter, wrap up well and never let your kidneys become chilled. If your kidneys ever feel inflamed or you suffer from genitourinary problems, applying a castor oil pack over them will bring instant relief. A summer kidney cleanse is often advisable—see chapter 6.

The Adrenal Glands

The adrenal glands are found just above each of the kidneys and are, in effect, part and parcel of kidney function. When our adrenals are low and exhausted, our whole being becomes depressed in a variety of ways. Severe mental dysfunction can be attributed to their depletion, and many diseases and conditions, from allergies to chronic illness, can have their roots in adrenal dysfunction. Their depletion can be either inherited or produced by other factors.

One group of hormones produced by the adrenals helps to build, fuel, and regulate growth and repair within the body. These hormones also work to control and instigate inflammation, which is vital when infection or tissue damage is apparent. They are known as natural steroids. Another group of hormones produced in the adrenal glands acts to maintain the appropriate ratio of potassium and sodium, helping to inhibit loss of sodium and water through the kidneys. This function is important because waterlogged tissue strains the heart. Finally, the adrenal cortex produces sex hormones, and it is the balance of these that creates gender differences.

The adrenal medulla is associated with the flight-or-fight response, and is really part of the nervous system. Varying amounts of adrenaline are released into the bloodstream, circulating and preparing the body to react to particular situations. Should this adrenaline reaction become a constant stress norm, however, the body will become exhausted, and digestive problems, among others, will manifest themselves (digestion is temporarily shelved during this response). Adrenaline reaction is a useful response in cases of genuine danger, rapid breathing patterns, and varying responses to allergens. Unfortunately, the body can often become trigger-happy and, apart from being subjected to a physical toll, may produce confused emotions— for instance, anxiety and paranoia may occur. Exhaustion, depression, and the potential for acute or chronic diseases of the digestive system, pancreas, spleen, liver, thyroid, and colon could ensue. Blood sugar levels will also be badly affected. Entire endocrine support will be vital to help remedy the problem.

NUTRITION

Food and one's physical focus should be similar to those recommended for hypoglycemia and diabetes in chapter 10. For the adrenal medulla, all foods for the nervous system can very often help, particularly oats.

HERBS

Plant hormone precursors are invaluable for feeding exhausted or trigger-happy (that is, underactive or overactive) adrenals. They are present in wild yam root, Chinese licorice root, and Siberian ginseng root. Marshmallow root, *Astragalus* root, and *Schisandra* berry also provide bedrock tonic support. Take chamomile flower and skullcap leaf tea at bedtime. Drink one cup of parsley leaf tea a day.

NATURAL HEALING

The advice that applies to the kidneys is also applicable to the adrenal glands. On the whole, the body requires appropriate exercise and rest. Burning the candle at both ends should be avoided. Good sleeping habits are vital as well as catnapping, which can be a very useful habit to develop, as it conserves and restores energy.

The Reproductive System

Without hormones, the whole intricate network of our beings would cease to exist, not just sexually and reproductively but in a more widely functioning sense. As hormones surge through the bloodstream, they continuously send vital instructions to all parts of the body. In fact, the word *hormone*, describing this active and constant transmission, comes from the Greek word meaning "to excite."

We all seem to know about testosterone, estrogen, and progesterone—hormones that have a particular influence over our reproductive systems. But there are many more hormones—fifty located by science so far—influencing many aspects of our metabolism (see chapter 8).

Women have a very complex reproductive system. Consequently, a great deal of their daily energy is drawn toward its functioning and upkeep, from monthly menstruation to childbirth, breast-feeding, and menopause. The end result is that women are statistically three times more immunally vulnerable than men are. They constantly need to tend their bodies in a way that is not so vital for men. Men and women store hormones, semen, and other vital essences needed not only for their sexual and reproductive lives but also for general vitality and strength, especially of their immune systems. Therefore the hormones—and the body as a whole—must be nourished and rested accordingly.

NUTRITION

Avoid foods that contain synthetic hormones and steroids, such as dairy products and meat. It also helps to avoid fast foods wrapped in plastics that contain synthetic hormones. Stop or drastically reduce your tea and coffee intake, because they disrupt hormone regulation. Eat a generally diverse, wholesome, and, if possible, organic diet. For more detailed dietary advice, refer to chapter 4.

HERBS

American engineer Galen Hieronymus, with Dr. Ruth Drown and others, collaborated to make a machine that detected what appeared to be the plant equivalents of the seven human endocrine glands: pineal, thymus, pituitary, adrenals, thyroid, ovaries, and prostate. Plants are rich in hormones that, unlike their synthetic counterparts, are subtle in their interaction with the human body. They can switch on and off, go where they are needed, and generally act in a responsive way. Plants and trees need hormones for exactly the same reasons we do, and the wealth of hormones found in plant life is incredible and highly effective for its varying properties and usage. Whether for tempering adolescence, balancing menstruation, aiding fertility, helping menopause, supporting the prostate, or balancing an estrogen dominance in the case of some cancers, plants contain the rainbow of hormones and hormone precursors necessary. They are known as phytosterols and can be used by human recipients as building blocks for their own hormones. Between four thousand and five thousand plant species are believed to contain hormones. Among them, sarsaparilla root, chaste tree berry, *dong quai* root, and saw palmetto berry are just four herbs commonly used to tone, regulate, and balance the endocrine system in men and women.

NATURAL HEALING

To keep both male and female reproductive systems healthy, we must eat well, exercise, be happy, and breathe properly. Deep breathing stimulates vital hormone secretions, while sitz baths encourage an increase in circulation to the womb, ovaries, or prostate. Take hot and cold showers, as they will benefit the entire endocrine system. Massage with geranium and ylang-ylang essential oils diluted in a suitable base oil. (For more general information, see chapter 8.) Colon, liver, and kidney cleanses will all be beneficial (see chapter 6).

The Thyroid

The thyroid is part of the endocrine system and is found in the front of the neck, on both sides of the Adam's apple. Its main job is to produce the hormones thyroxine T4 (75 percent) and L-thyronine T3 (25 percent), but it also stores iodine, and should the correctly balanced amounts change, problems will occur.

A common reason for thyroxine output problems is if the adrenal glands or the pituitary gland and hypothalamus are unbalanced and unable to stimulate the thyroid correctly. The thyroid gland is the body's internal thermostat, and the hormones it provides are in charge of this job. If it fails, the body can initially overburn calories, and then underburn calories.

The two major dysfunctions of the thyroid are hypothyroidism (underproduction of the thyroid hormones) and hyperthyroidism (overproduction of the thyroid hormones). Energy is low for both conditions, and frequent illness can occur from the resulting impaired immune function.

There are thyroid self-help tests in which temperature taking can assess underactive conditions. Your basal body temperature can be determined by placing an old-fashioned mercury thermometer under your arm for ten minutes first thing as you wake in the morning. For women, this test is best taken during the menstruation week. Plot your temperature on a chart in order to determine your average trend. It would naturally fluctuate but be around 97.4° to 98°F. Low basal temperature readings (below 94.4°F) over a month could indicate not only an underactive thyroid but also low adrenal function, so it is always advisable to take your results to a physician or nutritionist to get them further analyzed. There are also thyroid blood tests that can ascertain hyperthyroid problems, when thyroid stimulating hormone (TSH) levels are too high. Refer to chapter 10 ("Overactive Thyroid" and "Underactive Thyroid") for symptoms.

An overburdened or overheated liver is known to affect thyroid function, so liver foods and herbs will often help. Liver conditions frequently occur during pregnancy, leaving many women with short-term or long-term deficiencies that, if left untreated, may become chronic. It is, therefore, important to support the liver and adrenals in order to assist the thyroid, as well as, of course, the entire endocrine system.

NUTRITION

Refer to "Overactive Thyroid" and "Underactive Thyroid" in chapter 10.

HERBS

Refer to "Overactive Thyroid" and "Underactive Thyroid" in chapter 10 for appropriate choices of herbs and include Siberian ginseng root and, occasionally, echinacea root. All endocrine and liver herbs such as dandelion root, barberry root bark, milk thistle seed, and chaste tree berry, will indirectly and directly support the thyroid.

NATURAL HEALING

Castor-oil packs (see chapter 3) placed over the thyroid can help to regulate its function. Hot and cold showers will encourage circulation to the area. Exercise and practice deep breathing. You will need to cleanse the colon, liver, and kidneys (see chapter 6).

The Spleen

The health of the spleen relies on good stomach and pancreatic balance because it is part of the supporting tissue of the stomach (see the section on the pancreas, above in this chapter). This supporting role means that the spleen plays a valuable part in the digestive function. In Chinese medicine, the spleen and liver have a special relationship—again related to digestion. Many traditional models of medicine place the main emphasis on its digestive function, its job being to extract nutrition and, therefore, energy from food. The spleen transforms our food, changing the impure to the pure. It is also a major component of the immune system, so when the role of the spleen is hampered, its immune function becomes restrained. It loses its force, and this impairment is often accompanied by chronic fatigue. Digestion also becomes badly affected. You may experience pain upon eating, bloating, gas, constipation or diarrhea, and weight loss. Support of the entire endocrine system is vital.

NUTRITION

Seaweeds, vegetable juices, and superfood made up as energy drinks are ideal, as they require very little digestion. A few examples are algae, wheat grass, and kelp. Otherwise, use foods for the pancreas, as stated. Slow cooking of foods helps aid digestion. Excessive worry or obsessive behavior can overburden the digestive process.

Note: For those who are chronically ill, such as those suffering from cancer, an excess of raw foods—which are usually vital for the healing process—can produce a deficiency in the spleen and hamper the immune system. Therefore let the practitioner keep an eye the behavior of the spleen—an acupuncturist can do this by feeling the pulse.

HERBS

Those herbs that are supportive to the pancreas are also appropriate here, along with herbs like echinacea root (as long as autoimmune problems are not present) and burdock root to support the immune system.

NATURAL HEALING

See liver and colon cleanses in chapter 6 and general advice for the pancreas.

The Circulatory System

Heart attacks and circulatory disorders are often a "disease of the knife and fork" (a key phrase often used by natural healer Richard Schulze). It may not have been our own knife and fork, it may have been our parents'—but diet is, nevertheless, very frequently the cause. In America, cholestrol-conscious diets are having a positive effect. If we were to give heart and circulatory fatalities as much attention as we do AIDS or even cancer deaths, we would be faced with the reality of examining what people in the industrialized nations eat. Most people don't want to look at this connection or to change their habits, so the high death rate continues. We create problems for our children and our children's children by passing on our bad habits via our genes, creating burdened circulatory systems at birth that, according to surgeons, are giving rise to heart problems in younger and younger people. In Britain, women are four times as likely to succumb to general circulatory disorders as men, though actual heart attacks are higher in men.

Dr. Christopher healed hundreds of people with minor heart problems and circulatory diseases in the 1930s using natural healing methods. Now angiograms and CAT scans are able to prove the value of this kind of work to other medical professionals, showing that through diet, herbs, and changes in lifestyle, coronary plaque in the arteries can be greatly reduced, thus ultimately making surgery unnecessary.

The heart, to all poets, painters, spiritual guides, and those who really know, is the key to emotional well-being. "Open" your heart and you will feel loving, caring, compassionate, and at peace with life. Should your general disposition be low and your nervous system stretched, or should you feel depressed or angry, your heart will be affected. In many ways, the heart and the way we feel, or rather how the mind feels, are interconnected. Singing, chanting, movement, dance, meditation, and food can all "open" and get to the "heart" of the matter.

In Asian traditions, the small intestine is connected with the heart. This partnership gives the male role to digestion (small intestine) and the female role to the heart, the rhythmic, perpetual beat. If one side of the partnership is disharmonious, then its partner will feel it.

There are, of course, many drugs for these conditions—drugs to prevent spasm, to dilate arteries, to strengthen heartbeat, to drive out excess water and salt, to block beta cell receptors, to slow down clotting processes, to help decrease cholesterol levels—but all carry deleterious side effects, especially if they are used for long periods of time. It would be much better to avoid them if at all possible. Sometimes they provide first-aid measures, but finding alternatives is really worthwhile.

NUTRITION

The Chinese teach us that bitter foods are very supportive and strengthening to both the small intestine and the heart and, in our present sugar-oriented society, I think this is an ever more important point to remember.

Avoid eating excessive amounts of meat, in order to lower cholesterol levels and homocysteine levels. High homocysteine levels cause plaque to build up in the arteries. Folic acid and other B vitamins will greatly help lower cholesterol and homocysteine levels.

Fats should be avoided in general, while saturated fats, found in meat, should never be used. Moreover, when you are shopping, read all the labels on the foodstuffs you buy and, whenever you see oil or fats mentioned, consider that product undesirable. Olive oil, heated at a low temperature (not above 90°F) or used raw, is the safest oil to use, along with flaxseed oil, which is also rich in omega-3 and other fatty acids. Be sure to use a cold-pressed oxygen-free oil such as Udo's Oil (available at www.iherb.com).

Salt is okay if you use a high-quality variety—if possible, hand-harvested and sun- and wind-dried. These salts have the correct balance of minerals and naturally tend to be lower in sodium. Used sparingly in cooked food, they are acceptable. Raw food does not need extra salt flavoring, but explore the use of herbs and spices, which often negate the need for salt. Consider using coriander seeds, bay, thyme, and fennel fronds.

Avoid alcohol, as it increases the strain on the circulatory system and heart, breaking open veins and expanding the arteries. It also increases free-radical damage and oxidation. Oxidation is what happens when something is overexposed to oxygen. Like a piece of rubber when it gets older, veins and arteries go hard, lose their elasticity, and will finally crack or sag.

Basic positive foods include beets (the color of blood). Taken raw, juiced, or cooked, they will clear, cool, and strengthen the blood and heart. Use them mixed with apple or carrot if the taste seems too intense. Onions and garlic are master cleansers and coolers of the heart and whole circulatory system. Whole wheat (the whole organic grain of wheat) is another good heart strengthener. It will also help to cool and clear the blood, easing any inflammation. You can sprout the grains and eat the grass with salads—a preferable choice for the many who need to avoid cracked wheat. Following a mainly juice-oriented vegan eating program for just one month can go a long way toward normalizing blood pressure and removing cholesterol buildups. Use plenty of garlic (three to six cloves a day). You should also add plenty of medium to hot raw cayenne. As a guide, take a minimum of one small teaspoon per day, but two teaspoons per day would be better, and nine teaspoons would be excellent (but check with your stomach).

Most fruits are rich in salicylate, and this plant constituent helps to keep the blood from becoming sticky and clumping together to form dangerous clots, so eat plenty of bilberries, lemons, oranges, peaches, prunes, figs, grapefruit, rhubarb, cherries, melons, nectarines, plums, apples, and pineapple, always eating the skins (except, of course, those of melons, pineapples, and grapefruit). The inner skin (pith) of lemons, grapefruit, and oranges is an excellent source of bioflavonoids (vitamin P), which really strengthen the veins, arteries, and capillary walls. All the above fruits are also rich in vitamin C and will aid the structure and elasticity of the veins, as well as protecting arteries from oxidation and diminishing the growth of plaque on the vessel walls. Most fresh fruits and vegetables are rich in antioxidants that keep all cellular structure healthy and functioning as required. In modern life, we are increasingly becoming deficient in vitamin C because stress and pollution rob us of this vital vitamin, which we are not capable of making for ourselves. If you have cold extremities, add raw black pepper or ginger to the fruits to add fire and warmth for yourself. Meadowsweet leaf and flower and willow bark are rich in salicylate, which is helpful for digestion and aids the whole small intestine and heart partnership.

Cholesterol is a vital part of cell membrane structure. It is needed for bile formation, hormone production, and vitamin D synthesis and is transported from the intestine to the liver in order to perform these functions. Any excess that cannot be metabolized will be deposited in the linings of the arteries. Cholesterol-like particles called lipoproteins can cause the growth of plaque, which gradually builds up to such an extent that it constricts blood flow. Vitamin C helps to reduce the risk of these lipoproteins binding to the wall of the artery. The amino acid lysine also helps enormously, as it reverses the plaque buildup.

A cholesterol test kit will give you a quick guide to your cholesterol count, or you can ask your doctor for a test. Always do the test before you eat in the morning. If it is high, here are some ways to help reduce it:

- Eat a generally good and balanced diet (see chapter 4), and make sure that you have enough vitamin E. Avoid eating sweet pastries, cakes, savory snacks, and any other foods of this kind.

- Eat plenty of lightly steamed green vegetables, green salads, and su- perfood, as you need higher levels of vitamin C, potassium, and magnesium to maintain the vascular system in general.

- Increase fresh garlic intake (also onions, leeks, and chives).

- Take black currant seed oil or evening primrose oil capsules (GLA), as they help the metabolism to rid the body of cholesterol. Gamma linoleic acid (GLA) capsules are rich in omega-6, which is an essential fatty acid for this job.

- Eat oats and oat-based foods.

- Eat pineapple and papaw *(Asimina triloba)*, which will cool and calm the liver and gallbladder while also addressing the problem of plate- let stickiness.

- Make sure you have good vital stomach and bowel flora, as acidophilus and other beneficial bacteria lower cholesterol levels.

- Check your thyroid function through a blood and temperature test (see the section on the thyroid, above in this chapter).

- Refer to "Heart Disease" in chapter 10 for extra dietary advice.

HERBS

Apart from garlic and cayenne, hawthorn is perhaps the most important single herb to use in healing the circulatory system. It is a "heart" food capable of protecting, buffering, and repairing the heart muscle. You can make hawthorn teas and hawthorn syrup. Collect your own hawthorn leaves and blossoms in the spring and berries in the autumn when they are bright red. Research has shown that compounds in hawthorn adhere to the heart cells, making them absorb oxygen more efficiently thus preventing a heart attack. It can equally well restore those who have sustained a heart attack and miraculously remove palpitations and murmurs. It does so particularly by buffering beta cell receptors and is a more sophisticated version of the class of drugs called beta-blockers, as it is also able to "unblock" as required. Hawthorn is also an antioxidant, being rich in chemicals called flavonoids, which are useful for removing plaque from the circulatory system. If you are taking hawthorn leaves, flowers, and berries and you do have a heart attack, your body will repair itself three times more quickly than usual.

Dandelion root, made as coffee, aids the dispersal of water retention, which can be a problem with heart and vascular blockages; swollen ankles are often a sign of water retention. Repairing and cleansing the vascular system via diet and herbs will drastically alter this waterlogged situation as the blood slowly begins to move more and more freely around the body.

Cayenne, which has already been mentioned under the section on nutrition, is a wonderful supplement for any heart and circulatory disorders, just like garlic, and both should be used daily to thin cholesterol and maintain blood pressure. They can both be taken as tinctures or capsules.

It is as vital for the bloodstream to be clean as it is for it to be rich in iron and uncongested with plaque. Should the blood constantly carry infection, debris, and toxins (often from a constipated bowel), the whole body will feel sick and depleted. Red clover is particularly good at cleaning the bloodstream, thanks to its high beta-sitosterol content. Sitosterol is poorly absorbed but competes with cholesterol for absorption, thus reducing blood cholesterol. Other chemical constituents in red clover help thin the blood, and thinner blood allows better, less-inhibited circulation. Nettle leaf, licorice root, burdock root, dandelion root and leaf, plantain leaf, sarsaparilla root, prickly ash berry, yellow dock root, barberry root bark, and garlic are also prime blood cleansers, while burdock root has the added advantage of being able to deal with high cholesterol levels. Lime tree *(Tilia)* flowers can help remove plaque from the system and at the same time calm the nerves and heart. Motherwort leaf also needs a mention as a useful heart herb, its Latin name, *Leonurus cardiaca*, showing how useful it has been for centuries.

A clean bowel is essential for clean blood. Look at the three-stage herbal colon cleanse in chapter 6 in order to clean the bloodstream properly. The liver should also be cleansed.

NATURAL HEALING

Cleanse and cool the blood, taking care of general circulation, liver, gallbladder, stomach, and bowels via cleanses.

A little sweating (through hot showers, baths, saunas, and exercise), as long as it's not exhausting or too heated, is beneficial, as cholesterol can be sweated out through the skin.

Smoking will similarly stress and inhibit the body, therefore *do not smoke*. Smoking accounts for a large proportion of cases of heart failure and circulatory diseases (see the discussion of the respiratory system, below in this chapter).

Exercise is vital, particularly with reference to the heart. It should be taken daily and carefully paced. At some point during the day, ideally after a period of gentle exercise, push the heart to a rapid beat for five minutes;

this will really make it pump and flex. **If you experience heart pains, stop immediately and take a few drops of lobelia leaf tincture to relax the muscles, including the heart, and remove the associated pain. Then tell your health professional.**

Hydrotherapy will greatly help the heart and circulatory system; adjust the temperature of the water according to your individual strength and tolerance. Train your body gradually over a period of time to tolerate the extremes of hot and cold, which will be extremely beneficial.

A castor-oil pack placed over the sternum is excellent (see chapter 3); make one half the size of a tea cloth and place it slightly toward the heart side. A compress made from ginger, cayenne, and mustard powders will also help; it can be a great relief to the circulatory system because it gets the blood moving. Increase the strength of the herbs according to your own strength and use once or twice daily.

Massage and meditation will enhance the circulatory process. Essential oils of hyssop and ylang-ylang are particularly good for either massaging in or adding to the bath.

The Respiratory System

Modern society truly underestimates breathing and its key role in the well-being of our bodies. Older cultures and societies understood the role of breath much more than we do. They used it as emotional and physical nourishment for the body. A freely and fully breathing body is healthier and better equipped with natural defenses against negative effects including pollution, infection, and nutritional deficiencies. One of the most potent ways of stimulating the lymph system, thus aiding the immune system, is by deep yogic breathing.

Yogic breathing and other breathing techniques devised and practiced in other parts of the world have been used for centuries to allay hunger, heal sick bodies, balance strong emotions, and explore different states of consciousness. Anybody at any time can explore breathing this way; it is an attainable goal. What usually happens to our breathing is that we forget it and generally get so mixed up with our emotions that we literally stifle, repress, and contort its healing potential and daily life-giving properties.

After our first breath as babies, we generally continue for roughly the next three years breathing deeply into our bellies, expanding and pushing our diaphragms and filling our lungs. About the age of two to three years old, this pattern changes as the ego asserts itself more. A colorful range of more advanced emotions come into play, and breathing moves from the round cherubic belly up into the chest during the day, returning at nighttime to the more relaxed belly area. Practicing and remembering how a baby breathes can be a tool for life, helping emotionally and physically at any time there is stress or strong emotion—or indeed coughs and asthma. (For more on breathing, see chapter 5.)

Whatever age you are, when threatened, your breathing may become rapid, uneven, shallow, and jerky, and when panic takes over breathing can collapse altogether. A reaction to emotion—any emotion, good or bad—generally tends to be breathing that is shallower and higher in the chest. Negative emotion usually creates an added restriction in the belly area and even a temporary paralysis of the air sacs in the lungs, creating a kind of physical and emotional suffocation. Relaxed breathing and a calm feeling always come from the belly. Laughter comes from the belly and is one of the most potent lung healers of all.

In Chinese medicine the lungs are said to be the female side of a partnership with the male colon. As with everything in this universe, upset one side of a partnership, and the other will be in imbalance. If the lungs are not working well, the colon will falter, and constipation, diarrhea, and other symptoms can easily develop.

NUTRITION

Avoid dairy and wheat products if you have respiratory problems; the excessive mucus production caused in your body when these are eaten will clog and inhibit proper lung, sinus, and other related mucous membrane function. Nutritional deficiencies also affect the respiratory system; low hydrochloric acid levels in the stomach and a lack of zinc and magnesium are often found in people who suffer from respiratory diseases, so eat cabbage and garlic. Garlic should be eaten on a daily basis to create and then maintain digestive equilibrium. Other important nutrients that will assist respiration are those for immune-system function and include selenium, vitamin C, and vitamin A.

HERBS

Lobelia is a key herb to help alleviate and relax overburdened lung function. Known as the lung herb, lobelia helps release mucus congestion, and relaxes and opens the tiny air sacs of the lungs, making it easier to replenish oxygen. An overdose, however, will make you vomit. Ancient laws have victimized this plant and modern governing laws still restrict its access and dose, but if used sensibly, it is a wonderful and very useful plant. Seek advice from a herbal practitioner. Other useful herbs include horehound leaf and flower, garlic, raw chiles, horseradish root, and mustard seed.

NATURAL HEALING

Adopt and practice a program of belly breathing (see chapter 5). Exercise and try hot and cold showers, which are essential for circulation and lung air exchange. Colon cleanses will help maintain the health of the lungs.

Saunas, if taken for short periods of time alternating with cold showers, will be beneficial to lung health, but avoid them if pregnant, weak, or elderly.

Essential oils can really help breathing, and different ones will produce a wide range of effects. Eucalyptus and camphor will clear and open the lungs, and the majority of people will find this mixture most effective. Some asthma sufferers, however, may find it makes things worse. In such cases, use essential oils like frankincense and mandarin that will calm and regulate the breathing.

Nicotine affects the central nervous system, particularly numbing autonomic ganglion blockers, which is partly why it's addictive. However, nicotine and the herb lobelia are similar in some ways (lobelia contains lobeline, which is similar to nicotine, both of which raise serotonin levels in the brain), so for anyone wishing to give up smoking, the lobeline-rich plant lobelia would be an ideal substitute, with no side effects if used properly except thoroughly positive ones. When you stop smoking, bowel function is often affected, as nicotine is a stimulant and laxative. You may feel sleepier with less stimulation and, if this presents a problem, use prickly ash berry, which will almost instantly bring oxygen to the brain. Cigarettes inhibit the circulatory system; they force the heart to beat faster and create a constant oxygen deficit in doing so, because the carbon monoxide from cigarettes releases oxygen from the bloodstream. One cigarette creates a six-hour reduction of blood supply to the hands and feet. With this in mind, healing of wounds, internal and external, is inevitably slowed down by smoking, and so too are all the vital functions of oxygen and blood. Blood sugar levels are also severely affected by tobacco, creating low blood sugar.

You may compromise by smoking herbal cigarettes, but any plant material will contain smoke and tar, which both clogs and inhibits the bloodstream and lymphatic system. Short-term choices could be red clover flower, honeysuckle flower, mullein leaf, elecampane root, American ephedra leaf (not Chinese ephedra), and lobelia leaf.

The Nervous System

This system affects both our emotional and our physical well-being. Without feeding and sustaining it with a positive lifestyle and nutritious foods, we can feel stressed and emotionally unstable and exhibit a range of ill-health patterns, from epilepsy, shingles, insomnia, hyperactivity, and poor memory to learning problems.

There are two principal divisions of the nervous system: the central nervous system, which includes the brain and spinal cord, and the peripheral nervous system (PNS), which includes the cranial and spinal nerves. Our nervous system is similar to the electricity network of our homes, our nerve fluid acting like the electric current. When the nerve endings get worn down and the protective covering is no longer in place, these naked nerve endings spark and leap like live wires, and we feel as frazzled as they look. In fact, excessive electrical charge does build up in the body during the course of each day if we live predominantly on concrete and are constantly exposed to synthetic materials such as nylon carpets, manmade fabrics, and so on. The cure for this problem is to ground and earth ourselves, just as all electrical systems need to be grounded. The remedy of walking barefoot when feeling hypernervous, unable to sleep, unstable, or burned-out really does work, and many a patient has found relief and benefit from a barefooted night foray into the back garden!

NUTRITION

Nerve foods that actually repair and feed the nervous system are nonactive yeast flakes, spirulina, and whole grains, particularly organic oats and wheat germ, which are very rich in B vitamins. B vitamins are vital because the immune system "eats up" the acetylcholine receptors that are neurotransmitters, and B vitamins are able to remake them. Spirulina and nonactive yeast flakes enter the bloodstream very quickly, need little to no digestion, and quickly make these vital components. Soy foods naturally contain lecithin, which is an excellent nerve-building food. Celery, zucchini, avocados, lettuce, carrots, and pumpkin are supreme nerve foods and can be juiced, steamed, or used raw in salads. Almonds and sesame seeds are rich in calcium and will feed the nervous system. Kitchen herbs and spices such as mint, rose petals, marjoram, rosemary, basil, and aniseed will also help.

Daily nerve food suggestions include 1½ quarts of carrot juice; avocado and romaine lettuce soup; and 2 cups of soaked oats with 12 almonds, 1 tablespoon sesame seeds, and ½ tablespoon wheat germ with added cinnamon powder, honey, bee pollen grains, and lemon juice to flavor.

Vitamins and minerals and other components connected to the well-being of the nervous system are essential fatty acids, calcium, potassium, phosphorus, sodium, all B vitamins, vitamin D, magnesium, and chloride. Foods rich in phosphorus are vital as a partner to calcium for bone and tooth formation; they are cabbage, bilberries, and pumpkin seeds. Avoid tea and alcohol as they stop thiamin (a B vitamin) assimilation, which is vital for the nervous system. Drink plenty of water as it helps the body in many ways, not least by balancing the function of the entire nervous system; it also greatly helps elimination on all levels.

HERBS

Herbs that specifically help the nervous system will also tone and aid the whole body. Circulatory, respiratory, digestive, glandular, reproductive, and skin problems could all benefit from the nourishing treatment of the nervous system—which explains why nerve herbs are found so often in many other formulas. Nervous-system herbs have an array of effects according to the type of action required. For instance, with depression, one would use nerve stimulants, nerve foods, and nerve tonics, but not nerve sedatives; whereas with insomnia, one might choose nerve sedatives, nerve relaxants, and nerve tonics. Depending on any prescribed drugs being taken, nerve stimulants may also be appropriate in the short term. Adaptogenic herbs that help us to adapt to situations by supporting and encouraging equilibrium, which may well also feed the adrenal glands, are also important when looking at the whole body and its response to stress.

Nerve herbs are nutritionally rich in particular vitamins, minerals, trace elements, and other components that help feed and connect the body in a better way; examples are valerian root, *pau d'arco* inner bark, cramp bark, nettle leaf, Irish moss, and wood betony leaf and flower, all of which are extremely rich in calcium and magnesium, apart from their other supportive chemistry. Plantain leaf and flaxseed are rich in choline, which plays an important part in neurotransmitter pathways. Another herb that helps these pathways is St. John's wort flower, as a stimulant and relaxant it helps to produce "happy chemistry" by producing serotonin in the brain. Siberian ginseng root helps neurotransmission in the brain, and this particular plant can be given to anybody quite safely, unlike St. John's wort, which has some contraindications that must be taken into account.

The following are some herb categories that can be combined as needed.

Nerve tonics strengthen and feed the nervous system, restoring the tissues and cells to good condition. One such repair can be to the myelin sheath covering nerve endings, which can become worn away and produce breakdowns and stress. Once encouraged to regrow, the whole network of the nervous system can be made to interact efficiently. Nerve tonics that help are skullcap leaf, *Schisandra* berry, vervain leaf, and wood betony leaf and flower. Skullcap and *Schisandra* are perhaps the best choices and should be taken for at least four to six months. Skullcap takes times to build up and then needs time to consolidate and repair. Nevertheless, initial effects will be noticed within a week or less. Skullcap is also a nerve sedative and will help with nervous tension, sleeplessness, seizures, epilepsy, drug withdrawal, and much more. A good food nerve nutritive, similar to nerve tonics, would be oats, which nourish, balance, and stabilize.

Nerve relaxants are herbs that quickly calm the person to a state in which the body and mind become relaxed. Chamomile flowers are a familiar herb for this purpose, ideal for babies, children, adults, and the elderly alike. Lime tree *(Tilia)* flowers are taken on an everyday basis in France for headaches or migraine, or simply to soothe away a fraught day. In the United States, California poppy flowers are used in a similar way. Other herbs include hop strobilus (a very British option), black cohosh root, vervain leaf, wood betony leaf, cramp bark, lavender leaf and flower, passionflower, St. John's wort flower, and skullcap leaf. Wild yam root is a digestive nervine, relaxing muscle fibers, soothing the nerves, and providing pain relief for the bowel, stomach, gallbladder, and uterus. Valerian root is a very strong herbal relaxant and is useful if all else has failed. But please note that it should be used only for a few weeks, during the initial crisis, otherwise it can become overly sedative. Other food nerve relaxants include nonactive yeast flakes and spirulina.

Nerve sedatives are the strongest form of nerve relaxants and are illegal in Britain, though used legally by herbalists in some countries. They are opium poppy and marijuana. Opium is very strong, as it contains codeine and morphine. Both are traditionally used in the treatment of multiple sclerosis (although, with this disease, nerve sedatives can sometimes be replaced by nerve stimulants), cancer, and AIDS. Marijuana has recently gained popularity for its medicinal benefits as a pain reducer; but as with any herb, correct dosage is important. In the case of this herb, excesses can cause paranoia, hyperventilation, and panic attacks. Pain relief herbs like corydalis tuber and poppy leaf or resin can be tried, along with willow bark or cramp bark.

Nerve stimulants are traditionally the least-used nervines and are probably underused in diseases in which there are neurological breakdowns, like multiple sclerosis, muscular dystrophy, and myasthenia gravis. They are an absolutely invaluable category of nervine herbs, as they directly stimulate nervous tissue. A famous one is kola nut. Common daily nerve stimulants like tea and coffee are, of course, completely overused and therefore lose their potential as effective herbs for the above diseases. Guarana is a popular nerve stimulant; it contains three times the amount of caffeine as coffee, and was used to keep jungle hunters alert in South America. A herb for more daily usage that is ideal in times of great stress, especially around exam times, is rosemary, which wakens the brain and also acts as a nerve relaxant and calmer. Prickly ash berry really moves the blood and has an almost instantly recognizable effect on a fuddled brain. Kava and coca leaves are other nerve stimulants used among traditional peoples around the world. Cayenne pepper, as well as being a nerve stimulant, will aid circulation and blood supply. So we have many choices. Among the safest are rosemary leaf and flower, peppermint leaf, and cayenne pod, but for stimulating yet calming effects, rosemary is the best. Other fine nerve stimulants are oat seed and straw, and skullcap leaf. Whenever you use nerve stimulants, you must also take in a lot of B vitamins to replace those that the nerve stimulation uses. (Foodwise, blue-green algae is an excellent nerve stimulant.) This whole category of nerve-stimulant herbs is useful in treating addiction to neuro-stimulants like cocaine and amphetamines.

Lobelia (Lobelia inflata): The Peacemaker

Lobelia fits into all of the above-mentioned categories and was traditionally smoked in the peace pipe by Native Americans. Herbalist Dr. Christopher called it the peacemaker of all formulas and the "thinking herb," thanks to its amphoteric action. He put it into almost every formula for two very good reasons: first, so that all the other herbs in the formulas could be directed to where they were most needed, and second, because usually when people are sick for whatever reason, their nervous systems need equilibrium. I have personally seen lobelia deal with a wide number of situations; I try to never be without it, having seen it work more quickly and effectively than the drug Neurofen for chronic menstrual cramps and for calming and supporting those coming off antidepressants, as well as in many more instances. Just a few drops of tincture go a very long way. It can also be combined with valerian and cramp bark for an all-around cramp and pain relief remedy for adults only: four parts valerian root, three parts cramp bark, and one part lobelia leaf; take one to two teaspoons two to three times a day.

NATURAL HEALING

Rest is vitally important for the nervous system, and it comes best of all in the form of sleep. Going to bed early enough improves the quality of sleep; indeed, sleep taken between the hours of 10:00 P.M. and 2:00 A.M. is actually reckoned to double its value in terms of quality. Meditation will repair, calm, and bring peace to the day, so give this simple practice daily time if you can. Just sitting under a tree concentrating on or being aware of your breathing for ten minutes has a tremendous impact. Those who travel, work, and generally lead a high-intensity life need to guard their resources and avoid burning the candle at both ends; catnapping can help. For those with insomnia, it is important to use hydrotherapy and other natural healing routines, including internal cleansing, in order to stimulate the body and thereafter produce sleep. This is especially wise if you rely on sleeping tablets, and it could well help you finally to do without them.

Nerves are dependent on blood and circulation for proper function; therefore maintain a good blood supply via exercise and hot and cold showers. Saunas alternating with cold showers also create a beautifully relaxed state.

Skin brushing will stimulate the nerve endings and is a great rejuvenator, especially to those who are low, depressed, and sluggish. And try using nerve sedative and nerve stimulant essential oils, as appropriate, in massages.

Creativity through, for example, dancing, painting, singing, or writing is an important expression of emotion, and the nervous system will thrive when pursuing such activities with pleasure and in a relaxed manner.

In times of extreme nervous stress, use equal parts of skullcap leaf, black cohosh root, and lobelia leaf powders to make a poultice. Place it over the head and neck and down the entire length of the spine. For a more instant version, simply put lobelia tincture over these areas.

Add a few drops of chamomile, frankincense, or geranium essential oil to your bath—or a couple of chamomile tea bags. A very good sedative is hop essential oil. This is useful for insomniacs, and it is well worth the high price you'll need to pay for it. Lavender is another (and much cheaper!) soothing essential oil, and is suitable for children and most skin types.

Liver and colon cleanses will be vital for the good health of the nervous system. These alone have made particularly overwhelming situations radically improve.

The Skin

The skin is the outer covering of the body, protecting us from external influences, such as toxins, infections, dirt, light, heat, and cold. It is our external immune system and ecobarrier.

Skin is also a very important excretory organ when it is functioning properly. It helps us rid ourselves of a quarter of our waste products. If the skin is inhibited by eczema, psoriasis, or other conditions, this function will be only partially carried out. Should the skin be underfunctioning, the lungs, kidneys, bowel, liver, and bloodstream will have to deal with the burden. When skin is unable to excrete, these organs will, in turn, feel the strain. It must be remembered, however, that these organs and systems could be the cause of skin problems, their own dysfunction giving rise to a stagnated skin.

Touching your own and other people's skin can be a truly sensuous experience; there's nothing more gorgeous, for instance, than a baby's skin. We touch, feel, and exchange both emotionally and physically, sharing our feelings, thoughts, and love through our skin. This emotional connection can be seen even more clearly when we note that, as fetuses, our skin develops from nervous tissue cells. Skin diseases can be the result of internal, emotional upset, and accordingly, a loving touch can heal and mend like nothing else.

NUTRITION

Avoid foods that are not typically digested efficiently, or that you know you are allergic to, such as dairy and wheat products. Reactions to foods can be reflected through the health of your skin, so keep an eye on your food intake and observe your skin's reactions. Skin needs essential fatty acids and water in order to maintain its good health, visually and otherwise.

HERBS

Many herbs are useful, but those that clear the blood and lymph systems will be of particular value. Blood cleansers (alteratives) are red clover flower and burdock root, while lymph-system herbs (lymphatics) like mullein flower and the much stronger pokeweed root will clear obstructions. Antimicrobial herbs such as chamomile flower and echinacea root will help rebalance any microorganism overgrowth. Diaphoretic and sudorific herbs will help you sweat; for instance, yarrow leaf and flower induce perspiration and cleanse directly through the skin.

NATURAL HEALING

Never use chemical deodorants; they clog the skin and destroy natural bacteria. Use essential oil–based products and wash frequently. Try crystal stones (available in health-food stores) as deodorants.

Make sure all the eliminative organs are working, so that the skin is not burdened. Explore colon, liver, and kidney cleanses—refer to chapter 6.

Avoid conventional detergents, cleaning equipment, dishwashing liquid, and so on. Instead, research ecofriendly and body-friendly products. Propyl alcohol, PCBs, and other toxic ingredients should not be used in your household and bathroom cleaners.

Do not wear manmade fibers. The skin needs to breathe, and nylon and other synthetic fibers create temperature extremes, putting undue strain on the skin thermometer and immune responses. Use cotton, silk, or wool—wear these at bedtime or sleep naked, if it is warm enough. Use cotton sheets and preferably an all-cotton mattress, such as a futon. Air futons and natural-fiber duvets by hanging them over windowsills on sunny days. Leave futon mattresses rolled up one day a week, to refluff and aerate.

A little sun is fine, but protect your skin from excessive exposure so that drying out does not occur and natural oils are not lost. Paler skin, which does not contain sufficient pigment for safe exposure to the sun, will, of course, need more protection than darker shades. Jojoba oil is a natural protector, with a sun protection factor (SPF) of sixteen, making it ideal for many adults with medium- to darker-pigmented skin. Those with very pale skin, children, and babies will need more strongly protective sunscreens. Go up to a factor thirty-five or fifty, depending on the strength of the sun. With at-risk skins, covering with a sunscreen on exposed skin from April to October in northern temperate climates is important.

Drink plenty of water to allow the skin to excrete and function correctly. Balance the drying effects of central heating by placing bowls of water containing essential oils next to hot spots in the room.

Low body temperature can affect skin problems, so create more body heat via exercise. Take care of your adrenal glands and thyroid in case your low body temperature is a result of imbalance there—if it is, use cayenne pepper.

Make contact with your body via your skin, through massage and barefoot walking on the earth or sand. If possible, swim in lakes, streams, or the sea. If swimming in chlorinated pools, clean off the chlorine by bathing afterward with lavender essential oil. Hot and cold showers are vital; problem skin often becomes overheated, and a cold shower or bath can bring instant relief. In general, exercise to promote good circulation and to ensure that lymph and lungs are moving.

Dog hairs, cat hairs, fleas, ticks, household dust, and pollen can provoke skin irritations. If afflicted, remember to support the immune system, cleanse the colon, liver, and kidneys, and get the lungs to work better. You must not lose sight of internal processes, even when there are external causes or outcomes.

The Muscular and Skeletal Systems

The skeleton is the support structure of the body. Muscles and ligaments interconnect and work together, facilitating the movement of the bones. As we become older (and as people in Western society live to a greater age), brittle bones will become an increasing problem. Therefore finding ways to maintain and support bone health will become more important.

NUTRITION

The well-being of our muscles, bones, tissues, and joints doesn't just depend on how much wear and tear or stagnation they receive in daily walking, running, lifting, bending, sitting, or lying. It also relies on our internal health and the food we use to create and support this moving structure. Sugar, sweet drinks, processed foods, tea, and coffee will strip magnesium, calcium, and vitamin C from the body. All of these elements are vital for the formation and repair of bone, muscle, cartilage, and synovial fluid. Magnesium, calcium, and vitamin C can be found in dark greens, seaweeds, and whole grains and should be eaten daily. Also note that iron is vital to structural well-being. Night twitching can be a result of a lack of iron, so the nettle leaves and red raspberry leaves used to meet calcium requirements will also provide copious and assimilable amounts of iron. Vitamins A, E, B_6, and B complex and zinc are all important for the synthesis and maintenance of good structure. Ensure that you eat foods that are rich in zinc and the vitamins listed above, such as red peppers, whole grains, pumpkin seeds, and carrots. Essential fatty acids and water are also vitally important lubricants.

For postmenopausal women, kidney health and estrogen and progesterone levels should be maintained in order to guard against osteoporosis and brittle bone disease.

For serious injury, stop all food immediately and switch to superfood, juices, and herb teas in order to allow the healing process to begin quickly.

HERBS

Use lobelia leaf tincture both internally (if legally possible) and externally for muscle strains, broken bones, and the like; it will quickly relieve the associated spasms and pain. *Pau d'arco* inner bark, oat straw, and nettle leaf, which are rich in both calcium and magnesium, make ideal choices, while skullcap leaf and peppermint leaf, rich in zinc, will give general support to the muscular, skeletal, and nervous systems. Echinacea root and the zinc herbs listed above, along with vitamin C, will help the immune system fight any breaks, strains, or bone porosity.

Elasticity and mobility can be a problem with diseases like osteoarthritis or simply old age. Devil's claw root and both the European and Chinese angelica roots *(Angelica archangelica and Angelica sinensis)* will greatly help here. So will *pau d'arco* inner bark and black cohosh root. Turmeric rhizome and meadowsweet leaf and flower will soothe joints and muscles—both can be used internally and externally for painful inflammation.

Boneset is a favorite herb of mine. Perhaps one of the nicest accounts of its bone-mending abilities is to be found in Tom Brown's book *Guide to Wild, Edible and Medicinal Plants.* He tells us that he broke his hand quite badly and was informed by his doctor that it would take six to eight weeks in a cast to mend. A Native American healer helped him. He pointed to the boneset plant, showing him the new little leaves at the top that grew separately, and then the lower leaves that grew together, almost as one. "That," he said, "is what the boneset will do for your hand!" Tom drank a tea made from the fresh, larger leaves twice a day for the first week. During the second week he cut down to half a cup, twice a day. He felt an almost immediate difference, a kind of tingling feeling, as if the knitting process had started, while the dull ache and pain also went away and the swelling subsided overnight. If it weren't for the likes of Dr. Christopher and Tom Brown and their links with the wise and knowledgeable Native American healers, no one would be using boneset for healing bones. Scientific analysis can find no reason why boneset should heal bones, but it obviously does.

My personal knowledge of boneset also goes back years, and I have many stories of bones that have mended very quickly. In addition, I have noticed in my family (which is not disposed to bone breaking) how quickly it delivers calcium to the body. Weak, broken, and torn nails can be made into strong ones, and growing pains can subside in hours. Comfrey leaf used to be a favorite herb in Europe for mending bones, but the recent public ban on its general internal use has meant that it is not possible to use this plant in this way anymore. It can still be used externally, however, and it is very effective as a bone-mending poultice or ointment.

NATURAL HEALING

Much benefit can be derived from practitioners who are able to manipulate, massage, and cajole muscles, bones, and joints into correct positions. These include osteopaths, chiropractors, massage therapists, and many other kinds of bodyworkers, from acupuncturists and physiotherapists to yoga teachers. This sort of work is sometimes vital for the well-being of external functions but also for the proper working of all organs and systems as well as the neurological pathways radiating from the entire length of the spine that service them. In fact, the well-being of the spine alone is crucial, and much is rightly made of this concern in yoga. It provides an ideal way to service and tune one's framework and internal organs at the same time.

A poultice made from turmeric rhizome is a handy kitchen option for treating injuries such as bruises, fractures, swellings, and sprains. Mix enough powder with a little hot water to make a thick paste that will stay in place, and apply to the affected area. St. John's wort flower oil is another wonderful herb for bruises, sprains, and general injuries; it deals with the pain of pinched and damaged nerves.

Cold temperatures are important when swelling and pain are acute. Once they have subsided, continue treatment using hot and cold compresses, showers, and poultices.

For muscular and skeletal damage, such as broken bones, torn ligaments, damaged muscles, and weakly structured joints, use Dr. Christopher's bone, flesh, and cartilage formula internally and externally. It is invaluable used as a tea or made into a paste or ointment. For a soothing, numbing, and supportive massage oil, use Dr. Schulze's deep tissue oil. (See chapter 11 for details of both of these treatments.)

When an injury feels as though it is starting to mend, start gentle exercise to strengthen the muscles. Begin with armchair exercises or gentle movement in the bath, then graduate to swimming, walking, and body work in the gymnasium.

Book List

Common Sense Health and Healing by Dr. Richard Schulze (Santa Monica, California: Natural Healing Publications, 2002)

Guide to Wild, Edible and Medicinal Plants by Tom Brown (New York: Berkeley Publishing Group, 1985)

Healing Colon Disease Naturally by Dr. Richard Schulze (Santa Monica, California: Natural Healing Publications, 2003)

The School of Natural Healing by Dr. John Christopher (Springville, Utah: Christopher Publications, 1976)

Tissue Cleansing through Bowel Management by Bernard Jensen (Los Angeles, California: Bernard Jensen Enterprises, 1981)

❧ 10 ❦

Diseases

When treating any illness holistically, you need to employ more than just one or two therapies in order to treat the whole person. It goes without saying that herbs will form a major part of any suggestions, and that their incredible range of plant constituents will be instrumental in honing, healing, and revitalizing. Good food and drink are vital requirements because these are the daily input on which the body thrives. Regular internal whole-body cleansing is also important, especially as we get older. Just as a car needs regular servicing, so do we. Seasonal food cleanses can be an excellent way to achieve this. If you are sick, you must take appropriate steps according to the severity of the problem.

It is important to ensure that all your organs and systems are working freely and effectively, so one by one they will need special support, nourishing, aligning, and cleansing. Massage provides a loving touch and encourages blood and lymph flow, all of which will help organs to pump, squeeze, and relax more efficiently. Acupuncture can tune, direct, stimulate, or placate organs and systems—an acupuncture pulse-taking gives a good idea of exactly what needs attention. Iridology can also provide a health assessment, giving clues to one's constitution, strengths, and weaknesses. If any part of your spinal column is damaged (it may be eroded, a disk may be trapped, the hips may be out of alignment), any resulting misalignment can affect other systems, from bowel function to menstruation, liver function, or digestion.

Note: There are many herbs suitable for treating diseases; however, there are too many to list for each disease. Therefore, a small selection of the most suitable herbs is given. Any reference to dosage indicates adult dosage—age 16 years to 60 years.

In "An A to Z of Diseases and Treatments" on the following pages,

- 🍎   refers to diet
- 🌿   refers to herbs
- ✋   refers to natural healing

In general, this chapter does not specify exact doses for herbs or herbal formulas; neither have the contraindications of herbs been included, as they are numerous and specific (contraindications and recommended dosages for these herbs are available at www.herbshandshealing.co.uk). Those who are pregnant are in the highest category for avoiding certain herbs. Consult your physician and a qualified herbalist for all treatment.

All the herbs mentioned in this book can be used by qualified herbalists or can be sold over the counter in line with British laws. However, laws do vary from country to country; therefore, discrepancies may occur.

An A to Z of Diseases and Treatments

ANEMIA

If the body does not have high-quality blood containing enough iron, oxygen, and other nutrients, the body cannot sustain itself. Iron deficiency very often does not show up on tests for anemia, as it is possible to have normal hemoglobin levels and still be deficient in iron. Symptoms include pale, ridged nails; brittle, wiry hair; constant fatigue; a sore tongue and cracks at the corners of the mouth; poor general growth; a weak appetite in children; and a weakened immune system, which leaves one open to infection. The individual can feel tired and low. For a quick hemoglobin test, look at the inner palm of your hand. Look at the lines — are they pale or even white, or are they a good pink to red? Pale or white will indicate low levels of hemoglobin. Women will be most likely to suffer from anemia because of menstruation, so these symptoms should be watched for and a good daily diet ensured. An average iron loss at menses is 15 mg to 30 mg. Pregnant women need 130 mg daily, coupled with relatively high amounts of folic acid, in the region of 700 mg. These nutrients are best obtained from food and herbs because iron–folic acid pills frequently cause zinc deficiency. This deficiency can cause a host of problems, just as with iron and folic acid deficiency. It should be noted that supplements of synthetic ferrous iron from the drugstore have a tendency to constipate and are often unassimilable. Natural iron sources are able to burn up toxic wastes in the body, flushing the poisons out. Vegetarians are often low in iron.

- Foods rich in both iron and vitamin C help the absorption of iron from food. They include cherries, black currants, apricots, grapes, bananas, beets, globe artichokes, red kidney beans, watercress, blackstrap molasses, and carrots.
- Tea and coffee drinking is very disruptive to iron absorption.
- Yellow dock root, chickweed leaf, mullein flower, and pennyroyal leaf are rich in iron.
- I have used nettle leaf and red raspberry leaf tea with carrot and beet juice for patients who have been told they need a blood transfusion to save their life but refuse to have one owing to their religious beliefs. In one case, days into the herb treatment, anxious hospital staff carried

out tests and evaluated the patient physically, especially for pallor and energy. They were pleasantly surprised at the outcome and eventually discharged the patient after convalescence with no major concerns.

🖝 People with low copper levels often have lower iron levels; take skull-cap leaf.

APPENDICITIS AND RUMBLING APPENDIX

Appendicitis is an acute inflammation of the appendix that, if left untreated, can result in a rupture causing peritonitis. Symptoms can include stomachache; intense, sharp pain on the right-hand side; or tenderness to the right and below the navel, which is increased by pressure and movement. There may also be nausea, constipation, rapid pulse, vomiting, and slight fever (100°F to 102°F). It is most commonly caused by fecal impaction in which the feces have become compressed and immobile owing to a faulty bowel. Occasionally, foreign objects like buttons and safety pins are to blame.

For a rumbling appendix

🍎 Fast on mono-juice (drinking only apple, grape, or carrot juice), with a glass of prune and lemon juice in the morning for two or three days. Ease into a mucus-free whole-food diet, starting with potassium broth (see chapter 4), sweet fruits, and steamed vegetables. Build up to raw vegetables, grains, and legumes. For children, try one or two days of liquids—including juice, potassium broth, and pureed vegetable soups.

🍎 Drink plenty of water at room temperature.

🖝 Once the attack has subsided, take a tincture made from equal parts of marshmallow root, slippery elm inner bark, licorice root, chamomile flower, and barberry root bark. Dandelion leaf and root, as a tea will help.

🖝 Take herbs to ensure the bowel is moving, such as barberry root, fennel seed, and even senna leaf. Subsequently, for the next two to three days, take one teaspoon each of wild yam root and echinacea root four times a day, and three teaspoons slippery elm inner bark mashed into a ripe banana twice daily.

🖐 Massage the abdomen with ginger essential oil or make a fresh hot ginger compress. Massage the abdomen and feet each night with gentle movements. Castor-oil packs will also bring relief.

🖐 Take hot and cold showers.

🖐 Childhood rumbling appendix is said to be associated with the fear of life. Nighttime is a prime time for this to flare up, as with other illnesses. Place pillows and blankets snugly around the child at bedtime.

Then put a few drops of lavender and sage essential oils on the pillow; or the plants themselves, placed at the head, can help calm fears. Talking with children about recurring dreams and nightmares may also help this affliction.

For acute appendicitis

🖐 Call for an ambulance or your doctor. They can take a long time to arrive; the following procedure will help in the meantime.

🖐 Use a hot ginger compress or a castor-oil pack over the area for pain relief.

🖋 If no help is at hand, then stop food immediately and quickly administer a hot enema of chickweed leaf, catnip leaf, spearmint leaf, or wild yam root, or just plain hot water if nothing else is at hand. This treatment may have to be repeated several times until the worst symptoms have subsided. At the same time, put compresses of the same herbs over the area, using ginger packs and the hot and cold treatment, or a castor-oil pack.

ARTERIOSCLEROSIS AND ATHEROSCLEROSIS

Both arterioscleorosis and atherosclerosis conditions involve hardening of the artery walls. The arterial walls lose their elasticity and become blocked with debris. This debris can consist of yellowish-white clumps called *plaque*, which is made up of cells, connective tissue, and large quantities of fat. At the same time, the arteries absorb calcium from the bloodstream, becoming gritty, hard, and narrowed, much like old encrusted pipes in ancient house plumbing. This calcium debris produces arteriosclerosis. The flow of blood is restricted by the plaque, with dangerous implications. This process of artery encrustation isn't exclusively the province of the old. A much-quoted study of soldiers killed in the Korean War showed that nearly three-quarters of these young men already had some arteriosclerosis in their coronary vessels.

Read up on calcium balance and cholesterol care in chapter 4.

🍎 Take beet and grapefruit juice with cider vinegar to dissolve deposits.

🍎 Refer to the dietary advice for heart disease, below, and stop all alcohol and sugar intake.

🖋 Garlic cloves and burdock root will help to dissolve fatty deposits.

🖋 A good combination of herbs to help with calcium removal is three parts hydrangea root; two parts each turmeric rhizome, gravel root, parsley leaf, and marshmallow root; and one part each licorice root, dandelion root, gingerroot, Siberian ginseng root, buckwheat leaf, and ginkgo leaf. General heart herbs for maintenance would be hawthorn leaf, berry, and flower, and ginkgo leaf tea.

✋ Inhale and massage with rosemary, eucalyptus, and juniper essential oils.

✋ Stop smoking.

ARTHRITIS AND RHEUMATISM

There are several types of arthritis and rheumatism. Arthritis is the inflammation of one or more joints, causing stiffness, swelling, pain, and a reduction in mobility. Osteoarthritis is the most common form, occurring in those over forty years of age and causing a degeneration of cartilage, muscles, ligaments, and joints. Rheumatoid arthritis and juvenile arthritis are much less common forms and are autoimmune diseases. The body wrongly identifies the lubricating fluid in the joints as foreign matter and produces an immune response, which in turn induces an inflammatory response coupled with the destruction of, or damage to, the joints by the immune system itself.

The whole subject of arthritis in its various forms is complex. Sometimes bacterial, fungal, or viral infections of the joints are to blame. Here are some general tips:

🍎 Drink plenty of water to lubricate the system.

🍎 Eat plenty of garlic.

🍎 Cut out dairy products, red meats, salt, and sugar.

🍎 Do not eat any foods from the Solanaceae family, such as potatoes, peppers, and eggplants, as they interfere with muscle enzymes.

🍎 Avoid oxalic acid–rich foods, as they make matters worse. Avoid tea, coffee, wine, spinach, rhubarb, tomatoes, gooseberries, oranges, strawberries, black currants, and red currants. Some of these may eventually be reintroduced without incurring pain and inflammation.

🍎 Use juice cleanses and superfood. Use lots of pineapple with both of these; it will help reduce inflammation.

🍎 Take apple cider vinegar on a regular basis, as it works on a similar principle to lemon juice.

🌿 For excessive inflammation and to help mobility, use three parts Siberian ginseng root, two parts wild yam root, two parts tumeric root, and one part plantain leaf.

🌿 For general help, use St. John's wort flowers, meadowsweet leaf and flower, marshmallow root, *Astragalus* root, licorice root, garlic, burdock root, and red clover flower.

🌿 To aid sleep, consider the short-term use of valerian root, and drink chamomile flower tea.

✋ Take essential fatty acids in the form of GLA capsules, as they will help any inflammation.

❦ Perform liver, kidney, and colon cleanses.

❦ If overweight, start a serious weight-loss program, as this will relieve joint strain.

❦ If there is a lot of conflict and disharmony or emotional friction and pain in your day-to-day life, try to ease the strain by taking time away from the conflict.

❦ Exercise is vitally important, but build up slowly; do not overdo it.

❦ Take hot and cold showers to relieve stiffness and promote healing. Saunas will give similar relief; always finish with cold water.

❦ Massage St. John's wort flower oil into the afflicted area, and then apply a bag of frozen peas.

❦ Use a warming oil of ginger, chile, lavender, and rosemary if circulation is poor and you feel cold, stiff, and achy. Dr. Richard Schulze's deep tissue repair oil is supreme—see chapter 11. Avoid if the area is highly inflamed.

❦ Add to your bath a cup of Epsom salts, two cups of apple cider vinegar, and St. John's wort and lavender flowers tied in a muslin bag.

❦ Use lukewarm castor-oil packs on inflamed areas overnight.

ASTHMA

Asthma is a lung condition. During an attack, spasms cause the lung muscles to constrict, and the resulting lack of air flow causes coughing, wheezing, and gasping. It can develop because of irritants such as pollution, fur, or house dust and mites. Strong emotions, lifestyle, and diet can produce tension, congestion, and immune breakdown. Research suggests, however, that 80 percent of asthmatic children have insufficient hydrochloric acid levels, indicating that poor digestion and assimilation may lie at the bottom of this allergy. Low hydrochloric acid levels leave the person open to fungal and other infections, with other allergies also being a possible outcome.

🍎 Follow a mucus-free diet (see chapter 4).

🍎 Look at digestion, absorption, and gut flora levels.

🍎 Include one to three cloves of garlic in your diet daily.

🌿 If in spasm, use a few drops of lobelia leaf tincture. It breaks the spasm, reduces shock, and feeds the nerves while gently and safely opening up the air sacs.

🌿 Use meadowsweet leaf on a daily basis to help establish sufficient or balanced amounts of hydrochloric acid and pepsin. Also use apple cider vinegar.

🖋 For the anxiety and tension preceding the spasms, which make breathing difficult, take daily teas, capsules, or tinctures of chamomile flowers, hop strobilus, skullcap leaf (in the long term, for excellent results), lime tree *(Tilia)* flower (which must be fresh, as old stock is dangerous), vervain leaf and flower, wood betony leaf and flower, and lavender leaf and flower.

🖋 A herbalist may wish to prescribe valerian root in the short term. It helps to break the tension quickly and usually gives much-needed sleep. But this herb does not actually feed the nervous system, as other herbs do.

🖋 Cayenne pepper capsules and raw chiles will increase circulation.

🖋 Take Siberian ginseng root, *Pfaffia* root, or *pau d'arco* inner bark, or a combination, which will feed badly exhausted adrenals, giving long-term support and, at the same time, will act like hydrocortisone, helping to reduce any inflammation.

🖋 Immune herbs to help fight infection and bolster your immune system include *pau d'arco* inner bark and echinacea root.

🖋 General lung herbs include mullein leaf and flower, horehound leaf, lobelia leaf, and eucalyptus root as tea or tinctures.

🖐 Cleansing programs will help, especially of the bowel.

🖐 Practice breathing exercises.

🖐 Exercise.

🖐 Useful essential oils for baths, inhaling, and massage are cubeb, eucalyptus, peppermint, and tea tree, which open up the bronchi and help to rid them of any attendant infection.

🖐 Use chest poultices based on essential oils and mustard—these are very warming. A drawing compress could be made from a base of two parts bentonite clay and two parts slippery elm inner bark, with one part each pokeweed root, mullein flower, garlic, and red clover flower. Put all of the dried herb powders into a blender with warmed castor oil and mix. Daub onto the chest and back. This will relieve the chest from a buildup of mucus and, in some severe cases, blood clots from bleeding lung tissue.

🖐 Hot and cold showers over the chest will open it up—especially if they are combined with a few drops of lobelia leaf tincture before and after.

ATHLETE'S FOOT

Athlete's foot is a fungal infection that thrives in damp conditions, living on the dead skin cells of the feet, especially between the toes.

🖋 Drink *pau d'arco* inner bark decoction.

🖋 Dust the feet with equal parts of any of the following finely sieved powders: neem leaf, lavender flower, chickweed leaf, garlic, and black walnut leaf or goldenseal root.

🖐 Follow all the general advice for candidiasis, including the dietary advice.

🖐 Whenever possible, wear only cotton or silk socks. Otherwise, wear natural-fiber shoes.

🖐 At night, soak your feet for twenty minutes in 1 tablespoon black walnut inner hull tincture or decoction, 10 drops tea tree essential oil, 2 teaspoons cider vinegar, and 1 quart hot water in a foot bucket or basin; then use cold water to rinse.

🖐 Avoid swimming pools and changing your socks or walking barefoot in public areas.

BOILS

Boils are pus-filled nodules caused by staphylococcus bacteria infection. Found generally on the buttocks, face, neck, or under the arms, they are very painful and often contagious. Children and adolescents are commonly affected. Boils need both internal and external treatment. They are a sign of toxicity and low immunity, leading to bacterial overload. You need to work on the immune system, lymph system, bloodstream, and any elimination channels that may be causing or contributing to the situation.

🍎 Avoid most beverages, but drink plenty of water with fresh lemon juice.

🖋 Use a formula of nettle leaf, burdock root, echinacea root, and barberry root bark as a tincture.

🖋 Use eczema herbs as an ointment.

🖐 Home remedies include placing baked onions and pummeled raw white cabbage leaves over the boil.

🖐 Use a drawing poultice: ½ cup bentonite clay, apple cider vinegar (enough to make a paste), 2 drops tea tree essential oil, 2 drops lavender essential oil, ½ clove garlic, mashed.

BRAIN CLARITY

Forgetfulness can sometimes come with old age or simply be a result of stress and overwork.

🍎 Drink plenty of water.

🍎 The brain uses a lot of essential fatty acids. Superfood contains them and a glass taken morning and afternoon can keep your brain alert and blood sugar levels up.

🌿 Use a combination of three parts prickly ash bark, two parts ginkgo leaf, and one part each rosemary leaf, gotu kola root, and lobelia leaf as a tincture or tea.

✋ Keep your vascular system clear of plaque, be it composed of calcium or fatty deposits, as this clogs and slows circulation, hampering the thinking process. A lack of blood flow, oxygen, and nutrients to the brain can have disastrous results, and toxemia can result as the body deposits toxic substances in the brain.

✋ Liver and bowel cleanses can do much to encourage brain clarity and alleviate forgetfulness.

✋ Exercise is vital for proper brain function and oxygenation.

BREAST LUMPS — CYSTS, FIBROIDS, AND MASTITIS

We are taught to feel around our breasts after each menstruation to see if anything lumpy can be found. If lumps are movable and come and go with the period, then, we are told, they are generally nothing to worry about. By contrast, if they are solid but not particularly painful, if at all, and do not come and go with menstruation, you should seek further help.

Breast tissue is fatty and is intended to produce milk for babies. The breasts change shape and content throughout our lives, according to fluctuating levels of the hormones estrogen and progesterone. It is these hormone fluctuations that can cause swelling and water retention, pain, and even fibrocystic lumps that painfully move around in the breasts. These symptoms generally occur premenstrually, settling down with the onset of menstruation; pregnancy and menopause can also make breast lumps decrease. It must be remembered that most lumps are benign (nonmalignant) and that many thousands of women — almost one in three — have them at some stage.

For noncancerous conditions

🍎 Avoid tea and coffee, as the caffeine they contain is estrogenic and will encourage unwanted cell growth.

🍎 Drink plenty of water daily.

🍎 Eat soy-based foods, especially tofu.

🍎 Take chlorella tablets or superfood, or both.

🍎 Follow the dietary and cleansing program suggestions for endometriosis and for ovarian cysts and uterine fibroids.

🌿 Take evening primrose oil or some other source of GLA daily.

🌿 Throughout the month, use herbs to strengthen liver function, balance the hormones, and maintain the lymphatic and immune systems. A good formula would be equal parts of squaw vine leaf (and other aerial parts), chaste tree berry, milk thistle seed, olive leaf, and mullein flower.

🌿 Sometimes extra progestogenic herbs can help during PMS, especially if the premenstrual time is difficult (anything from 7 to 10 days before the period). Take one teaspoon chaste tree berry tincture on its own early morning in addition to the monthly formula—see "The Hormone Arrival" in chapter 8.

🌿 Drink three cups of dandelion root tea daily, as it will alleviate water retention. If water retention is excessive, add corn silk and other kidney herbs.

✋ Exercise to stimulate the circulation and give greater energy—for instance, power walking, dancing, and cycling.

✋ Warmed poultices from powdered herbs can be used in extreme situations: two parts slippery elm inner bark and one part each of bentonite clay, pokeweed root, cayenne pepper, fresh garlic puree, and charcoal crushed into a powder and moistened with castor oil. Apply at nighttime and leave on.

✋ Take hot and cold showers, especially over the breasts.

BRONCHITIS

Acute bronchitis is an infection of the bronchi. Chronic bronchitis is caused by frequent irritation of the lungs from cigarette smoke, pollutants, cold damp weather, or tissue damage from old infections; it can also be caused in part by excessive mucus buildup in the lungs. Symptoms include pain in the chest, coughing, fever, chills, and sore throat.

Refer also to "Coughs" and "Sinusitis" in this chapter, and to "The Respiratory System" in chapter 9.

🍎 Remove wheat and dairy products from your diet. Depending on the severity of your bronchitis, get professional help to tailor your diet beyond these general suggestions.

🌿 Mullein flowers help to reduce mucus and soothe inflammation. Add a little eucalyptus leaf (using a three-to-one ratio) and drink as a strong tea, three times daily.

🌿 Take a few drops of lobelia leaf tincture every few hours.

🌿 Other herbs to use include pokeweed root, cleavers leaf, *pau d'arco* inner bark, elecampane leaf and flower, edible lichens, fennel leaf and seed, pine needles, thuja leaf, and echinacea root.

🌿 Additionally, Iceland moss and Siberian ginseng root are antimucus and antiviral, and they will help to support the body generally.

❦ Use essential oils of eucalyptus, lavender, peppermint, rosemary, and cubeb in the bath, for massage, or inhaled.

BURSITIS

Bursitis is a condition in which the small water-filled cushions between the tendons and bones in various places on the body—especially the knees, elbows, hips, and shoulders—become inflamed. It can be caused by an accident, wear and tear, a tendency to arthritis or rheumatism, allergies, or even calcium deposits.

❧ Should the problem become chronic, adopt the same dietary program as for arthritis and rheumatism.

❧ Helpful anti-inflammatory herbs include *pau d'arco* inner bark, turmeric rhizome, and *dong quai* root.

❦ A compress using St. John's wort flower oil and a hot castor-oil pack, followed by a cold shower and cold packs, can bring relief.

❦ Stop or limit any activity that aggravates the inflammation and pain.

CANDIDIASIS AND ORAL THRUSH

Candidiasis, a parasitic, yeastlike fungal infection, is something that many women (an estimated one in three) have had or will have at some time in their life. Men frequently harbor it too, but without being so aware of it as women. Increasingly, children are becoming prone, sometimes from birth or after vaccination—especially if they are given the triple or multiple vaccines when they are very young, when the immune system is vulnerable and easily overwhelmed. Antibiotic usage also compromises the immune system and thus invites fungal infestation. Parasitic invasion often goes hand in hand with it, especially flatworms called flukes, introduced via pets, undercooked meat, and other sources.

Low hydrochloric acid levels and general poor digestive powers are very often a strong causal factor in candidiasis. Candida infestation can occur anywhere in the body and is frequently found in the mouth, stomach, bowel, vagina, or anus. But it is by its very nature a problem, infesting the entire body. It thrives in damp, humid conditions. Disease and hormonal changes in the body, such as during pregnancy, can instigate an imbalance in the gut and bowel flora, allowing the fungus to proliferate. Visits to countries with very different standards of hygiene can also instigate its appearance. Very often, allergic reactions to foods are simply a sign that candida is present.

The symptoms include weight gain that will not shift (whatever the diet or food restrictions); low blood sugar; alcohol intolerance; constipation or diarrhea; premenstrual syndrome; depression; bloating and gas; fatigue; irritable bowel; joint swelling and pain; itching and heat in the hands and feet; reddish-pink blotches of varying sizes on the face, torso, hands, legs, feet, or abdomen; anal itching and athlete's foot; fungal nail infections; night sweats; kidney and bladder infections; and pains across the chest, mimicking angina. A blood test will confirm whether candida is present.

- Weak digestion will cause chronic candidiasis, so refer to dietary advice for correct digestion.

- Consume nothing that contains antibiotics—most meat and fish do. Choose organic meat and fish.

- Eat organic vegetables and fruit.

- Cut out alcohol, tea, coffee, carbonated drinks, and tobacco.

- Eat no fruit or sugar for a period of at least two weeks. Then have occasional fruit, but no fruit juice initially, because the concentration of sugar is attractive to candida fungus. Avoid fruit concentrates and frozen juices. Instead, drink fresh lemon juice in plenty of water—two to four quarts daily.

- Consider leaky gut and other digestive weakness, as it may be the initial root cause, and liver problems and bowel congestion or constipation—and treat accordingly.

- Eat food with plenty of uncooked, cool spices and herbs. Do not eat cooked chiles or other hot foods. The heat will attract candida fungus.

- Cut out all yeasty or fermented foods, including mushrooms and Marmite or other yeast-based spreads and sauces. However, practitioners in Germany and recent trials in Britain have shown that shiitake mushrooms actually help eradicate candida.

- Avoid all refined carbohydrates—that is, any processed junk food.

- Eat only whole grains and raw foods—vegetables, seeds, and nuts.

- Avoid the apple cider vinegar normally suggested for poor digestion and low hydrochloric acid levels. Instead, take daily meadowsweet leaf, gentian root, and others.

- Use two parts valerian root, one part chamomile flower, and one part passionflower as a tincture if sleep is a problem. Daytime nervines may also be required (see "The Nervous System" in chapter 9).

- Take two parts squaw vine herb, two parts chaste tree berry, and one part red raspberry leaf to balance the hormones. Add two parts Siberian ginseng root as an overall tonic, especially for adrenal and thyroid restoration. Take as a tincture.

🖋 The use of the premenstrual herbs will help mood swings and emotions that are aggravated by candida at that time of the month.

🖋 Take immune strengtheners: olive leaf, echinacea root, and, particularly, *pau d'arco* inner bark. Drink two cupfuls of *pau d'arco* as a decoction once a day. (If you have leaky gut, *pau d'arco* can aggravate it — cease using it if this is the case.)

🖋 Include three to four whole cloves of garlic daily, in addition to that which is added to cooked food. Treat it as a medicine rather than a food source. It will decrease the levels of fungus.

🖋 Grapefruit extract is also very useful; just a few drops daily will go a long way toward eliminating candida.

✋ Take good quality probiotics, which will establish gut flora and kill parasites. You can also consider using aloe vera juice to repopulate the bowel with beneficial bacteria capable of overpowering the fungus. Capsulated oregano oil and *Lactobacillus salivarius* can be extremely useful.

✋ Avoid tinctures because of their alcohol content. However, pouring boiling water over the tinctures and leaving them to stand for five minutes removes 98 percent of the alcohol; they will then be acceptable to use.

✋ The three-stage herbal colon cleanse and the worming program in chapter 6 are very much designed to help eliminate candida, as it commonly infests the large intestine. (You may also consider a high enema; see chapter 6.) Continued use of barberry root bark for bowel maintenance will be vital after the cleanse. If you are pregnant, do not attempt the colon cleanse; consult a herbalist, and on his or her suggestion use instead bowel capsules based on barberry root bark, with additional supplements like oregano capsules and probiotics.

✋ Perform a mild liver cleanse.

✋ Highly diluted tea tree oil can be used to treat external fungus, but be careful to dilute it thoroughly because if used pure or overly strong it can cause deep, angry flesh burns. Use ½ teaspoon tea tree oil to 1 cup safflower and olive oil.

✋ Use pure lavender oil on fungus. It may tingle or even burn a little, but it will not actually cause harm.

✋ Use candida pessaries (see chapter 3).

✋ Have a daily bath with a few drops of lavender essential oil.

✋ If possible, avoid oral contraceptives as they can upset the microorganism balance in the body. Instead, use alternative contraception.

🖐 Saunas help—but it's vital to have long, cold showers during and after the sauna, otherwise the warm, damp atmosphere will encourage fungal growth and make matters worse.

🖐 Take hot and cold showers—always finish with cold water. Never go to bed straight after a hot bath, only after a cold shower.

🖐 Get plenty of sleep, and use cotton sheets. Underbedding and quilts should also be of natural fibers as these breathe, allowing moisture to escape, and will prevent further incubation of the fungus.

CELIAC DISEASE

Celiac disease is an intolerance to gluten (which is mainly found in wheat and wheat products). More specifically, the allergy is to gliadin, a protein found in gluten. The condition manifests itself as uncomfortable bloating, gas, and diarrhea caused by chronic inflammation. A specialist will need to confirm this disease by testing for gliadin intolerance.

Follow the treatments described below for colitis.

🍎 There is plenty to enjoy—whole grains like brown rice, quinoa, buckwheat, and millet, all of which have a greatly reduced gluten content. A gluten-free recipe book will give you further insight.

🌿 Herbal astringents may be necessary if diarrhea is persistent. Include yarrow leaf and flower tea with grains of bentonite clay if diarrhea is persistently watery.

🌿 Herbal demulcents that will soothe and heal may be needed if the inflammation is severe, but this can be individually gauged. Mash up some slippery elm inner bark and arrowroot into a ripe banana, or simply add to cold water and drink.

CHICKEN POX

Chicken pox is a highly contagious viral infection that starts with a headache, tiredness, and fever. The glands around the neck will probably be swollen, and some spots may be apparent on the body, face, scalp, or mouth. The spotting period can last for ten days, and then the scabs should fall off.

The worst thing a child can do is pick the spots. Get the child to wear gloves to prevent scratching and picking, especially at night; regular application of herbal powders to the affected areas will often dispel any itching.

🍎 Keep the child on light foods—fruit, juices, vegetable juices, soups, and the like. As Dr. Christopher always said, chicken pox thrives in a medium of excessive mucus—remove this, and the virus finds it hard to survive.

- Use echinacea root tincture with red raspberry leaf, yarrow leaf, or boneset leaf tea, sweetened with honey.

- Use equal parts of chamomile flower and skullcap leaf to calm and soothe the child. Take as a tincture with honey added, or as a tea.

- Three parts dandelion root, two parts burdock root, and one part echinacea root will help flush the skin through. A composite, sweetened tincture of these three herbs is probably the easiest method of administration, given five or six times daily—seek advice on dosage.

- Two warm baths a day, with a few drops of lavender essential oil added to the water, will relax the mind and cool the skin.

- After the bath, dust down with lavender flower and marigold flower powder. If available, use neem leaf powder.

- Use only cotton next to the skin and only breathable clothing or bedding over it, if necessary.

COLD SORES (HERPES SIMPLEX)

The cold sore virus is a very common problem and a sister to herpes zoster and chicken pox. It can remain latent in the body for years, but stress, other infections, strong sunshine, hormone swings, bad diet, constipation, and many other conditions can trigger it.

- Vitamins B complex, C, and A and zinc must be included in your food program. Use equal parts of carrot juice and lemon juice, including its white pith. Eat whole-grain rice with spirulina, chlorella, and other algal seaweeds or superfood and Engevita for B vitamins.

- Avoid arginine-rich foods; examples are wheat products, carob, chocolate, animal gelatin, coconut, oats, peanuts, and soybeans.

- Avoid coffee, alcohol, sugar, fried foods, and hot cooked spices, as they will worsen the attack.

- The chemical lysine helps and is found in all fruits and vegetables, especially beans and bean sprouts.

- Immune-system herbs and tonics will be vital to support the body generally: olive leaf, echinacea root, *pau d'arco* inner bark, and Siberian ginseng root.

- Work on all the elimination channels—at some point you will need to perform liver, kidney, and colon cleanses.

- Nervous-system support is often necessary here (see chapter 9).

- Get plenty of rest.

✋ Put organic honey mixed with turmeric rhizome powder on the cold sore during the weeping stage (it will stain, so take care). Use a lavender and tea tree essential oil rub, and continue use for three days after the sore has visibly gone. Internally, large amounts of the antiviral herb lemon balm will greatly help, as it is specific for disarming the herpes virus.

✋ Saunas are helpful and encourage the cold sore to come out, peak, and die down.

COLITIS

Colitis is inflammation of a section or sections of the colon, mostly in the mucous membranes. It is a very common problem, and is perhaps the most common of all bowel complaints. It appears to be a precursor for many other diseases, such as ulcerative colitis, which can ensue when ulcers develop as a result of chronic inflammation. It can be caused by intense stress, anxiety, or fear, or by bacteria, especially if antibiotics have been overused. The nervous system and adrenal glands need support if stress is a factor; but the food you eat also has a major influence on this disease.

🍎 No coffee, alcohol, tea, milk, or cheese should be consumed.

🍎 No cooked spices should be eaten; the cooler, raw spices and culinary herbs like thyme and marjoram should be used instead.

🍎 Fibrous foods should be avoided at this point. Instead try fruit purees (always cook with stones, pips, and skins and then strain), vegetable purees, pureed soups, and generally soft steamed or baked foods. Continue until the inflammation has subsided.

🍎 Often six small meals a day will be easier to digest than three larger ones.

🍎 Eat plenty of garlic in food and let it do the main work on bowel putrefaction for you.

🌿 Use equal parts of marshmallow root, cramp bark, lobelia leaf, barberry root bark, wild yam root, and red clover flower to help soothe and relax any spasms and reduce the inflammation.

🌿 Drink meadowsweet leaf tea for bouts of diarrhea and to establish balanced hydrochloric acid and pepsin levels. Chinese licorice root tea would help any constipation. (In this condition, the two often alternate.)

🌿 Use the herbs recommended for diverticulitis along with bayberry as a blood cleanser, because it will help the colon wall regain elasticity and encourage peristalsis.

🖋 Blessed thistle leaf tea helps reduce excessive mucus production and stimulates digestion. Dr. Christopher also pointed out that it improves the tone, structure, and elasticity of the bowel walls, as well as aiding detoxification.

CONSTIPATION

The results of constipation are far-reaching—not only does it distort the colon and build up toxins but the thyroid can also become underactive as the entire metabolism slows down. The liver and, in particular, the gall-bladder can become stagnant and diseased; vice versa, a poorly functioning liver can cause constipation. The stomach and pancreas can also suffer, and even the kidneys can become alarmingly involved. Brain function becomes clearer and sharper with a clean colon. Conversely, a congested colon can produce all kinds of memory and brain function problems. Skin eruptions, swollen glands, general fatigue, and a consistently and increasingly inoperative immune system are some of the possible effects of constipation. The body will become more and more intolerant to specific foods as general toxicity builds up. The whole emotional pattern becomes depressed, tense, angry, and, of course, uptight! As with many things, because of the complexity of their hormones, women tend to suffer much more from constipation than men do. The female abdominal structure has a part to play in this as well. Check that you do not have candida, as it can cause constipation. Surgical scars or a malfunctioning colon caused by adhesions where the walls of the colon are growing together may initially cause constipation, so always consider these factors. Tumors and cancers cause blockages, but so does ballooning. Good bowel cleanses and detoxification programs can give you some answers to where the difficulties lie if conventional diagnosis is inconclusive. See also the sections on the colon in chapters 6 and 9.

🍎🖋 Correct any lack of nerve nourishment with appropriate food and herbs, especially paying attention to magnesium (and calcium).

🍎 A low-fiber diet will hamper natural peristalsis; eat plenty of raw foods and whole grains.

🍎 Mucus-forming, binding foods such as eggs, cheese, potato starch, and other starches such as white bread, and pasta must be avoided, because they gum up the colon.

🍎 Take plenty of beneficial flora–rich foods: make rejuvelac (see chapter 4) and eat sauerkraut.

🍎 Plant proteins and fats, for example nuts and avocado, are important and should form part of your generally balanced diet.

- 🍎 Drink plenty to enable the bowel to move properly. Urination following a bowel movement signals that the bowel is completely empty. Two quarts of fluid, mostly water, a day is a minimum requirement for good bowel movements. Always drink a cup of water and fresh lemon juice first thing in the morning.

- 🍎 Soups made with whole-grain organic wheat and lots of onions, garlic, black pepper, and raw chiles will help.

- 🌿 Everyday bowel management with herbs will be helpful; see discussions about the use of strong herbs to get the bowel working and about the softer bowel herbs, like barberry root bark, in chapter 9 and the three-stage herbal colon cleanse featured in chapter 6. Your bowel may be in need of a combination of these herbs from time to time—even with a good diet and plenty of drinking water and exercise. Often, constipated people become worse when they are sick, while others may get diarrhea when they are fasting, nervous, or excited. So use both types of formulas and recognize the interchangeability of the two. You need to find a balance that will work for you.

- ✋ Always go to the toilet when you need to, and if possible use a footstool to keep the bowel at a more natural height—more like squatting.

- ✋ Avoid excessive worry.

- ✋ Do not sit a lot. Take regular exercise, especially if you are elderly. Ensure that a regular walk is included in your daily routine. Cycling and horseback riding are both excellent for massaging the bowel.

- ✋ Hot and cold showers especially are beneficial. Cover the whole body but spend longer over the colon area.

- ✋ Do not use drug laxatives.

- ✋ Drugs, whether prescription or illicit ones like heroin and opium, often overstimulate or completely freeze peristalsis. Antibiotics can kill off beneficial flora, causing constipation. Even small doses of antibiotics can set the pattern for years of constipation.

COUGHS

Coughing is, in the main, an important reflex action provoked by various irritations in order to expel mucus. But the reflex also works when there is nothing to expel but the mucous membrane is irritated.

- 🍎 If it is a dry, hacking cough with little mucus and combined with sweating, then consume a lot of raw fruits and juices.

- 🍎 If there is a lot of mucus and congestion, avoid cold fruits and juices and use more warming foods, like garlic and onion soups.

- Take plenty of fluids — especially water and fresh lemon juice — and go directly to bed.

- Herbalist Dr. Richard Schulze has a wonderful kitchen home remedy for coughs and colds, and this alone can do the job. See "Homemade Immune Supporter and Fighter—'Hooch'" in chapter 7 for the recipe. Take between two and ten teaspoons up to five times daily; gargle with it, and then swallow.

- As a preventive measure in winter, drink homemade elderberry and elder flower syrup. It encourages perspiration and provides valuable vitamins and minerals (refer to chapter 3). Take one teaspoon at a time, three to six times daily.

- A tincture or syrup can also be made with wild cherry bark, myrrh resin, barberry root bark, licorice root, lobelia leaf, pokeweed root, cayenne pepper, and marshmallow root: this will promote the healthy removal of mucus and encourage productive coughing, while helping the lungs to expand and the immune system to strengthen.

- Use mullein flowers, plantain leaf, and red clover flower tea. Other useful traditional herbs that can be excellent are horehound leaf, elecampane leaf and flower, and yarrow leaf.

- For a prolonged, deep-seated cough, take a tonic herb like Siberian ginseng root for support and recovery.

- Soaking one's feet in a bucket of hot water with mustard powder added to it is a great way of heating and sweating the body, but for this treatment the individual must be naturally strong. Then massage an oil mix containing eucalyptus into the chest and soles of the feet, already hot and yellow from the mustard.

- A sprinkling of eucalyptus essential oil on pillows and sheets is very helpful.

CROHN'S DISEASE

Crohn's disease normally affects the small intestine, but any section of the digestive tract can be affected. Inflammation and ulcers occur and, after healing, slowly cause a narrowing of the digestive tract. The inflammation may be a result of bacteria, viral infection, or an allergic reaction that may be caused by dietary problems, environmental influences, drugs, or unbalanced enzyme secretions, rendering digestion incomplete. Usually the liver, pancreas, and stomach are equally involved and need treatment. Other recent theories suggest that Crohn's results from a genetic abnormality and is a hereditary pattern. Symptoms include abdominal pain, which can be excruciating, diarrhea, and symptoms similar to those found in appendicitis and fever. Abnormal weight loss can also be a factor, as can depression. A diet rich in nutritious, mild foods with herbs that fight infection and rebuild the intestinal tract will help.

- Drink plenty of water. Begin with a three-day carrot juice fast, juicing a bit of garlic and ginger with the carrots, and taking chlorophyll or algae powders and barley sprouts for three to seven days; or drink superfood, as it contains all of the powders listed.

- After the carrot juice fast, add salads (with olive oil and cider vinegar), plus fermented or cultured foods. Eat only mild fruit (very ripe papayas, bananas, mangoes, and steamed pineapple), and raw and steamed vegetables, such as yams and squashes—but avoid sulfurous vegetables like broccoli and cabbage.

- Do not use whole grains or other fibrous foods until after the fourth week of this program.

- Drink a potassium broth (see recipe in chapter 4) once or twice a day, and eat all fruit and vegetables as separate courses.

- Avoid hot or strong spices in cooking; eat the cooler, raw ones. Use fenugreek seed, cinnamon sticks, a little nutmeg, dill, cumin, coriander, basil, parsley, thyme, marjoram, and garlic frequently in cooking.

- Avoid dairy products, processed foods, chocolate, sugar, alcohol, tea, and coffee.

- Avoid harsh fibrous foods such as nuts and seeds, unless they are well soaked, freshly ground, or sprouted.

- A diet rich in nutritious, mild foods with herbs that fight infection and rebuild the gastrointestinal tract will help.

- Use acidophilus and drink aloe vera juice and apple cider vinegar to restore colon flora balance.

- Women should take up to 1,000 mg of evening primrose oil (an excellent source of GLA) per day—this helps to rebalance the system.

- Take Siberian ginseng root—it is a fine general tonic.

- Use 2 or 3 teaspoons of a mixture of two parts slippery elm inner bark and one part each of marshmallow root, plantain leaf, turmeric rhizome, and wild yam root powders. Mash into a ripe banana or mix with water to soothe the bowel; take two or three times daily.

- Use plenty of garlic, barberry root bark, and echinacea root to fight infection.

- Drink plenty of meadowsweet leaf, fennel seed, chamomile flower, or peppermint leaf tea.

🍂 Make sure the colon is functioning correctly by using gentle herbs such as barberry root bark and rhubarb root. If you are suffering from diarrhea, then refer to the appropriate section in this chapter for treatment.

✋ If you are in severe pain, drink aloe vera juice or administer aloe gel as an enema for immediate cooling and soothing relief. You will need a high enema (see chapter 6). For those with painful ulcers in the mouth and throat, use aloe as a gargle—swallow after gargling.

CYSTITIS AND PROSTATITIS

Cystitis and prostatitis very painful bacterial bladder infections that create a scalding pain before, during, and after urination. They also urge the bladder to try to empty constantly, even if there is no more urine left to expel. The urine may be cloudy and have an unpleasant odor. Cystitis is a common problem for women, partly because of their shorter urethra and its closeness to the rectum, making cross-infection more likely. A variety of spinal nonalignments can have an effect here, therefore a visit to a chiropractor could be worthwhile. Candidiasis often goes hand in hand with cystitis, and helping one often helps the other. Men also get cystitis, and then the prostate needs to be examined.

🍎 Avoid highly acidic food and drinks (coffee, tea, alcohol, chocolate); instead drink lots of alkaline fluids, like fresh lemon juice in springwater (lemon juice itself is acidic but becomes alkaline in the stomach). Cranberry is the only exception to this rule. Its special chemistry and acidity prevent the sticking of harmful microbes to the urethra wall, which rapidly diminishes the attack. Drink unsweetened cranberry juice or a drink made from dried cranberries soaked in water overnight, or use frozen ones. Try to avoid supermarket cranberry drinks, as they tend to be loaded with undesirable additives.

🍎 Put one tablespoon of apple cider vinegar into a little apple juice and drink four times daily.

🍎 Drink homemade barley water (see chapter 4 for recipe).

🍎 Raw foods and juices are alkaline, so concentrate on them; they will also strengthen your overall immune system if you are not a "cold" type of person and underweight. If you have difficulty consuming excess roughage because of bowel problems, consult a natural healer for alternative suggestions.

🍎 To help fight the bacterial infection, include garlic and thyme in your cooking.

🌾 Every two hours, drink a tea containing equal amounts of yarrow leaf, dandelion root, cleavers leaf, and marshmallow root. Should there be blood in the urine (and even if not), add corn silk because this will encourage rapid water release as well as soothing the inflammation and consequent bleeding. An equal part of juniper berry will help disinfect the area and act as a diuretic.

🌾 Take antimicrobial herbs like olive leaf, echinacea root tincture, and turmeric rhizome for fourteen days, depending on the severity of the cystitis. In the case of prostatitis, add saw palmetto berry.

🖐 Have regular baths and showers to keep yourself clean. Apple cider vinegar in the bathwater will help, plus a few drops of any or all of the following essential oils: cedar wood, eucalyptus, bergamot, lavender, or juniper. Don't stay in the bath too long; keep the water warm rather than hot.

🖐 Wear a long skirt or baggy trousers and no underwear, if possible. Alternatively, wear loose-fitting cotton or silk underwear. Avoid tight, constricting clothing made from manmade fibers.

🖐 Make sure your bowels are moving at least two or three times daily because your carefully selected fluid intake will disinfect and cleanse the bacteria from the system. If these harmful toxins are left to stay in the system too long, reinfection will occur, and healing will be a slow process.

🖐 Avoid being cold and chilled. Take time for yourself to heal, and spend time in bed, if possible with natural-fiber bedding.

DANDRUFF

Dandruff is commonly caused by an imbalance in the oil-secreting glands or by a slight fungal infection, so check that you don't have candidiasis or oral thrush. A hormone or endocrine imbalance may also cause dandruff.

🍎 No coffee, tea, sugar, or junk food should be consumed.

🍎 Switch to a whole-food diet.

🍎 Eat plenty of garlic, olive oil, cider vinegar, lemon juice, whole grains, fruit, and vegetables.

🌾 Consider hormone balancing and antifungal herbs.

🖐 A hair water made with ylang-ylang, rosemary, sage, thyme, and tea tree essential oils will help; or make your own rosemary water with ½ teaspoon rosemary essential oil per cup of springwater; use apple cider vinegar and water as a rinsing agent.

DEPRESSION

Depression is a subject too diverse to discuss here, but the following are some general tips.

🍎 Eat healthfully, drink plenty of water (especially if you are not using drugs to help with your depression), and increase your intake of zinc by eating, for instance, pumpkin seeds.

🌾 Use herbs to support the adrenal glands, as they are often exhausted in this condition. Ask a qualified herbalist if St. John's wort tincture would be suitable.

✋ Liver and colon cleansing will help.

✋ Exercise often.

DERMATITIS

The word *dermatitis* literally means "inflammation of the skin." This inflammation can be due to an infection or an allergic reaction, caused either by direct contact (as with some metals or animal hair) or through exposure —sunlight, perfumes, and paints. Atopic dermatitis is probably a hereditary allergy symptom; dermatitis herpetiformis is a very itchy type associated with intestinal problems and disorders triggered by intolerance of dairy products, wheat, and other foods. Another type of dermatitis, caused by a malfunction of the sebaceous glands, causes greasy skin. The vitamins B_6 and B_2 are vital, and deficiencies can cause dermatitis. With all forms of dermatitis, attention to the adrenal glands, nervous system, immune system, and all the eliminative channels, especially the liver and colon, is vital.

🍎 Follow a one- or two-day cleanse, eating only papayas or ripe bananas, under the supervision of a practitioner. Continue with large proportions of raw foods, including lots of garlic.

🍎 Eat whole grains, nonactive yeast flakes like Engevita, and B vitamins, as found in seaweeds.

🍎 Include virgin olive oil in the daily diet, and use flaxseeds or flaxseed capsules.

🍎 Eat plenty of raw seeds, nuts, sprouts, and beans, and sometimes cooked beans and seeds.

🌾 Take evening primrose oil (GLA) capsules.

🌾 Use blood- and skin-cleansing herbs. Try three parts burdock root, two parts red clover flower, and two parts dandelion root.

✋ Liver and bowel cleanses and detoxification programs are helpful; see chapter 6.

❧ Dr. Christopher often had patients wash in a soothing decoction of equal parts of burdock root, chickweed leaf, and marshmallow root. Alternatively, sponge yourself down using a mixture of plantain leaf and chickweed leaf.

See "Psoriasis" and "Eczema" for further herbal information.

DIABETES

More than 1 percent of people in the West are affected by diabetes. In America, the land of sugar and junk food, it is the direct cause of one in seven deaths. Diabetes manifests when the body fails to regulate the metabolism of glucose via a pancreatic hormone. If the pancreatic hormones are unable to convert a sufficient amount of glycogen into glucose, then other organs—primarily the thyroid, adrenal, and pituitary glands—will become involved, leading to their eventual decline. In some cases, diseases or dysfunction of these glands can actually result in diabetes. If there is a history of diabetes in your family, it is advisable to take preventive action through childhood and into adulthood.

Those who have diabetes before the age of twenty-five are classed as juvenile diabetics, and it is believed that autoimmune factors may be involved in their condition. After the age of forty it is classified as late-onset diabetes. Conventional treatment of the problem involves daily insulin injections, but those with less severe diabetes can measure their urine periodically and use tablets to control their blood sugar levels. If you suffer from hypoglycemia, then be aware that it is possible for this condition to develop into diabetes if it becomes severe.

High blood glucose levels (with glucose-starved cells) can lead to weight loss, thirst, and an increase in the amount of urine passed each day. If untreated, the person will begin to feel weak and can eventually pass out or even fall into a coma. Trauma, stress, and shock can push a person into late-onset diabetes.

🍎 Three to six large cloves of garlic per day would be a minimum requirement. Garlic balances the amount of sugar in the blood by producing more insulin.

🍎 Eating enough of the right things at the right time is important in the control of diabetes. At no time should the person ever fast. Diabetes is all about maintaining correct carbohydrate metabolism. Food should be high in fiber and complex carbohydrates, and should have the correct protein levels to balance the carbohydrate ratio.

🍎 No tea, coffee, alcohol, or fruit juices should be drunk.

🍎 All sugars are to be avoided. Use instead rice syrup in minute quantities, barley malt, unrefined cane juice, and sweet herb *(Stevia rebaudiana)*.

Very occasionally you can use small amounts of raw unheated honey. Also avoid fructose, dextrose, and molasses.

- Nourishing, "earthy" foods will be invaluable, but make sure you choose the right ones: seaweeds and whole grains like rice, millet, quinoa, oats, and barley are good. Avoid all processed grains. Try the sweeter vegetables, like Jerusalem artichokes, pumpkins, burdock root, onion, and parsnips. Avoid potatoes, yams, and carrots.

- Avoid bread but, if necessary, eat rye bread.

- Six small and easily digestible meals a day may be better than three large ones.

- Oats are rich in many vitamins and minerals and are generally very nourishing. They can slow the rate of sugar metabolism, thus aiding the work of the pancreas. Organic oats are best; they can be soaked overnight in springwater with cinnamon powder and eaten for breakfast.

- Seaweeds, especially hijiki, normalize blood sugar levels. Cook them with whole grains and add to salads and soups.

- Drink one cup of homemade barley water daily (see recipe in chapter 4).

- At least one or two apples per day are the best fruit for diabetics. Wild fruits like blackberries, bilberries, quince, and pomegranate, with their naturally sharp and bitter flavors, are also suitable. Do not drink fruit in juiced form; the sugar content will be too high. Other suitable fruits are pears, grapefruit, grapes (in small quantities), and bananas. Bananas are known to lower blood sugar levels, but use only overripe (nearly black) ones, and have only two or three a week.

- Dried figs, dates, raisins, and other dried fruits are best avoided by diabetics because of their high sugar content. If they are eaten, they must be soaked for at least twelve hours.

- Cut down on or cut out meat, especially red meat. Use vegetable protein sources instead (see chapter 4). Avoid milk and cheese.

- Drinks containing nettle leaf and hibiscus flower are invaluable, giving almost instantaneous energy (they are high in chromium, the blood sugar mineral) and providing good nourishment between meals. Additionally, drink superfood.

- Zinc levels must be maintained. Pumpkin seeds as well as alfalfa seeds and sprouted alfalfa are excellent sources of zinc.

- All vegetables, raw and steamed, are helpful, particularly those that are opposite to sweet in taste, namely, sour and bitter ones like like chicory, dandelion leaves, artichokes, and olives.

❦ Ideally, individual patients should seek more detailed advice from their own health practitioners, in order to address their particular needs, be they overweight or underweight, or have any other specific important traits.

🖋 Fenugreek seed and burdock root both contain a substance called inulin that is very close to insulin. Make strong teas (decoctions which are simmered for twenty minutes) using three parts fenugreek seed and one part burdock root; drink 1 to 3 cups daily.

🖋 Meadowsweet leaf tea or tincture will balance and heal digestive problems.

🖋 Individual herbal advice should be sought, but herbs like dandelion root, fenugreek seed (one month on, one month off), Siberian ginseng root, garlic, cayenne pepper, juniper berry, wild yam root, burdock root, and barberry root bark all help balance insulin levels.

🖋 Numerous other herbs are capable of beneficially activating the pancreas. Cascara sagrada aged bark is one example and has long been recognized by conventional medicine as being highly useful. All endocrine herbs will be invaluable and individual tailoring by a professional for the recipient will be required.

❦ Liver and colon cleanses and herbs will be necessary (see chapter 6).

❦ Take alternating hot and cold showers.

❦ Use juniper essential oil in bathwater or added to a massage oil.

❦ If the pancreas is swollen, try hot castor-oil packs (see chapter 3).

❦ Stress and shock (both in the past and in the present) are an emotional factor influencing diabetes, and such situations should be avoided, even if major lifestyle changes are necessary. Work on enjoyable exercise, relaxation, and meditation.

DIARRHEA

Occasional diarrhea lasting only two or three days is usually the result of an infection; it is nature's way of expelling the offending bacteria (or whatever) from the body. Therefore, diarrhea shouldn't be suppressed with drugs, as people so often wish to. The body needs to rid itself of digestive poisons as quickly as possible. If diarrhea lasts a long time, however, the body will become weakened; if this happens, the body will eventually exhaust itself through dehydration in its efforts to keep cleansing itself. If diarrhea lasts longer than three days and recurs between bouts of constipation, then it may well be advisable to talk to a natural healer or doctor; the cause might be irritable bowel syndrome, colitis, celiac disease, or a worm infestation (refer to the relevant sections in this chapter). If diarrhea is affecting babies, small children, or the very elderly, then special care must be taken. It should be closely monitored if it continues for longer than twenty-four hours, to prevent dehydration. Teething also causes diarrhea.

For Occasional Diarrhea

- Drink barley water (see chapter 4).
- If you are able to, eat chopped garlic cloves; dip them in honey to help with administration.
- Take acidophilus capsules to help the bowel flora, or homemade rejuvelac if no acidophilus is available.
- Raspberry leaf tea, meadowsweet leaf tea, and slippery elm inner bark powder mashed into a ripe banana will help slow down the diarrhea and provide nutrition. Arrowroot or grated apples that have been left to turn brown could replace the slippery elm inner bark.
- Take two parts echinacea root, one part chamomile flowers, and one part barberry root bark or turmeric rhizome as a tincture to help fight infection if any is present.

For Babies

- Chamomile flower tea and homemade barley water (see chapter 4), given by bottle or sippy cup, will help diarrhea. If the baby is not too young, you can also try other ideas mentioned in this section to help diarrhea.
- For very severe bouts, give oak bark or yarrow leaf tea, as their astringent qualities will help. Alternatively, use very small amounts of bentonite clay, but only with professional help, as it is very strong.

For a Fragile Colon

If you suffer from regular diarrhea or your colon is otherwise damaged, the following remedies might help.

- Use feeding and soothing herbs. Combine three parts slippery elm inner bark with one part each of the following powdered herbs: chamomile flower, marshmallow root, licorice root, and peppermint leaf. Add one to three teaspoons of this mixture to a mashed ripe banana, three times daily.
- Other useful herbs are red raspberry leaf, cramp bark, meadowsweet leaf, marshmallow root, yellow dock root, wild yam root, marigold flower, and Chinese rhubarb root.

❦ Massage—very soft movements are vital. Use essential oils of cubeb, chamomile, geranium, and lavender. You could also put them on an oilcloth and place under a hot water bottle atop the abdomen.

DIVERTICULITIS

Diverticulitis is a condition in which the mucous membranes in the bowel wall have consistently remained so inflamed that pockets have developed. If these pockets grow large, they become increasingly capable of catching the passing and occasionally sluggish fecal matter. These wastes will build up in the pockets, which will then become a toxic breeding ground for bacteria, and can lead to inflamed areas that very often bleed. It is usually this point of chronic inflammation that produces pain, bloating, and blood loss—all noticeable warnings that help must be sought.

🍎 Any fibrous indigestible pieces of food, particularly raw skins of fruits and vegetables or their seeds, can easily set off intense pain, and although the problem has usually started through a lack of raw fibrous and unrefined food in the diet, this is not the time to introduce it.

🍎 Nutritious baby food must be adopted—try stewing apples, with their skins, seeds, and core, in springwater, adding cinnamon and a pinch of nutmeg. Strain out the pulp and eat a bowl of this apple puree daily with a teaspoon each of arrowroot, powdered slippery elm inner bark, and marshmallow root stirred in, with an added teaspoon of cinnamon. Honey may be used for taste. Continue until the inflammation, bleeding, and pain subside.

🍎 Gently inch into more raw foods. Buy a juicer—juicing fruits and vegetables will give first-class nutrition and aid easy digestion. Superfood is another option and is perhaps the easiest method of providing an instant, nutritious meal.

🍎 When the colon has started to heal itself, try steaming your vegetables. Also try small amounts of very finely grated peeled carrot and beet as an initial means of introducing raw foods. Make vegetable purees in the blender, but leave the skins on.

🍎 After a few weeks, rice and all the other whole grains can be tried, but chewing has to become a must, so that all food arrives in the colon well mushed and its fiber content broken down.

Following the initial introduction of the apple puree mixture detailed above, continue with the following recommended regime as the new diet unfolds:

🍎 Drink alfalfa tea and superfood daily to support and replace vital vitamins and minerals.

🖋 Drink aloe gel daily to soothe and heal.

🖋 Take equal parts of echinacea root tincture for immune support and *pau d'arco* inner bark tincture for viral and fungal buildup, or choose olive leaf for all situations.

🖋 Daily supportive herbs would be Siberian ginseng root tincture and two cups of chamomile flower tea.

🖋 Use four parts slippery elm inner bark, two parts marshmallow root, two parts chamomile flowers, two parts peppermint leaf, and one part licorice root powders. Take two to three teaspoons daily, made into a smooth paste with water or mashed into a banana; it will help soothe, heal, and regrow the damaged tissue.

🖐 Colon cleansing with professional supervision will be required.

🖐 For acute pain, use sitz baths and castor-oil packs (see chapter 3).

DUODENAL ULCERS

Duodenal ulcers can often occur when the valve that controls the release of parts of the stomach contents into the duodenum gets a little stuck, thus allowing too much acid into an alkaline area, causing inflammation, pain, and eventually sores. The cause of the "stuck" valve is very often nerve-related, with stress being a large contributing factor.

See also "Gastric Ulcers."

🍎 Drink plenty of water. Dr. Shamim Daya (a physician, herbalist, and nutritionist) believes that drinking enough water daily is one of the simplest and best treatments for duodenal ulcers.

🖋 Add a percentage of astringent herbs like bayberry root or cranesbill (American true geranium) root to your everyday diet. Also include soothing ones like meadowsweet leaf, marshmallow root, aloe vera gel, and slippery elm inner bark.

🖋 Treat the nerves. Use chamomile flower tea. Take five drops of lobelia leaf tincture at high-stress times — up to ten times a day. Valerian root and passionflower tincture will be invaluable to calm quickly and to promote a peaceful, easy sleep. Take one teaspoon of skullcap leaf tincture three times a day for three to four months as well.

🖐 Practice deep breathing.

🖐 Take walks, practice yoga, or dance.

🖐 Use relaxing essential oils in the bath.

🖐 Watch funny, nonserious television programs.

EAR INFECTIONS

Common causes of inflammation and swelling in the ear canal are food allergies, especially to dairy products, bacterial invasion of the ear, or a buildup of earwax. Ear infections are common in babies and children.

🍎 Avoid wheat, dairy products, and sugar, if possible, and investigate any other food allergies.

🌿 Ear infections are best dealt with by using Dr. Christopher's B & B ear formula (see chapter 11). This formula helps to clear the actual infection as well as the lymphatic system and sinuses. Always warm the formula to body temperature before use. Mastoiditis, which is caused by an abscess or boil in the middle ear, can also be treated with this formula, as can ringing in the ears.

✋ Avoid swimming while suffering from an ear infection.

ECZEMA

Eczema is a skin condition that may make the skin hot or cold, dry or suppurating. Each type must be treated accordingly to its symptoms and, depending on its severity, may require more individual and specialized help. It can be caused by food allergies and is likely to indicate inefficient digestion, particularly low levels of hydrochloric acid and pepsin, and a sluggish liver. Stress will exacerbate the problem, as will a delicate nervous system. For more advice, refer to "Dermatitis" and "Psoriasis."

🍎 Cold, scaly skin will best be helped by keeping to a diet of slow-cooked, warming foods, including grains and root vegetables, with additional warming ingredients such as cinnamon.

🍎 Wheat and dairy products are common problem foods, but ensure that the soy foods and soy milk you substitute do not cause allergic reactions.

🍎 Drink lots of water daily.

🍎 Foods with oxalic acid can cause disturbances, so be aware of sources such as tomatoes, oranges, gooseberries, strawberries, and rhubarb.

🍎 Use virgin olive oil in cooking and raw on salads, the latter with apple cider vinegar; both are good for the skin.

🌿 Flaxseed oil (rich in omega-3 fatty acids) is a good supplement; also use evening primrose oil (GLA), for omega-6.

🌿 Immune- and nervous-system herbs will be important—olive leaf, echinacea root, chamomile flower, skullcap leaf, and a little lobelia leaf.

🌿 Digestive herbs like meadowsweet leaf and flower, blessed thistle leaf and flower, and aloe vera juice will be vital.

- Use blood-cleansing herbs, such as a mixture of two parts burdock root, one part red clover flower, and one part dandelion root.
- Use eczema ointment (see chapter 11).
- The liver, bowel, and stomach all need attention in terms of function, cleansing, and support.
- Destressing by dancing, exercising, and meditating is ideal.

Infantile Eczema

Sometimes babies are born with eczema—in which case, the mother, if she is breast-feeding, must be treated as above.

- Tea made with very small amounts of simple herbs like burdock root and meadowsweet leaf and flower can be put into a bottle and given to the baby separately, if the baby can drink from one. If not, then the mother should drink the tea two or three times daily.

EDEMA (WATER RETENTION)

Retaining excess water in the body is a problem that women in particular are prone to, especially premenstrually. Both men and women can be susceptible, however. Particular "holding" areas are the fingers, under the eyes, and (thanks to gravity) the ankles and feet. Water retention may be one of the many symptoms of a faulty or congested liver. It can also be connected to the hormone system, the heart, and the kidneys. When the liver becomes overburdened with toxins, it cannot keep up with its work and so passes on the job to the kidneys, which in turn may overload and stagnate. The same applies to an overburdened circulatory or lymphatic system. Constipation, diabetes, and thyroid problems can also cause edema, so individual diagnosis and treatment will be necessary.

- Avoid refined salt, unless you are told specifically not to do so by a practitioner. Avoid foods that exacerbate the problem, like dairy and wheat products.
- Include plenty of leeks, parsley, celery seeds and sticks, and cucumber. For fruits, choose apples, pears, melons, peaches, pineapples, and bilberries.
- Eat plenty of dark green vegetables, chlorella, and other algae, which are rich in B vitamins, particularly B_6. Drink superfood.
- Herbs that remove excess water are easy to find, the safest being dandelion root. Use in teas or tinctures. In addition, when in season, the leaf can go into fresh salads.
- A colon cleanse will help balance the water level in the body and relieve the edema.

❧ A liver cleanse will be useful along with a kidney cleanse; this combination will make the kidneys work much more efficiently.

❧ Massage the affected areas with one teaspoon of juniper oil in one cup of base oil, or add 4 drops of juniper oil to your bathwater.

EMPHYSEMA, PLEURISY, AND PNEUMONIA

Emphysema, pleurisy, and pneumonia are viral, bacterial lung infections that can be exacerbated or caused by pollution and stress. They all need professional attention, but the general directions in chapter 9 for home care are strongly advised. Refer to the "The Respiratory System" in chapter 9.

ENDOMETRIOSIS

Endometrial cells line the wall of the uterus and build up each month until being shed at the time of menstruation. Endometriosis is a condition in which this lining produces small nests of stray cells that are transported out of the womb and into the fallopian tubes, bladder, ovaries, and elsewhere—sometimes even reaching as far as the lungs. The tissue still behaves as if it were in the womb and continues to fluctuate with the cyclic hormonal changes. Wherever these stray cells settle, they will bleed monthly, coinciding with the menstrual cycle. This blood collects and stagnates, causing toxic buildups that eventually become inflamed and develop into blood-filled cysts (chocolate cysts). There is, of course, a great deal of pain associated with this condition.

The cause of endometriosis is unknown, but poor hygiene, the use of manmade fibers in underwear, repeated infections including pelvic inflammatory disease, dirty surgical implements, dirty hands and fingers, tampons, retained placenta, and all manner of outside poisoning sources create infections. Sluggish periods with inadequate emptying of the womb each month could also be a possibility. Endometrial cells have been found in young girls, however, which does suggest a genetic link. While the causes of endometriosis are not really understood, recent information suggests that a poorly functioning immune system might, in part, be responsible. If the immune system is not functioning properly, any invasive straying cells, which should be instantaneously killed off, are not. Instead they travel through the bloodstream or lymph system and are deposited in other organs, such as the lungs.

If this disorder is caught early, many positive steps can be taken, but treatment must be very committed and consistent. Orthodox methods of surgery and drugs can be used, but male steroid drugs like danazol, which prevent menstruation, have alarming side effects. Many patients feel very depressed on it, and an increasing number of doctors prefer not to use it. As in pregnancy (another suggested "cure" for endometriosis), it is designed to work by giving the body a chance to stop menstruating. Another treatment consists of giving synthetic progesterone, but this does not suit all women or even help the situation.

Symptoms can include pelvic pain—especially at the times of ovulation and menstruation—irregular or excessive menstrual bleeding; backache (lower back especially); painful lovemaking; infertility; discomfort in the stomach, small intestine, and large intestine; painful urination; prolonged menstrual bleeding; and constipation and diarrhea in fluctuation.

Areas that should be considered when treating endometriosis are as follows:

🍎 Maintain a good diet of whole grains, vegetables, and plenty of citrus fruit. Include superfood.

🍎 Avoid meats, dairy products, and eggs that have been produced using synthetic hormones.

🍎 Avoid coffee, tea, and chocolate, as they also produce extra estrogen. Avoid alcohol because it harms the liver, which must remain healthy.

🌿 For excessive bleeding, use equal parts of yarrow leaf and alfalfa leaf. (With the supervision of a qualified herbalist, the herb beth root could also be used.)

🌿 There is always a possibility that infection may be lurking. To deal with this, use barberry root bark at the beginning of the program.

🌿 Liver herbs like wild yam root, barberry root bark, cinnamon stick, dandelion root, and milk thistle seed will be essential.

🌿 The immune system should be functioning efficiently; include herbs like *pau d'arco* inner bark, chamomile flower, and echinacea root.

🌿 Use endocrine herbs to balance and tone the system (avoiding those that encourage estrogen production). Use a combination of two parts each of squaw vine leaf (and other aerial parts) and chaste tree berry; and one part each of nettle root, sarsaparilla root, Chinese licorice root, and red raspberry leaf.

🌿 For excessive cramps and pain, use equal parts of lobelia leaf, pasque-flower, black cohosh root, and cramp bark.

🌿 For pain herbs, try corydalis tuber and poppy petal tincture.

✋ The colon, liver, and kidneys will all vitally need to undergo cleansing.

✋ Lose weight if you need to, because fat stores estrogen. Take a daily dose of GLA and spirulina to facilitate weight loss and help with pains and cramps. Increase fiber in your diet; this also absorbs estrogen and helps remove it through the bowel.

❧ Use vaginal pessaries (see chapter 3) every third night and douche with herbs at least once a week — these methods will help the body to rid the area of localized infection and encourage the regrowth of normal tissue.

❧ Hot and cold showers and sitz baths will help to maintain circulation in the womb area; this is vital for the healing process.

❧ For pain, use a hot castor-oil pack over the area.

GASTRIC ULCERS

Ulcers are very often the culmination of long-term stomach problems that many doctors believe often result from untreated bacterial infection. The resulting excessive acidity can literally burn the stomach walls, leaving them inflamed and even bleeding. These problems can also mean that the mucous membranes of the gut wall are no longer able to function in a healthy way, so that acid and digestive enzymes come in contact with the wall and erode, disturb, and irritate. The result is an ulcer, which is very painful. A condition known as leaky gut syndrome can also develop, to which the body responds by increasing barrier protection. This "armoring" produces a further complication of larger-than-normal molecules being absorbed by the gut, which in turn creates an immune response and a generalized allergic reaction. Both conditions should be treated in the same way.

🍎 Start each morning with a glass of springwater and fresh lemon juice — this combination eradicates excess hydrochloric acid and removes any lingering food from the night before. It can also encourage the correct production of hydrochloric acid.

🍎 Foods should be easily digestible and nonfatty, with no highly fibrous food, nuts, or cooked spices.

🍎 Include culinary herbs such as fennel, garlic, caraway, tumeric, mint, ginger, and basil, to aid digestion and ward off bacterial opportunists.

🍎 Eat apple puree, rice, pureed vegetables, and all easily digestible foods (see chapter 4) while the healing process is taking place.

🍎 Eat pineapples and papayas for extra digestive help; include aloe vera juice as a drink to prevent any harm to the stomach walls.

🍎 Take one tablespoon of apple cider vinegar daily in half a cup of apple juice.

🍎 Food intake should be slow, unhurried, and calm. Chewing should be thorough and slow. Eating without talking can be helpful initially.

🍃 If a major cause of the ulcer is stress and worry, take chamomile flower tea to feed and calm the nervous system. Valerian root will be invaluable in the short term.

🐾 Daily meadowsweet leaf and gentian root will help to soothe and balance stomach acids and general digestive enzymes.

🐾 Besides bacterial infection, the cause of gastric ulcers can be nerve-related, so nerve soothers and feeders will be useful. Try equal amounts of chamomile flower, wood betony leaf, skullcap leaf, and wild lettuce leaves. On a short-term basis, take valerian root.

🐾 To heal the ulcer, use powders of slippery elm inner bark, marshmallow root, licorice root, and chamomile flower. These powders can be mixed with aloe vera gel and eaten as a mush sweetened with honey several times a day. These herbs will coat, heal, allow tissue regrowth, and sustain a lubricated seal between incoming food, stomach acids, and the painful ulcer.

✋ Liver and bowel cleanses will be vital (see chapter 6).

✋ Exercise, sing, dance, and meditate to relieve any stress.

GASTRITIS

Gastritis literally means "inflammation of the stomach." It may have a number of causes. Very often it is not so much an infection as a condition brought about by the fierce acidity of the digestive juices (which is usually enough to kill most bacteria). Often, poisons have been swallowed — sometimes in the form of bacteria on food or from improperly prepared or preserved foods. Alcohol, aspirin, and even tar from cigarettes are other causes of gastric inflammation.

🍎 Fasting is recommended in this situation to give the stomach as little to work on — or to revolt against — as possible. It is best to drink water at room temperature (that is, neither hot nor cold).

🍎 The first foods should be onion and garlic soup, alternated with slippery elm inner bark powder stirred into water or a ripe banana. (Or try the herbal formula of powdered slippery elm inner bark, marshmallow root, licorice root, and peppermint leaves.)

🍎 Take acidophilus capsules to help repopulate beneficial bowel flora.

🐾 When you are able to keep things down, take echinacea root tincture diluted in water.

🐾 Take cayenne pepper to rebuild the mucous membrane lining, and drink meadowsweet leaf tea daily.

GERMAN MEASLES — RUBELLA

Rubella is a viral infection, which, if you are lucky, can be very mild. Starting with a sore throat and swollen lymph glands, often accompanied by a reddening of the eyelids, rubella will graduate to a reddish rash of small pink spots starting on the face and spreading down over the body. The itching is difficult for about three days but afterward things generally improve.

Anyone with German measles should keep away from pregnant women.

- 🍎 Follow the diet recommendations for mumps and chicken pox.
- 🌿 Internally use immune-boosting herbs like echinacea root, barberry root, and garlic.
- 🖐 Treatment of the skin is very much the same as for chicken pox.
- 🖐 For swollen glands, treat in the same way as mumps.

GOUT

Gout is really a variation on the theme of arthritis and rheumatism. Uric acid builds up to high levels in the joints, causing inflammation and pain. The condition can be exacerbated by excessive intake of alcohol or acid-forming food.

- 🍎 Moving body fluids via the kidneys will help; use homemade barley water to help (see chapter 4).
- 🌿 Yarrow leaf, milk thistle seed, dandelion root, burdock root, and celery seed are all useful herbs.
- 🖐 Cooling and clearing the liver and making sure the bowel is cleansed will be important.
- 🖐 Castor-oil packs will relieve pain.
- 🖐 Hot and cold showers will encourage healing and relieve stiffness.

HAY FEVER

Poor digestion and a weakened immune system can lead to hay fever, a pollen allergy. Itchy, streaming eyes and nose along with sneezing are the unpleasant symptoms, which can progress to asthma. This allergy is starting earlier and earlier in the year in Britain with the warming of the climate. It is more common in the hay and summer season, but it can start as soon as the first flowers bloom.

- 🍎 Change your diet (see chapter 4). Start by cutting out wheat, dairy products, tea, and coffee. If your diet is already good, you are probably low immunally or simply have poor digestive abilities, stress, exposure to pollutants, or some other challenge to your immune system.
- 🍎 Taking local organic honey year-round can build your resistance to the pollens in your area. One to two grains of bee pollen daily, taken consistently, is the key, especially for the one and a half months prior to your particular pollen season.
- 🖐 Your immune system needs strengthening; refer to chapter 7 for advice.

🖐 Liver and bowel cleanses will be vital to address intestinal and digestive imbalances.

🌿 General herbs to address all of the relevant issues would include four parts of mullein flowers; three parts of echinacea root; two parts each of barberry root bark, elder flowers, marshmallow root, *Astragalus* root, St. John's wort flower, and eyebright leaf and flower; and one part each of gentian root, lobelia leaf, burdock root, cayenne pod, dandelion root, and licorice root. Many others will work for different reasons.

🌿 Plantain leaf is a natural antihistamine and soothes irritated mucus membranes as well as helping with actual infections. It also dissolves mucus, and being so common, like elder flowers, it's an easy plant to identify and collect away from car fumes.

🖐 Make your own rose petal oil — it helps all allergies.

🖐 If your sinuses are very congested, use snuff (see chapter 11) to relieve the pressure.

🖐 If your eyes are itchy, use the eye formula suggested in chapter 11 under "Eye Injury and Temporary Blindness." Refrain from rubbing them.

🖐 Rub castor oil around the eyes if itchy and swollen.

HEADACHES, MIGRAINES

Head pain can be of many types and have many causes. Among the most common causes are a toxic bowel, constipation, liver overload, premenstrual tension and other hormonal imbalances, high blood pressure, or a faulty diet rich in stimulants, chocolates, and sweets. Occasional headaches can often be part of a circulatory problem. A simple way of finding out whether they are is to test with a hot washcloth or ice on the temples (see below for details of these tests). An acid buildup can also produce migraines. Correct diagnosis of the type of headache you have will be all-important.

🍎 Dietary changes will be vital, particularly omitting dairy products, wheat products, alcohol, tea, and coffee. Drink plenty of water.

🌿 If a hot washcloth calms the headache, it means that the blood vessels are constricted and need dilating. Rosemary leaf tea will calm and feed the nervous system, yet dilate the blood vessels; ginkgo leaf and prickly ash berry will help get oxygen to the brain, if this is what is needed.

🌿 If ice on the temples relieves the pain, you need to calm and close down your overdilated blood vessels; in that case, use lime tree *(Tilia)* flower and chamomile flower made up as tea.

🌾 Herbs for the nervous system will help to relieve stress headaches, while other headaches may come from the liver, diet, or bowel — you may need some further diagnosis to determine exact causes and treatment.

🌾 Willow bark and meadowsweet leaf both contain salicylic acid, which helps to relieve the pain of headaches — make decoctions.

🌾 Feverfew leaf tea can particularly help migraines.

🖐 Liver and colon cleanses will be necessary if the headache originates from toxicity.

🖐 If you suffer from sinus headaches, you will need to use herbal snuff (see "Nose Problems," below) and inhalations of essential oils.

HEART ATTACK

Many circulatory and heart problems can lead to a heart attack. These episodes can be demoralizing and scary, and may leave permanent damage or impairment. Yet a warning can be just the jolt needed to get you to change your eating habits and lifestyle radically, with very beneficial effects, as many people have discovered.

High cholesterol levels and fatty and plaque deposits, with resultant severe blockages in the system, can cause heart attacks. Other causes can be high blood pressure, clotting of blood vessels (thrombosis), and blood stickiness, caused by platelets clumping together and blocking veins. Thus anyone who has any of these problems should be aware that there are some very useful herbal first-aid measures available; I have seen them prevent what could probably have been much more serious situations, time and again. The following first-aid measures can be used in cases of suspected heart attack or stroke, while waiting for an ambulance:

🌾 Cayenne tincture should always be the first step. It helps to relieve the heart spasm, partly because it is rich in magnesium. It also stabilizes blood pressure quickly. Always have some tincture at hand — in your handbag, car, or kitchen cupboard. Put one teaspoon in a glass of warm water and drink as much as possible immediately.

🌾 Next, take a few drops of lobelia leaf tincture. This will also relax spasms, relieve shock, and balance whatever extremes of the nervous system are being displayed. The patient will usually feel a difference in moments.

🌾 If you have it at hand and can remember to use it, place a drop or two of camphor essential oil over the patient's heart and under the nose. Camphor is a vasoconstrictor and increases blood pressure quite quickly. It's a useful item to have at hand for those in a risk category.

The following suggestions are useful for long-term treatment (see also chapter 9):

🍎 Eat an appropriate diet.

🌿 Long-term use of heart herbs such as hawthorn flower, leaf, and berry can make huge improvements.

✋ If you smoke, then *stop.*

✋ Good food, exercise, and a generally good lifestyle are essential (see "Heart Disease," below).

✋ Doctors often prescribe aspirin for people who've had a heart attack because it helps to thin the blood. Unfortunately, aspirin can really disrupt your stomach lining and your digestion. You may wish to include meadowsweet leaf and white willow bark tea—both rich in salicylate—or red clover flower tea, which is rich in blood thinners.

✋ Hormone replacement therapy (HRT) is often recommended as a protection against heart attacks in older women. In fact, a nineteen-year study by the department of family and preventive medicine at the University of California, San Diego, found no change in heart attack death rates among menopausal women taking HRT. Balanced hormone levels are important, however, including thyroid function, so women should use herbs to balance these—as should men.

✋ Massage oils made with lavender, frankincense, geranium, or ylang-ylang (grades 1 or 2) would also be useful, and a few drops in the bath would be calming.

See also the separate section on stroke, below in this chapter.

HEART DISEASE (ANGINA PECTORIS)

The pains across the chest experienced in angina are caused by a lack of blood supply to the heart, resulting in a lack of usable oxygen in the heart tissue. Nitroglycerin (an explosive!) is given to angina sufferers—the drugs used are often called calcium channel blockers because, just like many other muscle pains, a heart pain, or angina, is often due to a lack of calcium. This lack of calcium causes an uncomfortable tightening or tensing. Usually when the symptoms are diagnosed as angina pectoris (which simply means "pains across the chest"), no doctor knows what the specific cause is. Indeed, I have seen this diagnosis given to a variety of conditions, from simple emotional upset to sudden strenuous exercise, high cholesterol, or excessive plaque in the arteries. The clogging effect of excess cholesterol, general debris, or calcium (plaque) causes the arteries and veins leading to and from the heart to become blocked, occasionally only allowing a trickle of blood through at a time. This blockage results in chest pains. Another cause of circulatory blockage can be pieces of this plaque breaking off and floating around the circulatory system, perhaps finally lodging somewhere where a natural narrowing occurs, and blocking off the vessel to a greater or lesser degree. What makes it worse is the formation of fresh blood clots, which increase the size of the obstruction. These could be fatal, causing a heart attack. Angina can be a warning of that ongoing possibility. Stress can also cause a lack of oxygen availability to the heart (and chronic candidiasis and indigestion can mirror and cause angina pains).

For lesser problems, the vessels need immediate dilation to allow more blood through. For long-term treatment of the cause, the blockage—whether it be fat or calcium—must be cleared.

- Fats to avoid are polyunsaturated margarine, dairy products, and meat. Soy margarine would be safe. Virgin olive oil, either heated at low temperatures (not above 90°F) or raw, is also beneficial.
- Vitamin C and lysine will be vital.
- Avoid coffee, tea, alcohol, and spicy cooked foods.
- You need lots of garlic—at least two fat cloves of garlic for lunch and two for supper. There is no cheaper or more perfect medicine.
- Lots of leeks, onions, and spring onions would be good, too.
- You should take some source of GLA: evening primrose seed oil or black currant seed oil.
- If you usually feel cold, add cayenne powder to your regime. Take up to three capsules, three times daily. Start at a much lower dose than this and gradually build up as your body becomes acclimated. Continue for three months, then stop if you wish.
- A herbal formula that will immediately help the heart and will work long term would be two parts hawthorn berry, and one part each of ginkgo leaf, motherwort leaf, and cayenne pod. They can be used in tincture form if capsules are unsuitable.
- Herbs to calm and relax would be skullcap leaf, black cohosh root, oat straw, passionflower, gotu kola herb, lobelia pod, and, in the short term, valerian root.
- A nutritional herbal drink would be equal parts of alfalfa leaf, red clover flower, and nettle leaf tea.
- Cleanses and hot and cold showers will be vital.
- Exercise, but pace yourself. You will need expert help and guidance, because overdoing it could be dangerous. Taking no exercise at all, however, could be equally dangerous. You need to find the correct middle way for your own needs. Start with gentle walking interspersed

with frequent rests, making sure that you have someone else with you in case any problems arise. Increase as your heart and chest pains allow. You could eventually walk alone, but always let someone know you're out and roughly how long you intend to be. Eventually, cycling and a wider variety of exercise may be possible.

HEMORRHOIDS (PILES) AND ANAL FISSURE

Hemorrhoids are ballooning flaps of skin in the rectum or anus that are very painful, usually more so when passing a bowel movement, as they are irritated by the pressure. An anal fissure forms when weakened and stretched tissue has split, remaining as a wound that is constantly sore and difficult to heal. With hemorrhoids (or piles) it's important to consider the state of the whole digestive system, including constipation, diarrhea, bowel irritability, and liver function, which is often found to be faulty in this situation.

🍎 Drink plenty of water, and eat fiber in the form of fruit and vegetables.

🌿 Aloe vera juice and meadowsweet leaf and flower tea will be two basic herbs to start with.

✋ Use a mixture of black walnut hull, a little oak bark, and some yarrow leaf; marshmallow root to soothe; myrrh resin to disinfect; a touch of cayenne pepper in case of bleeding; and some Chinese rhubarb root as an all-round bowel balancer. Make this combination into an ointment using a base of olive oil and coconut butter, along with benzoin essential oil and witch hazel essential oil. Use the ointment very frequently, before and after bowel movements and in between if possible. The same herbs can be mixed as powders. Add equal parts to capsules and take daily. Pure or diluted witch hazel can help for quick relief.

✋ A slant-board treatment will be useful (see chapter 5).

✋ Take cold sitz baths, which can help severely prolapsed piles, as can sitting on bags of frozen peas at intervals.

✋ An anal suppository (see chapter 3) will help heal and support the area. Useful herbs would be barberry bark powder, black walnut hull powder, a pinch of cayenne, and witch hazel essential oil.

HEPATITIS

Hepatitis is a form of liver disease that has several different causal agents, its types currently labeled A, B, and C. Less common ones also exist. It takes the form of liver inflammation, usually caused by a viral infection, which leaves the liver enlarged and unable to function properly. Treatment before travel to countries where hepatitis is endemic is preferable to vaccination; I have known of many cases in which the patient felt that the vaccination was responsible for later symptoms and, occasionally, for the full-blown disease. Conventional medical practitioners will openly admit that vaccination does not necessarily stop one from contracting hepatitis. Symptoms include headaches, facial flushing, inflamed gums, tenderness from inflammation in the liver area, diarrhea, a yellow coating on the side of the tongue, a profound sense of fatigue and loss of well-being, and possibly migraine headaches. Hepatitis A is transmitted through food, blood, water, bodily fluids, and other sources of infection, and is usually acute and infectious. Hepatitis B is more likely to be transmitted by bodily fluids including blood. It has an incubation period of three months, and is usually chronic. Hepatitis C is also infectious, present in blood and in broken, weeping skin. Current treatment of hepatitis C involves prolonged doses of interferon, which can make the patient feel permanently ill with flulike symptoms while simply delaying the regeneration of the liver. Hepatitis is known to increase the likelihood of other liver disease in later life.

Hepatitis is called chronic when it lasts longer than six months. Chills, fever, and malaise accompany acute hepatitis. Although liver function tests can be useful, generally no specific treatment is recommended except rest for hepatitis A and B. Isolation may possibly be recommended, depending on the type.

Hepatitis needs different treatment depending on the type. But all types will respond to the following treatments:

- Bile needs to be decongested in this situation, and the "fire" and "heat" of the problem purged and cooled. Many herbs common to the kitchen and garden will help: dandelion root, turmeric root, mint leaf, oregano leaf, and burdock root. Avoid cooked and raw hot spices and alcohol at all cost.

- Gentian root is a bitter tonic to be taken before meals. It is an ancient European remedy for all digestive and liver and gallbladder problems. Meadowsweet leaf, common in Europe, will also be useful. Siberian ginseng root for tonic support will be vital, as may other tonic herbs depending on the symptoms displayed. Expert advice will be vital.

- Use milk thistle seed though cautiously and in small doses so as not to push the liver too hard. The silymarin it contains has been found to have protective and regenerative properties, making it effective in chronic and postacute hepatitis. Milk thistle is known to protect liver cells from injury, toxins, free radicals, and viral toxins, and to increase the population of liver enzymes—all of which encourage a quick recovery from injury, while stimulating regeneration of liver tissue. *Schisandra* berry and dandelion root will also be vital for their powerful and balanced liver detoxification abilities.

☙ The spleen will need to be assisted to perform better (it can occasionally show slight enlargement with hepatitis C). Use echinacea root, olive leaf, and turmeric rhizome to assist immunity.

✋ Under supervision, liver and gallbladder cleanses, along with a colon cleanse are essential. Use barberry root bark and other liver and bowel cleansers as well.

✋ Castor-oil packs over the liver will help.

✋ For more natural-healing practices, diet, and routines for the liver, gallbladder, and spleen, refer to chapter 9. A bland diet with steamed, stewed food is essential. Vigilance will keep this disease to a minimum, so that it neither recurs nor worsens.

HIGH BLOOD PRESSURE (HYPERTENSION)

Hypertension is a well-known and common condition in society nowadays, probably because of our diets and lifestyle. It can be hereditary or caused by individual habits and stress levels. Its physical causes can include heart and circulatory imbalance, troubled kidneys, sluggish or overactive hormones, a lack of calcium or defective calcium metabolism, obesity, clogged arteries, nervousness, and worry. The dangers of persistent high blood pressure are damage to the brain, heart, and kidneys. The brain, kidneys, adrenal glands, and autonomic nervous system control blood pressure. Refer to "Heart Disease" for more information. Also see "The Circulatory System" in chapter 9 in order to develop a general awareness of appropriate diet, natural healing, herbs, and cleansing programs.

🍎 Eat sensibly and cut out tea, coffee, salt, alcohol, sugar, chocolate, fats, and cigarettes.

🍎 Avoid hot cooked spices except for cayenne capsules, and take large amounts of garlic with cool herbs like thyme, chives, marjoram, coriander, fennel, and cumin.

🍎 Search out potassium-rich foods, such as bananas, dried fruit, nectarines, melons, potatoes (with skins), broccoli, pumpkins, and potassium broth (see chapter 5).

☙ Good oils to take internally are those rich in omega-3 and omega-6 fatty acids. These can be found in the form of flaxseed oil capsules, GLA capsules, and olive oil.

☙ Good basic herbs to support, buffer, elasticize, dilate, and clear blockages in the veins and arteries are ginkgo leaf, lime tree *(Tilia)* flower, and hawthorn flower, leaf, and berry.

☙ If your high blood pressure is known to be emotionally based, then learn to relax and breathe. Consider valerian root in the short term, and oat straw and skullcap leaf in the long term, in order to feed the nervous system.

🖝 If the body is physically tense, use three parts cramp bark accompanied by one part lobelia leaf.

✋ Exercise and hydrotherapy are vital for increasing circulation.

HYPOGLYCEMIA (LOW BLOOD SUGAR)

Low blood sugar is currently a very prevalent problem, especially among women, and is often at its worst when a woman is premenstrual. Men can also suffer, but they are in a minority. Sugar cravings can take the form of outright sugar bingeing with the consumption of unusual amounts of chocolate, or more discreet searches for dried fruit around the kitchen. Like diabetes, hypoglycemia is an imbalance of blood sugar levels, which often stems from imbalanced glycogen levels in the liver. To treat this problem, the liver and the pancreas will both need balancing and fortifying. It shows as a deficiency of sugar in the blood owing to overproduction of the hormone insulin in an attempt to provide much-needed supplies of energy. Excess insulin causes too much sugar to be driven into the cells, resulting in a sudden blood sugar drop. The brain is particularly affected; normal thinking will become difficult, as will talking, driving, or making sense. Never leave low blood sugar untreated, because when brain function is inhibited and therefore poor, the nervous system will deplete. The need to stop and sleep can be overpowering, should chocolate, coffee, cigarettes, or alcohol not be available to prop the situation up! Low blood sugar can also produce impatience and aggression.

So what causes this problem? There are many things—for instance, skipped meals and crash diets; unremitting stress; sudden weight loss; the intake of excessive amounts of refined carbohydrates, such as chips, cakes, snacks, and candy; excessive sugar intake; or excessive tea, coffee, and alcohol intake. In women, causes may include general endocrine imbalances, including premenstrual problems, menstrual imbalances, pregnancy, breastfeeding, and menopause. For both sexes pancreatic weakness and vitamin and mineral imbalances can contribute, including deficiencies of B vitamins, magnesium, chromium, manganese, zinc, and potassium. Poor liver function, digestive excesses and insufficiencies, and adrenal and thyroid function can also be factors. Candida is also a highly likely cause.

Many people do not know that they are hypoglycemic, but "swimming" feelings, shakiness, driven hunger, irritability, fatigue, indigestion, headaches, hyperactivity, anxiety, paranoia, sudden energy drops, even blackouts or "must sleep" times may all be indications of this. The list of symptoms seems endless—sweating, bad dreams, lack of libido, epilepsy, stomach cramps, and general allergies. It may be necessary to find a specialist to make a diagnosis for you. Very often the problem is constantly covered up and "supported" by increasing sugar intake when the worst feelings arrive. If left untreated, anemia, calcium depletion, immune deficiency, cancer, premenstrual syndrome, and many other conditions may arise. If too many refined-sugar foods and drinks are succumbed to, then protein requirements will increase. If this cycle continues, one often sees an alternating meat and sugar desire becoming stronger and stronger. A desire for sugar can also arise from a deficiency of protein, because of the controlling function that protein has on sugar; the metabolism decreases if protein is not provided, and consequently the sugar cravings increase. The conventional medical profession rarely diagnoses hypoglycemia, so many people are left untreated or confused. The truth of the matter is often seen when sugar in all its forms, apart from fresh fruit, is removed from the diet. At first this change will feel incredibly drastic, but by exchanging sugar for food and herbs that support blood sugar levels when they are very low, the problem will begin to even itself out. For sugar substitutes, see chapter 4. If you treat this condition carefully, you will avoid its possible development into something worse.

- Follow the diet and herbal advice for diabetes and look at the adrenal glands, as they need support. Pay special attention to the intake of garlic, fiber, and water.
- Superfood is wonderful for sustaining blood sugar levels between meals.
- Take evening primrose oil capsules (GLA).
- Take herbs to stimulate, tone, and support all digestive processes: meadowsweet leaf, aloe vera gel, gentian root, sorrel leaf, and dandelion root.
- Take acidophilus capsules.
- Liver and bowel cleanses are vital.
- Take gentle exercise; walking and deep breathing are initially the best until your balance and stamina are developed. Exhausting activities like swimming, saunas, and so on should be avoided until the body is stronger.

IMPETIGO

Impetigo is a skin infection caused by staphylococcus or streptococcus bacteria, which forms clusters of yellowing, crusting patches and small abscesses. Impetigo is a contagious disease and needs constant attention regarding hygiene: use separate towels, water, clothes, and so on.

- The food program should be of the highest level of vitality—whole foods, seaweeds, algae, nuts, seeds, beans, and fresh organic juices like carrot and apple. Drink plenty of water.

- Use immune and adrenal herbs, such as equal parts of echinacea root and Siberian ginseng root, for support internally.

- Chamomile flowers in quite high doses as a tincture or tea will kill off the infection very quickly and relieve the itching.

- In the long term or, better still, in the short term, liver, kidney, and colon cleanses will be necessary.

- Externally, use herbal ointments containing black walnut hull, neem leaf, plantain leaf, and marigold flower.

INCONTINENCE OR SLIGHT BLADDER WEAKNESS

A weak nervous system, genetic weakness in the area, stroke and paralysis, or old age are most likely to cause one to suffer from incontinence. Yet a surprising number of apparently healthy middle-aged people are also prone to such problems. Physical obstructions—like a swollen prostate gland in men—can be one common cause. Giving birth causes weakening of the pelvic floor muscles, and prenatal and postnatal exercises will help. Hormone disturbances, especially around menopause, can be a factor (special exercises can help enormously; see the section on pregnancy in chapter 8). A tumor causing pressure or even being overweight are other possibilities. Chronic constipation is yet another common cause. With help from a practitioner, one should find the cause and treat it, at the same time strengthening the sphincter muscle of the bladder and other muscles in the area.

- If fear, worry and anxiety are the cause, calcium- and magnesium-rich foods will help: seaweeds, almonds, barley water, sesame, and herbal teas or formulas including equal parts of valerian root and chamomile flower.

- Use equal parts of parsley leaf, *Rehmannia* root, black cohosh root, marshmallow root, gravel root, bearberry leaf, lobelia leaf, and gingerroot.

- Use chamomile and lavender essential oils via massage or in the bath.

- Carry out a one-day kidney cleanse.

INDIGESTION

The inability to digest food properly is a modern-day problem and the cause of many allergies and conditions. Among its many causes are tension or stress and unbalanced intestinal flora. When a poor balance of stomach flora is allowed to develop to the point that it cannot rebalance itself, constipation and other forms of bowel dysfunction can manifest. The small and large intestines are largely interconnected and are, therefore, unable to function properly on their own. A sluggish or overactive liver, weak spleen and pancreas, and overpressured heart can all disturb the harmonious function of the small intestine, resulting in indigestion.

Excess Acidity

- Avoid alcohol, fried foods, and cooked spices. Also avoid wheat, dairy products, and caffeine.

- Very fibrous foods can irritate.

- Foods that require a lot of chewing and digestion, like nuts, should be avoided for a while.

- A little rice may be tolerated after the one-day fast, with some cabbage juice; keep up the slippery elm. Slowly come back to other foods.

- Avoid acidic foods—except for lemons and apple cider vinegar, which are allowed unless you have an obvious reaction to them.

- Long-term use of antacid drugs will make the problem worse, as drug-induced suppression will eventually lead to increased excess acidity. Drink three cups of a tea made from meadowsweet leaf and blessed thistle leaf daily.

- A one-day fast using slippery elm inner bark powder may help. Mix one tablespoon of powder with water and drink, or if you prefer, you could mash it into a ripe banana.

Insufficient Digestive Juices

This condition is a lack or total absence of hydrochloric acid. Average levels stand at 3 percent in healthy people. Very often, lack of hydrochloric acid can denote a lack of ability to absorb vitamin B_{12}, along with a deficiency of another digestive enzyme—pepsin. A great many cancer patients (including those with stomach cancer) are found to be deficient in hydrochloric acid and pepsin; this is also true of children, especially those with allergies like candidiasis, asthma, and eczema.

- Avoid tea, coffee, fried food, alcohol, cooked spices or an excess of raw ones, salt, and smoking.

- Hydrochloric acid and pepsin production can be balanced by using apple cider vinegar. Take between one and three tablespoons daily in apple juice or honey and water.

- Eat pineapples and papayas for extra digestive help; the bromelain in the pineapple is good at breaking down half-digested food matter, and the papain in papaya digests proteins and starches, soothing the stomach as it does so.

🌿 Resurrect beneficial stomach flora with acidophilus capsules and garlic.

🌿 Meadowsweet leaf stimulates the parietal cells in the stomach to produce hydrochloric acid and pepsinogen, if necessary. Take this herb daily as a tea or a tincture.

🌿 Include digestive herbs as frequently as possible. Try using equal parts of cinnamon stick, angelica root, fennel seed, Chinese licorice root, wormwood leaf, and gentian root. Blessed thistle leaf is useful, as it stimulates all digestive juices as well as encouraging correct acid production.

🌿 Increase your general immunity if necessary through occasional use of echinacea root, elderberry, thuja leaf, or olive leaf.

INSOMNIA AND DISTURBED PATTERNS OF SLEEP

🍎 Follow a healthy diet, totally removing all dietary stimulants like coffee, tea, and sugar.

🌿 In the short term, take three parts valerian root with two parts passionflower and one part lobelia leaf. This combination will alleviate sleep disturbance whether it has short-term or long-term causes. Long-term use of herbs such as two parts skullcap leaf, two parts vervain leaf, and one part lobelia leaf will be needed to support and regenerate the nervous system.

🖐 Walk barefoot on grass, sand, and pebbles to ground and disperse any static electricity.

🖐 Do breathing exercises and meditation.

🖐 Take saunas and hot and cold showers, and practice skin brushing.

🖐 It is important to remember that we need stimulation in order to sleep. Therefore, go running or dancing, take a long hike or a swim in the sea, and then learn to relax. Sunbathe for short periods of time or take catnaps.

🖐 Cleanses will be of key importance in helping balance the body and restore correct metabolism.

🖐 Menopause can cause sleeplessness, and therefore using herbs to alleviate hormonal imbalance will improve sleep patterns.

IRREGULAR AND DYSFUNCTIONAL PERIODS

Early periods are those occurring eight or nine days prior to the expected cycle of twenty-five to twenty-nine days. Much variance outside the normal cycle will cause the body to feel tired and depleted. If your period is constantly early, you may feel consistently anxious. An early period can be caused by insufficient progesterone, shortening the second phase (the phase after ovulation). It is also possible that ovulation occurs early, in which case a little estrogen will help extend and complete the first phase.

Very occasionally, ovulation doesn't take place at all, in which case the general health of the entire body will need to be attended to, as other irregularities can occur (osteoporosis, for instance). Periods that are consistently late may be due to hormonal imbalance, congestion and stagnation, anemia, or bowel and liver conditions.

- 🍎 A dietary overhaul will be needed. Avoid tea, coffee, food containing synthetic hormones, and any foods that cause allergies.

- 🌿 If the cause is insufficient estrogen, use red clover flower, black cohosh root, hop strobilus flower, sage leaf, and licorice root.

- 🌿 If the cause is insufficient progesterone, use two parts chaste tree berry and one part sarsaparilla root.

- 🌿 If there is congestion, use equal amounts of warming, relaxing, and moving herbs like gingerroot, cayenne pod, pennyroyal leaf, black cohosh root, cramp bark, and lobelia leaf.

- 🌿 Lack of ovulation or general hormonal imbalance can be dealt with through cleanses (especially liver and bowel) and a good mixed herbal formula taken regularly. Dr. Christopher's female formula would be ideal in this situation: use blessed thistle leaf, cayenne pod, cramp bark, black cohosh root, gingerroot, barberry root bark, red raspberry leaf, squaw vine leaf, bearberry leaf, and chaste tree berry.

- ✋ Colon and liver cleanses will be necessary (see chapter 6).

- ✋ Use vaginal pessaries (see chapter 3).

- ✋ Take hot and cold showers.

- ✋ Exercise regularly.

IRRITABLE BOWEL SYNDROME

Irritable bowel syndrome is the most common bowel complaint seen by doctors. The bowel has irregular muscular contractions, which cause food and toxins to become trapped and stored, leading to bloating, constipation followed by diarrhea, and excessive mucus production, all of which will cause pain. This is often a precursor to other complaints. In general, follow directions for diverticulitis and colitis.

- 🍎 You will need to change your diet radically (see chapter 4) and repopulate colon bacteria by taking acidophilus.

- ✋ A bowel cleanse with appropriate herbs to suit the individual will be vital. A liver cleanse would also be advised. Consider using equal parts of slippery elm inner bark, marshmallow root, and meadowsweet leaf if diarrhea predominates.

✋ Gentle massage with essential oils of chamomile and ylang-ylang is helpful.

✋ Use a hot castor-oil pack with chamomile and ylang-ylang essential oil placed on the abdomen; reheat and replace till the pain has subsided.

✋ Get plenty of exercise.

JAUNDICE

Jaundice is a yellowing of the skin and eyes caused by discoloration from a buildup of waste products in the bloodstream that would normally be dealt with by the liver. It can be caused by a blockage in the bile duct, an infection, or liver disease.

🍎 Take carrot juice, wheat germ, lots of steamed broccoli, artichokes, cabbage, and rice, along with plenty of garlic and turmeric.

🍎 Temporarily, at least, use sources of protein other than meat or dairy products.

🌾 Daily burdock root, dandelion root, red clover flower, and nettle leaf tea will all help; try rotating them. Dandelion is one of the best day-to-day treatments for cooling and strengthening the liver. Both the roots and the leaves can be used.

🌾 Use equal amounts of barberry root bark, milk thistle seed, dandelion root, burdock root, yellow dock root, gentian root, and turmeric rhizome as a tincture daily.

🌾 If the immune system is weak, use echinacea root or olive leaf.

✋ You will need to do a liver cleanse and eventually a bowel cleanse.

✋ Chicory root enemas and castor-oil packs over the liver accompanied by hot and then cold showers with the water spray aimed directly over the area may help and reduce the bile.

KIDNEY STONES

The incidence of kidney stones has risen dramatically over the past century alongside a huge increase in the consumption of animal fats and proteins. Stones can be found in the kidneys, bladder, and ureter and can vary in size tremendously. They are generally composed of calcium oxalate. Normally the body controls the pH level of urine, and any deleterious components remain suspended in solution. With imbalanced pH levels or with lowered immunity, however, these mechanisms fail, the compounds crystallize, and the crystals start clumping together. The pain of stones, which radiates from the upper back down to the groin, is excruciating. Other symptoms include fever or a chill, or blood in the urine. The composition of the stones can vary; for instance, they may contain cystine (an amino acid). If diagnosis shows what type of stone or gravel composition you have, then a more exact diet can be tailored to your particular needs; but this is not easy to detect, nor do hospitals have the time or technology to do it very often, so general guidelines usually have to do.

Often people are unaware of stones until they have passed one, which is an incredibly excruciating experience. Where there has been one, however, it is likely that there will be more, so start treating them at first occurrence.

- Avoid tea, coffee, chocolate, peanuts, rhubarb, Swiss chard, spinach, tomatoes, strawberries, and beet, as well as any other foods containing oxalic acid.

- Avoid eggs and fish in particular, as they have very high oxalic acid levels, but also stop eating animal fats and protein because they will interfere with oxalate absorption.

- Avoid salt, alcohol, refined foods, fried foods, and sugars.

- Foods rich in natural silicon will help maintain a stone-free urinary system. Silicon is found in the skins of organically grown grains, fruits, and vegetables, particularly oats, radishes, and garlic; in unpolluted seaweeds; and in bee pollen. Foods rich in vitamin A will also help: melon, pumpkin, yams, and carrots.

- Drink plenty of water to ensure a constant flushing of the entire urinary system. Choose water with low or no mineral content. Distilled water is free from any minerals, so it flushes through at a faster rate. A good substitute for distilled water is springwater. Sometimes add quite large quantities of fresh lemon juice, as this will ease the pain.

- Drink barley water three times daily—see chapter 4 for the recipe.

- Occasionally, stone formation (or, indeed, urinary infections) can be caused when the urine flows backward because the bladder is not emptying sufficiently. Diuretic herbs like dandelion root and leaf will largely solve this problem.

- To start dissolving the stones and ease their journey through the body, use equal amounts of herbs like gravel root and hydrangea root, combined with demulcents like marshmallow root or corn silk; they help prevent inflammation and bleeding. You can soak the herbs in apple juice overnight and simmer them. Drink the liquid throughout the day—at least three tablespoons at half-hourly intervals. Continue for a few days. Even the hardest calculi will eventually turn into softer balls with no hard edges, which can then be more easily passed.

🪶 If your immune system is low, take olive leaf or echinacea root along with other immune-supportive herbs. Take Siberian ginseng root over the longer term.

✋ Take baths and massage with geranium, juniper, chamomile, and sweet fennel essential oils.

✋ A kidney cleanse will be vital (see chapter 6).

✋ A sedate lifestyle with little or no exercise encourages the accumulation of calcium in the bloodstream. Exercise will redirect it into the bones.

A stone stuck anywhere at awkward entrances and bends in the kidneys, urethra, or bladder is extremely painful. Most people contact their doctor or arrange to be taken to the emergency room immediately if the pain is unbearable, but while waiting for professional help to arrive,

🪶 Try drinking a diuretic fluid such as dandelion root tea, or if you have none, drink lots of water.

✋ A compress of lobelia leaf (see compresses in chapter 3) is soothing when placed over the kidney area, or substitute five drops of lobelia leaf tincture hourly (taken internally). Make the compress as hot as you can (a wet, hot rag with lobelia tincture poured onto it is quick), then put a hot water bottle over it.

✋ A cold compress on the forehead will ease any nausea or fever.

LIVER SPOTS

Liver spots are brown blotches that occur on the backs of hands and on the face and neck, generally in later life. They are sometimes referred to as age spots. They are an indication of a strained liver, so it is necessary to clear and regulate the liver and gallbladder. Excessive exposure to the sun can exacerbate their appearance. Liver "coat hangers" or liver "inflated spots" are the same, only three-dimensional, and can be a nuisance as they catch on clothing.

🍎 Increase intake of vitamins B complex, C, and E and appropriate foods to help the liver function better—see chapter 9.

✋ Colon and liver cleanses will be necessary, along with the herbs associated with them—see chapter 6.

✋ Treat the spots topically with a mix of equal amounts of lemon juice and castor oil nightly.

✋ Stay out of direct sunlight while treating this condition. Wear sunscreen.

LOW BLOOD PRESSURE (HYPOTENSION)

You can have naturally low blood pressure. It can be hereditary, and vegans and vegetarians certainly have naturally lower blood pressure than eaters of flesh and dairy products. A vegetarian's normal blood pressure is 110/70, compared to an average meat eater's blood pressure of 120/80. For an accurate indication of blood pressure health, note how you feel. Are you tired, lethargic, and regularly yawning? If you suspect or know that your blood pressure is very low, get professional help in examining your diet, exercise, and adrenal and thyroid function, as well as your bowel, lymph, and other systems, for signs of imbalance. Seriously consider the possibility of anemia (see "Anemia" and "Poor Circulation and Chilblains," in this chapter).

LUNG OR SINUS INFECTION, BACTERIAL OR VIRAL

The quality and quantity of mucus production are directly linked to the well-being of the lungs. If the lungs maintain a light, moist protective coating of mucus, they can be considered healthy. If the lungs are overcongested with mucus and the air passages are generally inflamed, infection will be attracted. Exercise can remove some of the excess buildup. Lack of exercise can make the situation worse, leading to a severely hindered and ineffective lung capacity. As a lot of lung problems manifest themselves with the onset of damp and cooler weather, special attention should be paid at this time. Some lung problems are a result of poor digestion, accompanied by low stomach and bowel flora from an enzyme deficiency.

- Adopt a mucus-free diet, especially avoiding milk, yogurt, cheese, and eggs.

- Take no alcohol, tea, or coffee.

- Avoid gluten-rich grains like wheat, or refined grains like wheat pasta.

- Avoid sugar, meat, and fried foods.

- If you already have what you feel to be a healthy diet, then excess mucus is probably an indication of general poor health, a cold body, and a weakened immune system. Your system will need to be generally sustained and strengthened with tonic and supportive herbs and foods. Natural food choices should predominantly be those that grow regionally and seasonally.

- Eat onions, leeks, spring onions, garlic, turnips, fresh lemons, limes, ginger, cinnamon, cloves, cabbage, cabbage juice, rice, and corn.

- Make and drink barley water (see chapter 4).

- The immune system may be low and in need of motivation and support, so use echinacea root and *Rehmannia* root.

- Dr. A. Vogel, a respected Swiss herbalist, says that weak lungs need plenty of calcium, an easily available source of which is daily nettle leaf tea, made from young nettles (preferably picked in the spring, and not later than July).

- Practice breathing exercises.

If the mucus is yellow, brown, or green, you need to cool the body down:

- Use plenty of lemons, limes, and garlic, alongside a little ginger, cinnamon, and cloves.

- Essential oils of lime and lemon with a little eucalyptus in a base oil could be massaged into the chest and back morning and night.

If you have white or transparent mucus, then you may feel more cold and shivery and need extra heat and energy:

- Use fewer fresh fruits and raw vegetables. Take plenty of horseradish, baked onions, and grated ginger in dishes, and drink ginger tea.

- Massage with marjoram, rosemary, and black pepper essential oils, or use them in the bath.

For any kind of mucus and blocked nose, sinus, or chest:

- Use the Ayurvedic method — chew twelve raw peppercorns.

- Plantain leaves, elder flowers and berries, edible lichens, nettle leaves, yarrow leaf, and pine needles can all be made into teas.

- Take some garlic syrup and elder flower and elderberry syrup.

- Lobelia leaf is a prime lung herb. A tremendous antispasmodic and expectorant, it is very useful for asthmatics who can learn to use it instead of prescription inhalers for calming and assisting breathing, as well as for bringing up excessive phlegm. A few drops at a time are generally adequate.

- Make sure your bowels are working properly; any bowel disorders will affect the proper working of the lungs.

- Exercise helps the lungs. Horseback riding encourages the diaphragm to push strongly up and down, particularly when galloping. Go cycling, swimming, running, and dancing. Strong emotions like apprehension and fear, which affect breathing, can be physically dissipated with these simple pleasures. An exception is when the air is heavily polluted; exercise should be avoided at such times.

- Take hot and cold showers. Direct the spray onto the chest and back, from the shoulders to the waist. If you are frail or weak, make sure this treatment is done under expert supervision. But if you have the go-ahead and adequate help, it is a great lung strengthener, and can help turn a chronic condition right around.

✻ Inhale a variety of essential oils, such as eucalyptus, lime, pine, lemon, fennel, or cubeb. If you find yourself coughing, take a break and try again in a few moments, or try leaving out the eucalyptus, which can over-exacerbate. The same oils can also be added to the bath or sprinkled onto handkerchiefs, pillows, sheets, and sleepwear. When lying down, the whole body becomes more clogged and congested, and these essential oils can work well at this time.

✻ Massage your chest. Your lungs practically touch your collarbone, so massage up to your shoulders and down to the bottom of your rib cage; and don't forget that both your back and front house your lungs.

✻ Try reflexology. You don't need to be an expert—just rub and stroke your feet. This is best done just before you go to bed.

✻ If problems are severe just before you go to bed, use garlic paste (see "Garlic Paste for Feet" in chapter 3). During this treatment, the body will bring the garlic very effectively into the lungs, helping to relieve any congestion, mucus, or infection. (The protective layer of petroleum jelly is vital to prevent burning of the skin; be sure to use plenty.)

MEASLES

Measles is a viral respiratory-tract infection that is highly contagious. It takes fourteen days to incubate from initial exposure, and the child (or adult) will be infectious on the seventh day after exposure until ten days after the appearance of the rash. It affects the eyes and skin as well, and is spread by coughing and sneezing.

The first signs are usually a cold or runny nose, followed by a fever. When one of my daughters developed it, however (she was not vaccinated), she went straight into a slight fever and rash, which was found in her mouth as Koplik's spots (white ones on the cheek lining), and on her body as brownish-red spots. The whole episode was over in three days, though doctors cite ten days as the normal duration of the illness. At times the reddish-brown spots can also be found behind the ears and on the face and neck, where they often originate before finally spreading to the body.

The fever generally increases as the rash develops; only fluids should be taken during this stage.

🖛 Take a few drops of lobelia leaf tincture every hour to ease the pain, and add drops of lobelia leaf tincture to bathwater.

🖛 Drink herbal teas like yarrow leaf, red raspberry leaf, red clover flower, mullein flower, and nettle leaf, as well as carrot juice or potassium broth (see chapter 4) and superfood.

🖋 Use herbs to enhance the immune system, especially antivirals and those that will help calm the fever and encourage the correct function of elimination channels—see "Chicken Pox," above.

🖋 Grapefruit seed extract in olive oil has been shown to neutralize the virus.

MONONUCLEOSIS

Mononucleosis begins with flulike symptoms—aches, tiredness, runny nose, and the like, as well as occasionally a rash similar to German measles. It is caused by a herpeslike organism called Epstein-Barr virus. The lymph glands in the neck swell and, very occasionally, there are rashes, a sore throat, or digestive upset.

A blood test will confirm mononucleosis, and early diagnosis can be useful, as it can last for months. It should be handled very, very carefully, as postviral fatigue syndrome can easily ensue if the body's energies are not supported and fortified. It has become a common precursor of myalgic encephalomyelitis (chronic fatigue syndrome)

🍎 Excellent food programs will be vital: start with juices and superfood.

🍎 Reduce protein intake (meat, eggs, fish).

✋ Perform colon, liver, and kidney cleanses, and use herbs for these areas (see chapter 6).

🖋 Siberian ginseng root or *Astragalus* root, or both, will be vital for general long-term adaptogenic support.

🖋 Immune herbs such as echinacea root, myrrh resin, and pokeweed root alongside blood cleansers like burdock root and dandelion root will be needed.

✋ Include very moderate exercise and massage.

MULTIPLE SCLEROSIS, MUSCULAR DYSTROPHY, AND MYASTHENIA GRAVIS

Multiple sclerosis, muscular dystrophy, and myasthenia gravis involve the slow destruction of the sheath covering the nerve endings—the myelin sheath—which then becomes replaced by scar tissue. We do not know what causes these diseases, but some speculate about a virus that encourages the immune system to kill myelin-producing cells using overzealous killer T cells—an autoimmune reaction. Muscular weakness, pins and needles, coordination impairment, and vertigo all complicate movement and produce intense pain. These diseases can be inherited, and all require professional help. Immune-system abnormalities are often the reason behind neurological breakdowns. Whether under viral, bacterial, or parasitic attack, the immune system must be supported; likewise the hormonal system.

❦ Good food rich in B vitamins and other nerve foods, must predominate. Include whole foods and plenty of water, but absolutely no dairy products or wheat. Herbalist Richard Schulze makes the point that nerve foods like spirulina and nonactive yeasts enter the bloodstream and are used very quickly, with little digestion required. Superfood would be ideal.

🌿 Take evening primrose oil capsules (or any source of GLA) and flaxseed oil capsules.

🌿 Take supportive and immune herbs like Siberian ginseng root and *Pfaffia* root, but do not ingest echinacea root.

🌿 Take nerve tonics, including lobelia leaf, as well as hormone-regulatory herbs (see chapter 9).

🌿 Dr. Richard Schulze uses a formula designed to build, stimulate, and awaken. It contains three parts each of oat straw, skullcap leaf, and St. John's wort flower; two parts each of lavender flower, celery seed, and kola nut; and one part each of coffee beans and lobelia leaf. The coffee in this formula is in stimulative, therapeutic quantities and should be organic; ordinarily it must not be consumed. You can substitute prickly ash bark if you prefer, or use it as well as the coffee — in which case, halve the amount of coffee beans used. Take small amounts initially, as this mixture will not suit everyone. (A few doses will let you know.)

✋ Take hot and cold showers, along with other hydrotherapy and massage.

✋ Liver, kidney, and colon cleanses are absolutely vital (see chapter 6).

MUMPS

Mumps, a viral infection, results from toxic mucus accumulation in the body. It takes two or three weeks to incubate and is usually caught from other children, indicating that your child's immune and glandular systems are a little low or clogged. The infectious time is one day before the glands swell until three days after they have gone down; they can be swollen for three to seven days. The face will look swollen because the glands around the tonsils and the salivary glands are highly inflamed, causing difficulty in swallowing, probably the most uncomfortable symptom.

🍎 Organic vegetable juices, such as carrot, are helpful during the acute attack and during recovery.

🍎 Drink plenty of water, followed by lemon juice and water when the throat pain is over. Take fresh vegetable and fruit juices during the swollen phase and then graduate to salads, raw foods, rice, and lots of garlic.

🖋 You may also like to use the herbal B & B ear formula in chapter 11.

🖋 Internally, a formula that aids the immune system, clears the liver, cleans the blood, and clears the lymph will be needed: use three parts of echinacea root; two parts each of red clover flower, pokeweed root, mullein flower, and cleavers leaf; and one part of lobelia leaf. Separately, mullein flower tea would be excellent.

✋ Frequent gargling is helpful (see the mouth gargle in chapter 11).

✋ A neck oil applied over the affected glands can be comforting: try a mixture of ½ teaspoon lavender, ¼ teaspoon eucalyptus, and ¼ teaspoon tea tree essential oils in a cup of base oil (olive oil is fine); warm it through, then apply and hold over the glands with a muslin cloth. You might add some mullein flower tincture to this hot compress, as it is an excellent lymph decongestant.

MUSCLE CRAMPS

Severe cramps can occur at any time, but they most commonly occur at night. They mainly involve the legs (especially the calf muscles) and feet. Muscle cramps often affect children and adolescents in the form of growing pains. Women also suffer from menstrual cramps. Pregnant women and the elderly also commonly suffer from cramps. They can be caused by many things, including calcium, magnesium, iron, and vitamin E deficiencies; anemia; dehydration; or poor circulation. For some people, cramps indicate a liver or gallbladder problem, so seek out a professional diagnosis if the cramps continue.

🍎 Eat foods rich in calcium and magnesium (see chapter 4); B vitamins, especially B_6; and vitamin E.

🍎 Take herbs and foods rich in iron. For further information, see "Anemia," above.

🖋 Use equal parts of lobelia flower, cramp bark, and pasqueflower tinctures. This combination will quickly relax the individual and reduce the spasms.

🖋 Include herbs that are rich in calcium and magnesium: black cohosh root, boneset leaf, cramp bark, nettle leaf, and red raspberry leaf; add valerian root for the first three nights to induce sleep. Chaste tree berry is also a relaxant and can beneficially balance the hormone system.

✋ Moderate or increased exercise will help, increasing circulation and oxygenation of muscles.

✋ Using a hot water bottle for womb and other cramps can help, or hot and cold showers over the affected areas.

NEPHRITIS AND GLOMERULONEPHRITIS

Nephritis and glomerulonephritis are systemic infections originating in the kidneys. They are very often accompanied by fever, so correct fever treatment is important. I've known dangerously high fevers to rage, in particular with nephritis, and permanent damage to eyesight and other areas may follow if it is not carefully treated with the help of a practitioner. All of these conditions require professional help, but prolonged use of antibiotics invariably makes the situation much worse, and they should be avoided after any initial use. The general recommendation is to rest and relieve the kidneys as much as possible.

- No salt, animal protein, dairy products, tea, coffee, or alcohol should be taken.
- Assess and correct individual nutritional deficiencies.
- Use lots of garlic when you are cooking.
- Plenty of barley water will help, as will nonroasted dandelion tea.
- Avoid sugar, as it encourages bacterial growth. Vegetable and fruit juices, raw foods, steamed vegetables, fruits, and springwater are needed here.
- Follow general guidelines and use herbs for cystitis, along with bearberry leaf and *buchu* leaf made as a tea; however, more personal, professional treatment is advised.
- Kidney cleanses will be vital (see chapter 6).

NOSE PROBLEMS

Along with an increase in asthma and catarrhal buildups as an allergic response to our diets and environmental pollution, blocked noses are also on the increase, often causing long-term and deep-rooted infections. External pollutants like benzine from car exhaust, chlorine gases from swimming, paints, and many others can lead to mucus production becoming extreme. Blocked nasal passages are often inevitable. Also look to a weakened digestive system caused by lack of enzymes and gut flora imbalances as a factor.

- Ensure that your diet is free from junk foods and mucus-producing foods, especially carbonated drinks, sugar, wheat, or dairy products — see chapter 4 for details.
- Eat onions, chives, and garlic, all of which are rich in sulfur.
- Horseradish, raw cayenne, and black pepper will also help.
- Avoid tea, coffee (including decaffeinated versions), chocolate, carbonated drinks, sweets, and cakes. Drink plenty of water.

🍎 Drink juices and eat light foods—rice, steamed vegetables.

🌿 Herbs that help the immune system in general and directly cope with pollen, exhaust fumes, and household irritations are mullein flowers, *Pfaffia* root (suma), gentian root, plantain leaf, barberry root bark, cayenne pod, echinacea root, lobelia leaf and pod, eyebright flower, juniper berry, burdock root, and licorice root.

🌿 Other herbs that help maintain the positive function of the lungs (helping to clear excess mucus and, in turn, to facilitate oxygen replenishment) are chickweed leaf, eucalyptus leaf, licorice root, horehound leaf, and elecampane leaf and flower. Use in equal parts. In the short term, small amounts of coltsfoot leaf can be used.

🌿 Dr. Christopher's B & B ear formula (see chapter 11) can be useful, because release in the ears can often help release the nasal passages.

🌿 Lymph herbs may help to decongest a very clogged system; use three parts mullein flowers, two parts pokeweed root, two parts cleavers leaf, and one part lobelia leaf.

🌿 Use herbal snuff, a mixture of powdered herbs in equal amounts: bayberry root, lobelia leaf, cayenne pod, horseradish root, turmeric root, and mustard seed. Put a tiny amount on the back of the hand and sniff into each nostril in turn. Hold as long as possible, then blow your nose. Repeat procedure twice daily. This mixture is also useful for nasal polyps.

🖐 Essential oil inhalers are helpful: Use one, more, or all of the following: peppermint, eucalyptus, pine, and camphor. Breathe in deeply until the nose feels clearer. An ointment can be made of these inhalant herbs (or bought ready-made) and used over the chest, back, and nasal passages, particularly at nighttime to help with the extra clogging that occurs during this static time.

🖐 Determine what kind of weakened digestive system you have, and treat appropriately—refer to "The Digestive System" in chapter 9.

OSTEOPOROSIS

Osteoporosis is a decrease in bone mass; it affects one-third of all women by the age of seventy. But younger people can be affected as a result of the body being unable to absorb and utilize nutrients properly (or during pregnancy, especially if you become pregnant frequently). Menopause can affect magnesium and calcium levels because of the reduction in estrogen, triggering a loss of bone mass; so pay attention to calcium and magnesium needs from the age of forty. Maintaining healthy level of these minerals will prepare and strengthen you in readiness for menopause, as well as supporting kidney function. A large meat intake will inhibit calcium absorption. Meat also contains large amounts of phosphorus, which ruins the calcium-phosphorus balance by inhibiting calcium levels. Any prolonged cortisone treatment will also take its toll; cortisone inhibits bone formation and decreases absorption of calcium in the stomach. Those with rheumatoid arthritis are often treated with steroids and may suffer from osteoporosis later on.

Early warning signs include broken nails, leg cramps, joint pain, and restless behavior. More advanced cases will exhibit loss of spinal movement and a decrease in height. There are machines able to measure bone density and structure without the use of radiation or a body scan. The test cost is minimal and involves placing your bare foot on a plate that is connected to a computer for data processing. The diagnosis is printed out in two minutes.

- Eat and drink foods rich in calcium and magnesium (refer to chapter 4).
- Cut out coffee and tea.
- Drink superfood on waking and at bedtime.
- Drink nettle leaf tea at bedtime, as bone mass is decreased the most while one sleeps. *Pau d'arco* inner bark also contains high levels of calcium and relieves inflammatory problems, as does black cohosh root.
- Herbs to help maintain hormone levels at menopause include *dong quai* root, chaste tree berry, black cohosh root, wild yam tuber, hop strobilus, fennel seed, and many more.
- Kidney cleanses will help balance calcium and phosphorous levels better, and estrogen output will remain balanced.

Hormone Replacement Therapy has been shown to increase the likelihood of osteoporosis by causing mineral deficiencies that, in turn, promote hormone deficiencies.

OVARIAN CYSTS, UTERINE FIBROIDS, AND CERVICAL POLYPS AND CYSTS

An ovarian cyst develops when an ovarian follicle fails to release an egg as it should. Instead it fills with a clear fluid and becomes saclike and slightly firm. Cysts are, some say, a defense system against serious toxicity or more malignant problems; 89 percent of them are benign. Some even suggest they are more like localized mini livers.

There is a similar view about uterine fibroids (benign tumors), which grow inside or outside the uterus wall. Very often they remain small, but they can grow, in which case they will often become painful and even bleed. If very large, doctors will want to remove them (occasionally they also remove the womb, but this procedure is becoming more unusual). Ranking as the most common female reproductive tumor, fibroids affect one-fifth of all women. They are almost never malignant (cancerous). Most fibroids grow inside a capsule, which acts as a barrier between the uterine wall and the fibroid itself. As they are heavily estrogen-dependent, the intake of estrogen, as with ovarian cysts, must be kept to a minimum.

Cervical cysts and polyps are completely harmless. They are found inside the uterus but can protrude through the cervix and bleed and are best dealt with quickly. They can be treated comparatively simply and effectively, and the bleeding can be stopped with herbs and natural healing.

Polycystic ovaries indicate a hormonal imbalance and are often connected to infertility.

- Decrease all estrogenic food and drink intake, including among others coffee, tea, chocolate, dairy products, and hormone-fed meat.
- Adopt a good food and cleansing program—see the general suggestions for endometriosis, above.
- Take one evening primrose oil capsule (GLA) daily.
- Use herbs to balance the endocrine system and especially ones that tend to be more progestogenic in action, such as chaste tree berry and sarsaparilla root; a more wellrounded formula is also fine.
- Pain or cramping can be alleviated with equal amounts of lobelia leaf and pod, pasqueflower, and cramp bark tinctures, along with castor-oil packs.
- If you are overweight, lose weight, as estrogen is stored in fatty tissue. Weight loss is enhanced by taking GLA and spirulina or superfood.
- Colon, kidney, and liver cleanses will be vital, as these growths indicate sluggishness and congestion.
- Use vaginal pessaries (see chapter 3).
- Have sitz baths and hot and cold showers to encourage blood supply and flow (see chapter 5).
- Exercise to encourage blood supply.

OVERACTIVE THYROID (HYPERTHYROIDISM)

When the thyroid gland overproduces thyroid hormones (as diagnosed by a blood test), the body's metabolism becomes overactive. The general symptoms include irritability, heat, increased perspiration, insomnia, and fatigue; less frequent are increased flow of menstruation, rapid digestion and bowel movements, and malabsorption of nutrients. Goiter can also develop. (Underactive thyroid is discussed below.)

🍎 Ground and support the body with "earthy" foods like barley, rice, millet, quinoa, and all the root vegetables, particularly the sweeter ones like carrot, parsnip, and sweet potato. Also eat plenty of cabbage, brussels sprouts, cauliflower, kale, mustard greens, and watercress to suppress excess thyroid hormone production.

🍎 Try eating six small meals rather than three large meals a day.

🍎 Avoid dairy products and all stimulants, including tea, coffee, and alcohol.

🍎 Avoid seaweeds, particularly bladder wrack and kelp, as they contain iodine which will overprovoke the thyroid.

🌿 The nervous system needs to be treated with sedatives to calm and feed it. Use chamomile flower, skullcap leaf, and even valerian root as a short-term measure. More specific treatments may be needed according to the individual situation.

🌿 Immune-system and adrenal debility is often the cause (or an added problem), so echinacea root and Siberian ginseng root are useful.

🌿 Take hormonal tonic herbs: chaste tree berry for both women and men, or saw palmetto berry for men (or both for both sexes) with fenugreek seed and a little Chinese licorice root.

✋ The liver, colon, and entire endocrine system will need individual assistance and support for overall balance (see "The Thyroid" in chapter 9).

PAINFUL PERIODS (DYSMENORRHEA)

Dysmenorrhea can be initiated by an inadequate calcium and magnesium supply; these are needed to flex and squeeze the uterine wall muscles in order for menstruation to begin. The womb can also be burdened with old toxic and stagnant discharge as a result of poor monthly flow owing to poor circulation or because of inadequate womb peristalsis. The resulting congestion can cause tremendous pain. Often, once a womb has expanded to hold a baby and gone through the huge peristaltic waves needed for childbirth, this problem diminishes. Some women can experience dysmenorrhea for the first time after childbirth, however, because of the huge drop in magnesium and calcium levels associated with pregnancy and breast-feeding. These levels need to be replenished. Occasionally, a uterus is positioned in a way that makes menstruation difficult. This possibility can be considered should all else fail, but the uterus is normally individually aligned and will change alignment throughout one's life. Women age thirty to thirty-five years old may suddenly develop an aching abdomen, legs, and thighs, which may be caused by a congestive buildup. Symptoms include sweating, fever, nausea, fainting, and intense physical pain caused by muscle spasms. Fibroids, endometriosis, hypothyroidism, and other problems should also be considered, and then professionally explored if simple treatments are failing to alleviate the problems.

🍎 You must increase calcium and magnesium intake: include seaweeds like wakame and hijiki, both from the kelp family, to ensure that your physical and nutritional needs in general are met.

🍎 Make sure that your intake of iron and folic acid is adequate.

🌿 Herbs to increase calcium and magnesium include *pau d'arco* inner bark, oat straw, nettle leaf, and Irish moss.

🌿 A useful mix of herbs for spasm, pain relief, and hormone balance includes three parts each of chaste tree berry, squaw vine leaf, *dong quai* root, and cramp bark; two parts each of black cohosh root, nettle root, sarsaparilla root, and blessed thistle leaf and flower; and one part lobelia leaf.

🌿 If you suspect congestion and stagnation in the uterus, use *dong quai* root and cayenne pepper capsules for general circulation.

🌿 Use general hormone balancers like chaste tree berry, sarsaparilla root, squaw vine leaf, and blessed thistle leaf and flower.

✋ Liver, kidney, and bowel cleanses will be vital.

✋ Practice deep breathing at all times, but spend a concentrated twenty minutes doing belly breathing in a warm bath to let go and really relax.

✋ Relax in a warm bath with a few drops of rosemary essential oil.

✋ Exercise regularly to increase circulation and decrease congestion.

✋ Gentle daily exercise should include yoga.

✋ Use a slant board (see chapter 5), or put your feet up as high as you can against a wall.

✋ Put a muslin cloth that has been soaked in chamomile essential oil and sunflower oil over the abdomen underneath a hot water bottle for extra relief.

PALPITATIONS

Palpitations are the erratic or fast beating of the heart. The condition is not necessarily dangerous, but it can be disturbing, especially if it is partially caused by (or occurs in conjunction with) anxiety, stress, anger, or other emotional outbursts. Checking your blood pressure will give you an insight into the effect these palpitations are having, and the results may suggest possible treatment. The condition can also be a symptom of food allergy or candidiasis.

- 🍎 Refer to suggestions under "Heart Disease" for dietary guidance.

- 🍎 Make sure your digestion is good, and if you're not sure, take a teaspoon of cider vinegar three times daily.

- 🌿 If you are feeling undue stress and nervousness, add valerian root and skullcap leaf for a limited period. Stop the valerian after three weeks, but keep using the skullcap for at least three months. Lobelia leaf tincture would also be ideal for any panic moments—take a few drops at a time.

- 🌿 Hawthorn berry would be an ideal herb to use every day as a general heart and circulatory balancer.

- 🌿 If you often feel cold, take cayenne capsules.

- ✋ Massage with lavender, ylang-ylang (grade 1 or 2), peppermint, and rosemary essential oils, or use them in the bath.

PANCREATITIS

Pancreatitis can be associated with alcoholism, trauma, or infection of the biliary tract. The biliary tract and the gallbladder share the same duct, and it is this duct that often causes the problem, especially if the duct is blocked with gallstones. This is by no means always the case, however. Inflammation of the pancreas by the potent digestive enzymes created by the pancreas itself can cause it to attack its own tissues.

- 🍎 Drink vegetable juices, but avoid fruit juices because of their high sugar content.

- 🍎 Drink plenty of water, because dehydration can often be the root cause of this condition.

- 🍎 Eat lots of garlic.

- 🌿 Eat powdered digestive herbs—slippery elm inner bark, meadowsweet leaf, fennel seed, and licorice root.

- 🌿 Long-term herbs for the pancreas include cedar berry (*Juniper monosperma*), fenugreek seed, and licorice root.

- ✋ Perform liver, kidney, and colon cleanses (see chapter 6).

- ✋ Use castor-oil packs directly over the pancreas (see chapter 3).

- ✋ Take hot and cold showers, especially directing the spray over the pancreas.

- ✋ Look at the advice for diabetes for extra tips.

PARKINSON'S AND ALZHEIMER'S DISEASES

Parkinson's is a degenerative disease in which neurotransmitters no longer function properly and motor functions gradually decrease. Alzheimer's disease is a chronic dementia that causes great distress for those around the patient; it is sadly on the increase. The patient becomes forgetful and disoriented, has mood swings, and becomes less and less able to walk, eat, and function normally. Some practitioners feel that the mercury from dental fillings is drastically increasing the risk of Alzheimer's disease. Aluminum from cooking pots and utensils is also suspected to be involved. Another theory is that the brain attacks itself in an overactive and misguided immune response. Mercury, aluminum, pesticides, and processing agents added to food are also felt to contribute. I have reason to believe that the bowel and liver have a huge effect on both of these diseases; when these organs and systems are cleared, I have seen fundamental changes take place.

- Refer to chapter 4 and adopt a good diet, free of foods that will harm the nervous system, such as stimulants like coffee, tea, and sugar. Malnutrition is felt to be a large factor in both Parkinson's and Alzheimer's diseases.

- Nerve foods like soaked oats, nonactive yeast, and spirulina will be important.

- Eat antioxidant foods (see chapter 4).

- Nerve sedatives will help to promote sleep: valerian root in the short term and skullcap leaf in the longer term.

- Nerve relaxants and tonics must become a daily ritual. Use equal amounts of gotu kola herb, vervain leaf, wood betony leaf and flower, lemon balm leaf, lobelia leaf, and St. John's wort flower.

- Time and again it has been shown that using herbal stimulants to treat the shakes experienced by Parkinson's sufferers is effective. In effect, the body needs waking up and rebuilding; refer to "The Nervous System" in chapter 9.

- Intensive cleanses for the kidneys, liver, and colon with the use of juices and organic food will be vital, as clearing the liver and colon helps the brain function more effectively. Many health workers feel that liver toxicity underpins both of these conditions.

- Relaxation methods, together with significant exercise, should be pursued.

- Use deep bodywork, reflexology, and massage.

- Persistent hydrotherapy can be helpful, according to the individual and the caregiver's time and abilities.

PELVIC INFLAMMATORY DISEASE (SALPINGITIS)

Inflammation of the pelvic organs is caused by infection from the uterus, which can sometimes be linked to or result from endometriosis. It may also develop independently. The uterus, ovaries, or fallopian tubes become congested, with fluid retention and puslike secretions. The pain, which can be treated easily if the condition is caught quickly, can become intense, and bleeding can occur. I've had patients who have endured it for years in severe and almost constant pain, sometimes caused in part by abscesses. Some people feel that it can be caused by initial bacterial infections like chlamydia, gonorrhea, and so on. Appendicitis, ectopic pregnancy, intrauterine contraceptive devices, fallopian tube twisting, abortion, gynecological procedures, and the use of tampons can be other causes. Look at the general routine recommended for endometriosis for extra information on diet and lifestyle.

🪶 Use immune herbs like *pau d'arco* inner bark, garlic, echinacea root, barberry root bark, and pine needle tinctures internally.

🪶 For pain and cramping, use equal parts of cramp bark, pasqueflower, lobelia leaf, and valerian root.

🪶 To balance the system, take endocrine herbs and uterine tonics such as chaste tree berry, squaw vine leaf, and wild yam root.

✋ The bowel and liver will be vitally in need of cleansing (see chapter 6).

✋ Make sure the kidneys are well flushed—drink fresh lemon water (this also cleans the bloodstream) and dandelion root tea. Take lymphatic system herbs like cleavers leaf and marigold flower, and consider a kidney cleanse.

POOR CIRCULATION AND CHILBLAINS

Cold hands and feet are quite common. They are really worth working on, rather than leaving them to simply make your life miserable or allowing them to turn into something more troublesome.

🍎 Eat horseradish, the hot English mustards, and gingerroot frequently.

🍎 Refer to the dietary advice for heart disease.

🪶 Take the following herbs in equal amounts: cayenne pod; prickly ash berry, and hawthorn flower, berry, and leaf.

✋ Stop or cut down on smoking.

✋ Exercise frequently.

✋ Take hot and cold showers.

✋ Use a hot ointment or massage oil containing mustard, chile, juniper, pine, cubeb, and rosemary essential oils.

PREMENSTRUAL SYNDROME

The range of symptoms experienced premenstrually is quite alarming: headaches, stomach bloating, breast tenderness, cysts, mastitis, general water retention, cramps, acne, joint aches and pains, depression, irrational anger, oversensitivity, lethargy, extreme tiredness, sugar and chocolate cravings, nausea, and many more.

Premenstrual syndrome (PMS) can often be caused by a congested liver. If the liver is not breaking down excess hormones effectively, transitional stress hormones can linger, making the person irritable, angry, or depressed. It is for these reasons that the liver is often associated with anger. The liver can also contain an excess of hormones that it is supposed to be able to deal with, but cannot for a variety of reasons. In this case, the heat caused by this excess must be purged; dandelion root and milk thistle seed will greatly help. The health of the liver has a strong connection to the female gynecological system. A congested, immobile liver often results in PMS tension and period pains, while a deficiency of cholesterol made in the liver leads to underproduction of progesterone, which is vital for women at this time of the month.

The whole endocrine system needs looking at, especially the estrogen and progesterone balance, along with levels of prolactin, and thyroid and adrenal hormones. Constipation or diarrhea will greatly affect PMS; therefore look for bowel problems.

- Do not eat red meat; all red meat is rich in excessive estrogen. Any other meat consumed should be organic, if possible.
- Include foods containing sulfur, like garlic and onions.
- Decrease intake of cabbage-family foods for one week before your period.
- Follow a wholesome diet, with particular attention to liver foods (see chapter 9).
- Eat plenty of fresh fruits, whole grains, olive oil, and lemon juice.
- No fats (with the exception of olive oil, which is wonderful to use), tea, coffee, alcohol, sugar, or chocolate should be taken.
- Take evening primrose oil capsules, or other sources of GLA.
- Take daily dandelion root and nettle leaf tea with fresh dandelion leaves in salads to meet iron, magnesium, and calcium needs. The dandelion can also be put with other kidney herbs like bearberry leaf and corn silk, made up as a tea, in order to alleviate any water-retention problems.
- General hormone-balancing herbs will be useful throughout the month. Combine equal amounts of the following herbs to make a

tincture: chaste tree berry, sarsaparilla root, black cohosh root, milk thistle seed, blessed thistle leaf and flower, licorice root, nettle leaf, wild yam root, and squaw vine root. Take one teaspoon of the tincture three times daily.

- Ten days prior to menstruation, replace the herbs listed above with herbs that will need to be individually chosen and tailored to your own particular chemistry. However, a general formula to help with many of the premenstrual discomforts and needs could be chaste tree berry, black cohosh root, wild yam root, milk thistle seed, lobelia leaf, red raspberry leaf, and *buchu* leaf.

- A liver cleanse and use of liver herbs should be a primary step, followed by colon and kidney cleanses.

- Exercise consistently but lightly. Avoid taxing physical exercise, and do more walking, dancing, yoga, meditation, and breathing exercises.

- Try special abdominal and pelvic exercises, and perhaps lie on a slant board.

- Take long relaxing baths and get to bed early to conserve energy.

- Hot and cold showers during the month will help, but avoid them just prior to and during menstruation.

PROSTATE ENLARGEMENT

Prostate enlargement is a common problem for men in later life. They experience pain on urination, and the constant urge to urinate can produce fitful sleep and become quite exhausting. One cause can be a bacterial infection invading the prostate. But herbalist James Green tells us it mostly affects men between forty and sixty years old, which suggests a hormonal imbalance or glandular stagnation. Sometimes a dull ache will be felt in the abdominal area, from the prostate pressing into the urethra. Occasionally, blood in the semen or urine is noticeable. Treating the condition quickly is important. If it is left untreated, retained urine that cannot be expelled can eventually cause cystitis or prostatitis as it flows back into the bloodstream, while the pressure on the bladder and kidneys can become very dangerous. The prostate gland is occasionally removed if the problem has been allowed to develop too far without proper attention. If left untreated, the whole prostate could become cancerous.

- Consume plenty of zinc-rich foods, as this mineral normalizes testosterone production. Use sea vegetables, organically grown pumpkin seeds, pumpkins themselves, sunflower seeds, garlic, bell peppers, mushrooms, bilberries, and soybeans.

- Steer absolutely clear of coffee, tea, alcohol, sugar, and refined foods.

🍎 Eat plenty of grains, fresh vegetables, and fruit.

🍎 Drink lots of barley water and water with lemon juice.

🌿 Do not buy cheap zinc tablets. Zinc can boost the immune defenses, but excessive intake in the form of zinc tablets can undermine and impede the immune system. Herbs that are rich in zinc include skullcap leaf, Siberian ginseng root, nettle leaf, and chickweed leaf, all of which can be taken for their general tonic properties.

🌿 A herbal formula that will generally help to balance the hormones and strengthen the kidney and bladder in the long term would be three parts of saw palmetto berry and one part each of damiana leaf, dandelion root, *Rehmannia* root, chickweed leaf, marshmallow root, lobelia leaf, ginkgo leaf, *Astragalus* root, burdock root, parsley leaf, and bearberry leaf. Saw palmetto berries will also help to relax the nervous system.

🌿 To ease inflammation, use tincture or teas of gravel root, hydrangea root, corn silk, and marshmallow root in equal amounts.

🌿 For infection, use garlic cloves and echinacea root.

🖐 James Green also suggests herbal enemas—this is well worth a try, and you can use the herbs mentioned below.

🖐 Some medical practitioners feel that the cause of the enlargement is an accumulation of testosterone in the prostate itself. Using up the testosterone is possibly an answer, so continue sports, sexual activity, and work with zeal, if you can. If the prostate feels hot and unbearably inflamed and urination is a nightmare, use a clay poultice over the area at nighttime. Use equal parts of the following: bentonite clay, slippery elm inner bark, barberry root bark, and lavender leaf and flower powder, with enough castor oil to turn it all into a paste.

🖐 Take regular exercise to increase circulation and oxygen to the area.

🖐 Hot and cold showers will also increase circulation and oxygen to the area.

PSORIASIS

No one knows quite how or why psoriasis appears. Some now believe, however, that it occurs when skin cells are produced about ten times faster than usual. Many practitioners suspect that the thinning of the small intestine's walls can allow poisons to enter into the circulatory and lymphatic systems. Theories as to the cause also include autoimmune conditions, digestive incapability, food allergies, constipation, candidiasis, and immunization. In severe cases, the thickened white, red, and silvery scaly skin (sometimes with yellowish pustules) can be very dry and itchy and constantly flake off.

It can be all over the body, including the scalp, but is most commonly found on the arms, legs, elbows, and knees. Read "Eczema," above, for extra tips.

- One-day, three-day, and five-day fasts should be done as directed by a practitioner, eating only fruits and vegetables appropriate to individual needs. Water intake will be vital at all times.

- Make sure that your hydrochloric acid levels are sufficient, and increase essential fatty acid intake via GLA and olive oil.

- Eat lots of apples, grapes, carrots, and garlic.

- Seaweed should be used both internally and externally, especially if the skin is hot, red, and producing pus.

- For hot skin, cooling foods will help: raw fruits and vegetables, bilberries, celery, grapefruit, spinach, melon, cucumber, and apples are all good.

- For cold skin and low body heat, warming foods will help: raw ginger, chiles, horseradish, garlic, and onion.

- Drink fresh lemon juice in distilled water—it will naturally cleanse and clear.

- Garlic will be one of the prime foods because of its immune-boosting qualities and its sulfur content, which cleans and clears the skin.

- Mahonia root inhibits the growth of skin cells, so bathe the affected areas with a solution of it and also take internally.

- Use equal parts of nettle leaf, echinacea root, lavender leaf and flower, burdock root, gentian root, cleavers leaf, skullcap leaf, red clover flower, barberry root bark, licorice root, sarsaparilla root, dandelion root, pokeweed root, plantain leaf, and yellow dock root as general liver, digestive, and blood cleansers and to provide immune-system support.

- Drink three cups of burdock root tea daily.

- Use three parts skullcap leaf and one part lobelia leaf as a tincture to nourish the nervous system.

- Clean and detoxify the eliminative channels—liver, kidney, and colon (see chapter 6).

- Aloe vera gel is absolutely brilliant at soothing and cooling. It has built-in antimicrobial abilities and is easy to apply from freshly cut leaves, if these are available.

- A seaweed and clay skin treatment is cooling, cleansing, and restorative. Mash bentonite clay powder with dulse and other crumbled seaweeds, then add enough virgin olive oil to make a paste. Apply liberally, and then bandage the area. If the psoriasis is on the scalp, treat during the evening and cover with a cotton bath cap, washing off before bedtime.

- For less severe psoriasis, use plantain leaf and chickweed leaf, along with other herbs, such as mahonia root, marigold flower, and black walnut leaf, in an ointment.

- A dusting powder can help alleviate itching. Use equal amounts of the following powders: lavender leaf and flower, chickweed leaf, marigold flower, yarrow leaf and flower, chamomile flower, and plantain leaf.

- Avoid all ordinary shampoos, and stick to those which are gentle and designed for such conditions or those containing low doses of appropriate essential oils with enriching, soothing, and pH-balanced soaps. Avoid any shampooing when not completely necessary, and do not use soap on the body.

- Skin brush; however, do not brush inflamed, scaling areas, only healthy skin.

- Sweating may give relief, so take saunas, but intersperse them with frequent cold showers, starting on the top of the head.

- Exercise is essential.

- Use clothing and bed linens made from natural fibers.

- Try to make sure no undue stresses and strains exist.

RINGWORM

Ringworm is a surprisingly common skin disease. It is a fungus that causes ring-shaped marks on the skin. Sometimes the middle of the ring heals, but not the outer ring. A common site is the scalp, but sometimes it occurs around the nails. This is the so-called true ringworm, but "dhobie itch" is also a form of ringworm. The name originated in hot tropical monsoon regions; it affects the area of the groin.

- Avoid sugar and yeasts until ringworm has cleared up.

- Drink *pau d'arco* inner bark decoction.

- Use a few of the following: marigold flower, lavender leaf and flower, chickweed leaf, black walnut hull, and other antifungal herbs as powders for dusting affected areas, including the scalp, groin, and nails.

- Keep the areas clean and dry at all times. Kidney cleanses will help clear the skin.

SCIATICA

Though classified as a neurological disease, sciatica is usually caused by poisons collecting in the kinks and pockets of the sigmoid section of the bowel, up to the descending colon and over to the rectal area. The poisons collect in the upper leg area and, in turn, irritate the sciatic nerve, eventually dislocating the sacroiliac joint. The resulting inflammation and pain around the nerves is excruciating. Eventually, muscle wasting will add to the problem.

- A colon cleanse will be a vital first step.
- Adjustment by a chiropractor or osteopath can help.
- Massage will ease the pain.
- Hot and cold showers over the area will help.
- Exercise.

SHINGLES (HERPES ZOSTER)

Shingles is a virus and a close relative of chicken pox. Stress and low immunity are two conspiring contributors that will strongly provoke an episode. It can also be triggered in adults by contact with children who have chicken pox, so if you are run-down and feel low, take care. The virus, once it has set in, can remain for some time if it is not treated. The nervous system, liver, and immune system need the most attention.

- Adopt a good diet—see chapter 4 on food and the "Chicken Pox" section in this chapter. Include plenty of garlic and water.
- Eat liver cleansers like dandelion leaves, globe artichokes, asparagus, olives, and olive oil.
- Ensure that you eat plenty of foods rich in magnesium, calcium, and B vitamins (refer to chapter 4).
- Consume plenty of superfood.
- Take GLA capsules daily (evening primrose oil).
- Take nerve restorative and tonic herbs like Siberian ginseng root, *Astragalus* root, skullcap leaf, vervain leaf, wood betony leaf and flower, and lobelia leaf, all in the long term, and valerian root in the short term.
- Immune-boosting herbs like echinacea root and elderberries will greatly help.
- Use marigold flower, chickweed leaf, and lavender leaf and flower in powder form to dust over the itchy areas.
- Liver, colon, and kidney cleanses prevent recurrences.
- Nourish the nervous system and immune system on a general natural healing level, relaxing and resting as much as possible (see chapter 9).

SINUSITIS

Sinusitis, or inflammation of the nasal sinuses, mainly affects the area around the eyes and either side of the nose. It can also affect the other systems in this area, with excess mucus building up because of allergies or viral or bacterial infection. If you have small sinuses they will clog up more quickly. Symptoms include headaches, earaches, and facial pain.

- Adopt a mucus-free diet, especially cutting out wheat and dairy products. Investigate any food allergies you may have, and address these to balance digestive enzyme action and so on.

- Take acidophilus capsules.

- You need to take small but consistent amounts of lobelia leaf in order to purge the lungs of old tissue, mucus, and other foreign materials. But be careful, as taking too much will cause vomiting.

- General respiratory herbs will help as a daily formula, including horehound leaf, wild cherry bark, mullein leaf, and elecampane leaf and flower. Also take immune-boosting and tonic herbs to help with infection: use equal parts of garlic, echinacea root, thyme leaf, and Siberian ginseng root.

- Inhale steam infused with essential oils like chamomile and lavender. Afterward take a cold shower and eat twelve raw black peppercorns; you will feel cleansed and soothed.

- Put two drops of eucalyptus or lavender essential oil into the bath. Inhale the water into each nostril, and similarly blow out of each nostril. This treatment really clears the nose, and can help first thing in the morning when the mucus blockage is usually at its worst.

- Use herbal snuff (see "Nose Problems," above). Sometimes the problem is so severe and deep-rooted that repeated use of the snuff will be necessary.

- Dr. Christopher's B & B herbal ear formula may be necessary (see chapter 11). Indeed, it may be worth using them even if you do not have earache.

- Avoid decongestants and surgery.

STROKE

Stroke is a very common neurological disorder. It occurs because of a blockage or rupture in a brain blood vessel, and it can affect movement and speech. High-risk people include smokers and those with diabetes, obesity, an excessive alcohol intake, high blood pressure, and high cholesterol. A tendency toward strokes can be genetic, but they can also be directly linked to lifestyle. A change in diet is probably the most important first step in treating or preventing them. Refer to "The Circulatory System" in chapter 9.

- ❧ Lobelia leaf is most effective when used immediately after the stroke and continued for several days afterward. Five drops at the base of the tongue every hour for an adult will be very beneficial.

- ❧ Cayenne pod and prickly ash bark or berry will help circulation (especially to the brain), and long-term use of skullcap leaf to nourish the nervous system will also be beneficial.

- ❧ Other choices of herbs include gingerroot, rosemary leaf, ginkgo leaf, and gotu kola herb. These are all especially helpful for the brain.

- ❧ Take hot and cold showers.

- ❧ Skin brushing will also be beneficial.

- ❧ Other natural healing procedures will help, including massage and all cleanses.

THROAT PROBLEMS—LARYNGITIS, TONSILLITIS, AND PHARYNGITIS

Problems can arise in the throat that are caused by the lungs, sinuses, mouth, ears, or even stomach and bowel. The glands in the neck (below the jawline and up toward the ears) may simply be swollen because of toxic overload from the bowel or allergic reactions in the stomach. The lungs or the whole ear, throat, and nose network may be congested.

Treat laryngitis, tonsillitis, and pharyngitis in basically the same way, paying close attention to the cause as well as easing the symptoms.

Read the sections in this chapter on mumps and mononucleosis, and refer to the sections on swollen glands and mouth gargle in chapter 11, and then combine recommendations as appropriate.

THROMBOSIS, PHLEBITIS, THROMBOPHLEBITIS

Phlebitis is inflammation of veins, while thrombosis is a blood clot. These conditions can be deep or superficial. Phlebitis is the more common and is often caused by pregnancy, standing for long periods of time, a lack of exercise, or smoking. Deep thrombosis is more serious because the veins affected are deep within the muscle. With thrombosis, blood clots can break off and travel around the circulatory system. Circulation and oxygen are impeded by the ensuing blockage, and surrounding organs served by blood vessels may be damaged, depending on where the blockage is. Thrombosis can be a very serious and potentially fatal problem. Occurrence of clots or ruptures in the brain is often referred to as stroke (see above), while in the chest it is known as pulmonary thrombosis (asthma can be an additional factor here).

Deep vein thrombosis often comes with no symptoms and can surprise all concerned; diagnosis can be difficult.

The aim is to clear the vessels, reduce the stickiness of blood platelets that are clumping together, and strengthen the vascular walls through the use of calcium and rutin (the latter a component of buckwheat leaves).

Refer to dietary and herbal advice for heart disease and the circulatory system, because it is crucial that you ensure that you have good circulation. Seek professional advice as well.

- ♥ Exercise and generally engage in sensible activities. For the bedridden, this can be a serious problem, so massage will be vital.

- ♥ If you smoke — *Stop*.

- ♥ If the inflammation or phlebitis itself is visible, use an external poultice made with equal parts of tincture of oak bark, horse chestnut, and comfrey leaf, plus a few drops of lavender essential oil in a little St. John's wort flower oil. It should be used ice-cold, so make the mixture strong, and then put it in the freezer. Apply twice daily for ten minutes. Depending on the cause of the phlebitis, other essential oils could be chosen.

- ♥ Take regular hydrotherapy and use a slant board.

TINNITUS AND MÉNIÈRE'S DISEASE

Tinnitus is a fairly common condition that involves ringing or buzzing in the ears. It may be accompanied by dizziness, nausea, and balance problems. It may develop from an infection, an obstruction, an accident, or excessively noisy environments.

Symptoms of Ménière's syndrome include variable loss of hearing, loss of balance, dizziness, nausea, and vomiting. It is an inner-ear problem affecting one or both ears. Many believe it is rooted in the nervous system, while others believe it is a metabolic imbalance related to hypoglycemia. Others suggest that poor circulation and inadequate blood flow to the brain are to blame. Both conditions are initially treated in exactly the same way. According to the speed of recovery, treatment is either short-term or longer-term, up to nine months.

- 🍎 Maintain or develop a good diet with no dairy or wheat products; eat wholesome, nerve-feeding foods in small but frequent meals. Avoid tea and coffee.

- 🍎 Superfood will be invaluable for keeping good blood sugar levels and supplying plenty of B vitamins.

- 🍎 The ears are associated with the kidneys, so supportive kidney foods will also help (see chapter 4).

🍎 Drink lots of barley water and consume plenty of ginger which improves balance.

🌿 Use equal parts of the following nerve herbs to support and nourish: skullcap leaf, black cohosh root, lobelia leaf, vervain leaf, and passionflower.

🌿 Use Dr. Christopher's B & B ear formula (see chapter 11), which contains nervines, lymphatics, immune stimulants, and antispasmodics. Use the ear drops nightly, then choose other herbs from the recommended list above to use as a regular teas and tinctures.

✋ Colon, kidney, and liver cleanses are vital for long-term treatment.

✋ Hot and cold showers will stimulate the whole head, and the neck in particular.

UNDERACTIVE THYROID (HYPOTHYROIDISM)

A deficiency of thyroid hormones leads to general sluggishness, a sensitivity to the cold, and general low body temperature. It can cause, in particular, cold hands and feet; a slow heart rate; poor and slow digestion and a loss of appetite accompanied by weight gain; painful menstruation and other hormonal problems, sometimes including infertility; constipation, general low immunity; dry skin and hair; thinning eyebrows; and overall fatigue. Goiter may also occur.

🍎 If there is weight gain, still eat three very balanced but light meals a day; include rice, steamed vegetables, fruit, and raw vegetables. Juicing fruits or vegetables is excellent as part of this food program, especially those rich in digestive enzymes.

🍎 Avoid cabbage, brussels sprouts, kale, broccoli, watercress, turnip, cauliflower, and mustard greens, as they suppress thyroid hormone production.

🍎 Gently increase seaweed intake as part of your food program. Bladder wrack and kelp are especially beneficial incorporated into cooking.

🌿 Use three parts Siberian ginseng root, two parts skullcap leaf, and one part lobelia leaf to support the nerves and adrenal glands. Nerve stimulants like celery seed and oat straw will be vital. Take male and female hormones like chaste tree berry and saw palmetto berry. Heart, circulatory, and digestive herbs will be needed. Do not use herbs that sedate the nervous system, like valerian root. Use bladder wrack seaweed as a tincture or capsule to balance the thyroid. If the immune system is low, take echinacea root periodically (see chapter 9).

❦ Take hot and cold showers twice a day, directing the water over the thyroid area (the front of the neck).

❦ Massage, using light strokes.

UNUSUALLY STRONG MENSTRUAL FLOW (MENORRHAGIA)

Occasionally, and always when it's least expected or wanted, one's period can flood. Should the flood be of short duration, there is no problem; but if it continues for days on end, or repeats itself each month, hormone imbalances or displacement of the spine or hip must be considered and professional help sought. Sometimes menorrhagia occurs because there has been no ovulation; then the increased thickening of the uterine wall can cause congestive infection.

Follow the general tips in chapter 8 on menstruation. Professional advice should be sought if the problem persists.

🍎 An increase in dietary iodine is important (take kelp tablets or eat extra seaweed).

🍎 Consume plenty of superfood.

🍎 Keep the diet simple yet supportive, with just whole grains, vegetables, and fruit.

🌿 It is useful to take astringent herbs to stanch the flow. A classic choice would be red raspberry leaf—an astringent rich in iron and calcium. Other herbs would include lady's-mantle leaf, cranesbill leaf, or yarrow leaf. Yarrow is available for picking from spring to late autumn; use it to make a tea.

🌿 To balance the hormones, there are many herb options; an individual choice of plants will probably be necessary. Start with chaste tree berry and squaw vine root.

❦ Don't exercise heavily until the flow has decreased, and keep any water contact gentle and warm.

URETHRITIS

Infection of the urethra needs similar treatment to cystitis, but extra mucilaginous and soothing herbs are usually needed; for instance, increase your intake of marshmallow root.

🍎 Keep your diet simple yet supportive with whole grains, vegetables, and fruits initially.

🍎 Drink plenty of barley water, and water in general.

VAGINAL INFECTIONS — LEUKORRHEA, TRICHOMONIASIS, VAGINITIS, AND OTHERS

Friendly to invaders, the warmth and moisture of the vagina provide the perfect breeding ground for all kinds of undesirables. Tampons, vaginal deodorants, nylon pantyhose, sexual lubricants, dirty hands, and many other factors can tip the balance, causing an infection of some kind, especially if the immune system is a little low. Add to this a poor diet, stress, little exercise, and a congested bowel or sluggish liver, and you have the ideal circumstances for the growth of yeasts, microorganisms, protozoa, and so on. Orthodox medicine generally deals with these problems with the use of sulfa drugs and antibiotics, which do work to a certain extent. They also leave the cause uninvestigated, thereby leaving wide open the possibility of recurrence. Whether it is the white discharge of leukorrhea, the irritation of candidiasis and other yeast infections, or the tenacious bacteria-based trichomoniasis, there are basic rules to bear in mind. Be alert to vaginal itching, red swellings, discharge, and odors.

- Avoid all tea, coffee, cola, juices, alcohol, fruit sodas, sugar, and chocolate — yeasts thrive on them.

- Refined foods and fats should be omitted from the diet, along with nonorganic meats and fish; pesticides and synthetic hormones will not help.

- Refer to chapter 4 and eat well. Eat lots of garlic, and drink copious amounts of water.

- Take lemon juice and apple cider vinegar daily; you can dilute them in water.

- Take acidophilus and rejuvelac (see chapter 4).

- Use equal amounts of endocrine-balancing herbs: chaste tree berry, squaw vine leaf (and other aerial parts), and blessed thistle leaf and flower.

- Use some or all of these plants internally in equal parts: antibacterial or antimicrobial herbs internally like myrrh resin, echinacea root, barberry root bark, arborvitae leaf; and lymphatics like pokeeed root, cleavers leaf, and mullein flower.

- Bowel, liver, and kidney cleanses will be vital, over a period of time.

- Any blood-stained discharge should be reported to a doctor immediately.

- Wear cotton or silk underwear. Nylon pantyhose will retain moisture and produce the environment that infections love; over-the-knee socks and stockings are better, or wear a garter belt. If wearing trousers, stick to natural fibers like cotton, silk, or wool.

♥ Use cotton-based sanitary napkins. Avoid tampons.

♥ Discontinue internal lovemaking until the episode is over.

♥ Use vaginal pessaries (see chapter 3).

♥ Consider vaginal douches using oak bark and other herbs, like oak bark, cranesbill leaf, and *pau d'arco* inner bark.

♥ Make your own garlic vaginal suppositories by wrapping a whole peeled clove of garlic in two pieces of muslin with a pull-out string. Use during the day so that you can remove it if you experience any burning sensation: the delicate tissue of the vagina must not be damaged. Garlic is lethal to yeasts and stubborn bacteria like trichomonas. For further information on garlic, see chapters 4 and 7.

♥ Take only warm baths, and always finish with a cold shower. You must cool the area to discourage bacterial and fungal growth. Add five drops of lavender essential oil and one drop of tea tree essential oil to your bath.

♥ Sitz baths will encourage circulation to the area (see chapter 5).

♥ After the bath, use a herbal vaginal dusting powder or gel (see chapter 3).

VARICOSE VEINS

Veins have the job of assisting the arteries with the job of circulating the blood. If the tiny valves of the inner walls of the veins do not work properly, then blood accumulates and causes stretching and bulging. Varicose veins look lumpy and bluish and can ache and feel sore. They may be the result of constipation, thrombophlebitis, liver disorders, calcium and magnesium deficiencies, heredity, working in jobs that require a lot of standing, habitually sitting with crossed legs, wearing tight clothing, and being pregnant or having borne children, along with poor diet and smoking.

🍎 Refer to "Heart Disease," "Hemorrhoids," and "Thrombosis" for dietary advice on circulatory well-being, and "The Circulatory System" in chapter 9 for general advice.

🌿 Take flaxseed oil capsules (high in omega-3).

🌿 Take natural lecithin, preferably in capsules.

🌿 As a preventive measure, drink two cups daily of a herbal tea made up of equal parts of nettle leaf and ginkgo leaf.

🌿 Take three cayenne capsules three times daily.

- Take a mixture of equal parts lime tree *(Tilia)* flower (a vessel strengthener), prickly ash bark (to stimulate circulation), hawthorn berry and leaf (essential for heart and vascular support), and dandelion root (for water balance).
- Maintain good exercise routines.
- Use cold sitz baths over the legs, and follow warm baths with powerful cold showers.
- Explore and maintain skin brushing.
- Keep your feet above heart level when at rest.
- Massage the affected area using a rub made with equal amounts of oak bark tincture, chestnut tincture, and castor oil. Add half a teaspoon each of witch hazel and cypress essential oils to a cup of the base oil.

WARTS AND VERRUCAS

Warts are small growths found anywhere on the body, including the genitalia. They are caused by a virus and are highly contagious. Warts on the feet are often known as verrucas or plantar warts.

- Include plenty of fresh garlic in your diet.
- Avoid coffee, tea, sweets, and junk food.
- Use general immune-boosting and specific antiviral herbs like echinacea root, *pau d'arco* inner bark, arborvitae leaf, and elderberry. Vary as tinctures, teas, and syrups.
- Repeatedly apply the white juice from dandelion stalks to the affected area.
- Viral verrucas and warts need to be treated specifically to keep ahead of the virus. Apply a threesome of targeted essential oils, using one a week: start with lemon, then tea tree, then bergamot.

WORMS AND AMOEBIC INFESTATIONS

Parasites that live in the intestines are becoming more prevalent, owing to the poor health of factory-produced meats. They are opportunistic creatures and thrive in our modern-day immunally challenged bodies, which have been bombarded with antibiotics and drugs of all kinds. Parasitic threadworm is, and always has been, very common; probably one in five children will have it at some time, but adults also get infestations. More and more children are becoming infested with parasites, particularly after multiple vaccinations because of their overwhelming impact on the immune system. Travel can also lay one open to all kinds of unusual parasites, and parasitic diarrhea is a common occurrence. Intestinal parasites like giardia, ascarids, hookworms, and amoebas are now becoming very common too. They were once associated with visiting foreign climates, but they are becoming increasingly common in developed countries. Tapeworms have always occurred in Britain and the United States, particularly from cooked meat. The problem is that a lot of parasites are active only in hot temperatures, so baths, electric blankets, and saunas will encourage their proliferation. (Testing for them in a pathology laboratory is usually disappointing, because they hibernate in the cold, and at present few laboratories appear to take this into consideration. People are often "tested" for infestations but the stools are not kept hot, which is vital. Thus the organisms die or hibernate, and the results prove negative.) Colonics can give you good feedback on parasitic activity.

🍎 Eat lots of raw garlic, freshly capsulated for children if necessary.

🍎 Avoid clogging, sticky, mucus-forming food when you have an infestation, in particular wheat and dairy products.

🌿 There are many herbs that can be chosen to treat parasites, and they vary according to the type of infestation; but wormwood leaf, black walnut hull, and olive leaf with barberry root bark, cascara sagrada root, and other vital bowel laxatives and liver aids will work. Alongside this mixture, take freshly crushed cloves to kill the eggs.

✋ For more information see chapter 6 and additionally carry out the three-stage herbal colon cleanse.

🖐 In general, colon cleansing and colonics will be vital. Warm to hot water can be used in the colonic, enticing out the parasites with its heat. Colonics are not necessary for children with threadworm, but will be invaluable for those with parasites.

Worming Program

You will need clove capsules plus black or green walnut hull tincture and wormwood leaf tincture combined, half and half, for this program. Capsules filled with crushed cloves need to be taken on an empty stomach; please note too that the cloves must be freshly crushed (with morter and pestle) to act efficiently in killing parasitic eggs.

Capsules should be taken daily according to age and weight; for the average adult, three capsules daily for one to two weeks should suffice. The walnut and wormwood formula should also be taken (in water or juice) daily for one to two weeks—one-half teaspoon, 4 times daily, for adults. Drink chamomile tea daily to soothe the bowel and use bowel herbs (see chapter 6) to make sure the bowel is moving to ensure the disposal of dying or dead worms and parasites.

Cancer and Other "Incurable" or So-Called Terminal Chronic Diseases

Cancer requires a very comprehensive, individualized approach. The whole person will need to be carefully considered on all levels, physically, mentally, and emotionally. Many people should be involved with treatment, not simply one practitioner or just the hospital, but rather a team of practitioners and therapists and a network of friends and caregivers. Certainly, do not self choose herbs; get qualified help.

FOR THE VERY SICK

When there is no time to lose and conventional medicine has pronounced someone terminally ill, a thirty-day natural healing and cleansing program can be undertaken under the guidance of a qualified practitioner, hospital consultants, the patient's own doctor, and a team of two or three assistants or caregivers. Guidance on this routine will be very specific, with many individual considerations.

Herbs to support the body in general will be vital, and those called adaptogens (see chapter 7) will be specifically required. Siberian ginseng root taken as a tincture (one teaspoon three or four times daily) is a very good choice; *Astragalus* root is another. Adaptogens make sure that the body can cope with any incoming stress, helping the body to "adapt" when it is asked to do things, rather than "crash." Optimal adrenal function is vital, and those with low adrenal output due to low levels of corticosteroids will be disadvantaged. Strong adrenal function will help keep a person's weight stable rather than allowing it to fall off, as it often does with cancer. If you experience weight loss, drinking three cups a day of fenugreek seed tea will be very helpful.

Herbs used for cancer are called *neoplastics*, which means that they have a blocking or inhibiting effect on the new growth, or neoplasm. A simple and famous neoplastic is garlic, while others include mistletoe berry, pokeweed root, burdock root, and red clover flower.

Herbs that clean the bloodstream will also be vital for cancer and other chronic diseases, as they support the body through its process of releasing toxins shed from cancerous growths. A blood nourisher and general stimulator, vital for all chronic diseases, is cayenne. It is vital to use very hot cayenne. Herbs with liver-balancing or neoplastic abilities combined, like burdock root, red clover flower, yellow dock root, cleavers leaf, and dandelion root, should be used.

Other foods and herbs will be required to support and nourish the nervous system (see chapter 9).

Immune-system enhancers and lymphatic cleansers like echinacea root, grapefruit seed, olive leaf, barberry root bark, turmeric root, pokeweed root, mullein flowers, and lobelia leaf and seed will be crucial.

Detoxification

All eliminative channels (including the kidney, liver, and bowel) will need to be cleansed and balanced. For this you will need plants like artichoke leaf, milk thistle seed, *Schisandra* berry (vital to optimum liver function), cascara sagrada aged bark, and corn silk. Specific cleansing routines will be essential — see chapter 6.

Other Considerations

Some individual areas will need assessment — for instance, breast cancers will require an increase in progesterone-rich herbs to counteract the estrogen surge that can often cause the cancer. Herbs rich in estrogen, like red clover flower and hop strobilus, will need to be avoided.

The digestive system is a key factor in cases of cancer. This must work efficiently.

Many cancer patients have low hydrochloric acid levels. Therefore, use meadowsweet leaf and other digestives, like gentian root. Food programs, however individualized, will need to be centered on plenty of freshly juiced vegetables — 72 percent carrot juice, with the rest taken from cabbage family vegetables (avoiding beet and beet tops, and avoiding cabbage if certain thyroid conditions exist). In addition, take superfood and raw food in general, especially garlic. Precautions are necessary to ensure that plenty of raw food and juices are eaten and drunk without causing an excess of cold and therefore creating excess mucus, coldness, tiredness, and a less-efficient spleen. Listen to your body; if you overdo anything it will let you know.

Anti-inflammatory assistance for cancer is of vital concern, because inflammation and cancer cell proliferation appear to go hand in hand. Many of the previously mentioned adrenal support herbs will help, but also black cohosh root, chamomile flower, and marshmallow root.

Finally, as a natural bonus, many of the herbs already mentioned are rich in antioxidants, including milk thistle seed, turmeric root, and *Schisandra* berry.

Vaginal and anal suppositories (see chapter 3), poultices, compresses, and castor-oil packs will be vital to deal with the manifestations of the cancers and other diseases, such as tumors and cysts. This drawing-out and healing routine will either pull the toxins up and out to the surface or help flush them through the circulatory and lymphatic systems and finally the bowel. Flower remedies and essential oils will be part of the routine, just as the herbs in their other forms are.

Other requirements will be exercise, acupuncture, massage, reflexology, and lymph drainage and hydrotherapy routines, some of which are very specific to chronic diseases.

Of course, emotional support and therapy with plenty of laughter to encourage the healing process will be vital.

Book List

Common Sense Health and Healing by Dr. Richard Schulze (Santa Monica, California: Natural Healing Publications, 2002)

The Encyclopedia of Medicinal Plants by Andrew Chevallier (London: Dorling Kindersley, 1996)

Healing Colon Disease Naturally by Dr. Richard Schulze (Santa Monica, California: Natural Healing Publications, 2003)

Healing Liver and Gallbladder Disease Naturally by Dr. Richard Schulze (Santa Monica, California: Natural Healing Publications, 2003)

Herbal Healing for Women by Rosemary Gladstar (New York: Simon and Schuster, 1993)

The Male Herbal by James Green (Berkeley, California: Crossing Press, 1991)

The Women's Guide to Herbal Medicine by Carol Rogers (London: Hamish Hamilton, 1995)

Resources

The American Botanical Pharmacy, 411 Glencoe Ave., Marina del Rey, California 90292; tel: 800-Herb-Doc.

Blessed Herbs, 109 Barre Plains Rd., Oakham, Massachusetts 01063.

⇥ 11 ⇤

First Aid

Knowing how to give first aid in emergencies can and does save lives. Herbal remedies have their limitations, and the help of modern medicine should be enlisted for any serious injury or illness. In fact, trauma medicine and trauma surgery are the best kinds of so-called conventional medicine; make sure you call for help if necessary. Take a first-aid course to gain basic skills that can help until professional help arrives.

While following the fundamental rule, Do no harm, you must also accept the principle of calculated risk in first aid. Even if there is some risk, it is right to apply a treatment that will benefit the majority of casualties. You must not, however, use a doubtful treatment just for the sake of doing something.

Emergencies

BEE STINGS

Bee stings are painful and can cause fever and headache, allergic reactions (because of to the body's release of histamine), swelling, redness, and rash. With bee stings, the poison bag may still be attached to the stinger; remove the stinger with tweezers, without damaging the poison bag, then apply freshly crushed plantain leaf, lavender essential oil, or crushed garlic directly on the sting.

A cold chamomile compress made with diluted essential oil could be equally well applied. One undiluted drop of chamomile essential oil can be applied directly to the sting; repeat every few hours (or when irritation occurs) for two or three days. St. John's wort flower oil or tincture is also helpful used topically, as is echinacea root tincture.

BLEEDING

Dr. Christopher, as well as a number of other popular herbalists, have recommended the treating of a bleeding wound with cayenne pepper in order to stop the flow both internally and externally. Other herbs with predominantly styptic qualities are plantain leaf, yarrow leaf, cranesbill (American true geranium) root, slippery elm inner bark, oak bark, and ground ivy *(Glechoma hederacea)*. All these herbs are best used in powder form. Find out the cause of the bleeding and seek appropriate further treatment. For profuse vaginal bleeding that is persistent, try beth root *(Trillium erectum)*, but only under practitioner supervision.

BURNS

Burns can be divided into four groups:

First-degree—affecting the epidermis

Second-degree—involving the dermis (blistering falls into this category)

Third-degree—includes the epidermis, dermis, and underlying tissues

Fourth-degree—down to and including bone

With third- and fourth-degree burns, the pain may be less because there is often a loss of sensation from nerve damage. Third- and fourth-degree burns require immediate medical attention, thus no first-aid measures are provided here. Until medical treatment is obtained, keep the area submersed in cold water to prevent further deterioration of the flesh.

First- and Second-Degree Burns

Initially, some St. John's wort flower oil poured over the burn will ease the nerve pain. Make or buy a burn paste (see "Other Items" in this chapter) and pack the wound with it. The paste will gradually be absorbed during the healing process and should be reapplied when necessary—but do not remove the previous application. The paste will form a soft castlike bandage, but initially a light bandage or covering will be required in addition. The use of burn paste does not require the cleansing of the burned area to clinical standards; there have been no reports of infection with this treatment. It eventually falls off just like a scab that has healed.

EYE INJURY AND TEMPORARY BLINDNESS

An Ayurvedic remedy for eye injuries is simple: freshly squeezed lemon juice mixed into an eye bath. Plantain leaf, eyebright leaf and flower, and chamomile flower, either on their own or combined, are also very useful for treating eye injuries—make as a tea first and wash your eyes with the fluid using an eye bath.

Temporary Blindness Caused by Chemicals or Acids

Flood the eyes with cold water or milk in order to wash away and minimize the effect of the irritant. Follow by carefully placing a tiny amount of cayenne pepper in the eyes; only a very small amount should be used so as not to cause further pain to the eye. Cayenne pepper, as well as being a high-quality healer, is intended as an irritant, causing the eyes to water freely, for tears contain a number of healing factors that can begin to effect repair. The discomfort experienced by using cayenne in the eye is short-lived. (Midstream urine or breast milk can be used to flush out the eye in an emergency.)

GASHES AND LACERATIONS — DEEP WOUNDS

Use a few drops of lobelia leaf and cayenne tincture orally, and then pack with deep wound paste (see "Other Items" at the end of this chapter for a recipe). Renew the paste on a daily basis.

HEATSTROKE AND SUNSTROKE

The onset of these conditions is usually slow and is heralded by a confused feeling, headache, drowsiness, a raised temperature, discomfort in the kidney area, and a lower urine output than expected. The skin appears flushed, hot, and dry. This type of temperature needs to be brought down quickly. Feed plenty of liquids, ideally involving infusions from plants with a high sodium content, such as seaweed, lichen, or licorice root. If mineral salt has to be added, use minimal quantities only.

INSECT AND SPIDER BITES AND STINGS — SERIOUS

Calm the patient. Then immerse the affected area in a bowl of cold water containing ice cubes and a teaspoon of baking powder, which slows the circulation and helps prevent the spread of poison. Alternatively, apply fresh raw onion over the area or cover with wheat germ oil, put an ice pack on top, or apply calendula ointment. This should be done before anything else. Give Dr. Bach Rescue Remedy (a flower remedy available from specialist shops and pharmacies), arnica (a homeopathic remedy), or a few drops of lobelia leaf tincture. Serious allergic reactions need to be treated with cortisone or adrenaline, for which you must seek urgent medical help; administer coffee in the short term. If the patient loses consciousness, apply a few drops of lobelia leaf tincture to the lips. This very often brings them back.

Don't scratch or squeeze the wound, which can encourage infection. Use lavender, tea tree, or rosemary essential oil, or lemon juice. Also apply echinacea root tincture topically. When in natural surroundings, look for plantain leaves and either rub on fresh or prepare as an extra-strong tea (boiled for ten minutes) and apply it to the wound on cotton balls.

INSECT REPELLENTS

Elder leaves and flowers can be bruised and made into a concoction. Applied to the skin it will act as a repellent, but can also be used as a poultice for insect bites. Lemongrass and citronella also make excellent insect repellents.

SHOCK AND FAINTING

Use lobelia leaf tincture; a few drops on the tongue will help in any shock situation, from grief to a car accident. It also helps to revive patients suffering blackouts. The tincture only needs to be rubbed onto the lips in situations in which swallowing or access is limited. Dr. Bach Rescue Remedy will also work well in this situation.

SLEEPLESSNESS WITH EXTREMELY SHOCKED OR EXHAUSTED NERVES

To ensure good sleep, use valerian root tincture or capsules (an average adult dose) three hours before bedtime and then more just prior to retiring. More can be taken if waking in the night is a problem but a two-hour interval should have elapsed since the bedtime dose. This treatment can be used for a week or more but real nerve building is also required; for this, use skullcap leaf, chamomile flower, lime tree *(Tilia)* flower, and lobelia leaf long-term.

SNAKEBITES

Lavender has a long history of use against the venom produced by the European adder; however, lavender essential oil and echinacea root tincture applied externally together are more effective. Echinacea root should also be administered by mouth as a tincture in frequent doses. Echinacea root for bites by rattlesnake, copperhead, cottonmouth, and the Florida coral snake has also been used for centuries in Canada and the United States. Additionally, just a few drops of lobelia leaf tincture applied both topically and internally will help keep the body from going into anaphylactic shock. Do not suck the bite—any injury in the mouth would become contaminated; filled teeth can also harbor the venom and may cause the jaw to swell to an enormous size. You can buy antivenom treatments at pharmacies and camping stores. The shape of the snake's eyes can give a rough indication of its type: round-eyed snakes are nonpoisonous, but snakes with elongated eyes are poisonous.

UNCONSCIOUSNESS

Apply a few drops of lobelia leaf tincture and Dr. Bach Rescue Remedy to the lips and wrists. If the patient does not regain consciousness within three minutes, call for an ambulance.

WASP STINGS

For wasp stings, which are alkaline, it is best to neutralize the sting with cider vinegar or lemon juice first. Then treat with applications of lavender and chamomile essential oils for two or three days.

Nonemergencies

This is a brief outline of some of the more frequent everyday problems you may encounter, with suggestions on how relief may be obtained by herbal and other methods.

BLISTERS

Apply one drop each of undiluted lavender and chamomile essential oils. Apply gently and rub in thoroughly. Or use lavender spray, followed by finely powdered myrrh, and cover with a padded adhesive bandage.

BRUISES

Apply hot and cold packs to increase the circulation. Follow with applications of comfrey leaf ointment, to which calendula flower, hyssop leaf, or plantain leaf could be added. These herbs can equally well be made into a poultice. Tincture of arnica (*Arnica montana*) flower and marigold flower, applied directly to the bruise several times a day, can be equally soothing. ***Do not ingest arnica in any form, as it is poisonous if taken internally.*** St. John's wort oil would also be a good alternative.

CHILBLAINS

Chilblains are caused by poor circulation. I have heard many a tale of traditional remedies—including cayenne pepper in the socks and onions in the stockings—and they all seem to work. But ultimately you need to work on the problem internally, which means investigating the reasons for your poor circulation (see "The Circulatory System" in chapter 9).

DIARRHEA, STOMACH ULCERS, BOWEL PAIN, AND OTHER DIGESTIVE DISORDERS

Mix slippery elm inner bark or arrowroot with cold water into a drinkable gruel. This is excellent as a convalescence food too.

INFECTION OF A DEEP CUT OR WOUND

Use echinacea root, because when each dose it is ingested, the white blood cell count will increase dramatically. The best course of treatment is to take it for ten days, have four days off, and then, if necessary, continue with another ten-day course. In the first few days you can take half-hourly doses of ten drops of tincture, and this dosage can be reduced as you feel better. Echinacea root can also be very effective when put directly on an infected cut. If you do not have any echinacea, use something like garlic and turmeric, which can be very effective when made into a paste, added to mashed potato, and applied directly to a wound. You should also eat some! Chamomile flower tea will also help because of its antimicrobial qualities.

SPRAINS AND STRAINS

Use a cold compress soaked in a strong decoction made from all or some of the following herbs: gingerroot, thyme leaf, lavender leaf, marigold flower, St. John's wort flower, plantain leaf, and chamomile flower. This compress will reduce swelling. Alternatively, soak the affected area in a hot decoction made from chamomile flower, comfrey leaf, rosemary leaf, and wormwood leaf. Alternate this treatment with cold soaks and rub the area with trauma oil (see the formula under "Other Items" at the end of this chapter).

TOOTHACHE

Make an immediate appointment to see the dentist. Meanwhile, chew a clove for a while and then spit it out, or put a little clove oil on a cotton ball and gently apply to the affected area. Take echinacea root tea or tincture, in case an abscess has begun to form. Frequently gargle with herbal mouthwash containing oak bark, myrrh resin, and St. John's wort flower (see "Other Items" at the end of in this chapter).

Contents of a First-Aid Kit

MATERIALS

- a selection of bandages: at least four elasticized, four crepe, tubular bandages with applicator, and gauze of various sizes
- a selection of sterile dressings
- plastic wrap
- cotton pads: bandages can be made using cotton pads and open-weave or gauze strips
- dental mirror
- dextrose tablets
- eye bath and small mixing container
- first-aid manual
- flashlight
- hot and cold packs — available from drugstores
- magnifying glass
- notepad and pencil
- plasters and butterfly stitches (homemade or purchased slim pieces of sticky, bandage tape that act as stitches)

- plastic gloves or disposable gloves (to wear when dressing wounds and handling waste)
- pointed and flat tweezers
- rubbing alcohol
- safety pins and clips for securing bandages
- scalpel
- scissors
- selection of sterile dressings
- space blanket (or a wool blanket if there is room), or an insulated plastic survival bag
- tape
- triangular bandages
- venom remover
- whistle
- wooden spatula

Bandaging primarily protects and supports, but it can also be used to apply pressure, thus arresting bleeding. It can support a fracture, help with pain control, and give psychological relief. The actual technique of bandaging is a vast subject and has been more than adequately covered in any number of first-aid and survival manuals often available in normal book stores and camping shops.

HERBAL FIRST-AID ITEMS

All items must be labeled clearly. All items except tinctures should be in plastic containers.

- 1 teaspoon cayenne pepper tincture—for bleeding, shock, and cold
- 5 teaspoons echinacea root tincture—topical and internal use for bites, cuts, and so on
- 1 teaspoon lobelia leaf tincture—for shock
- Dr. Bach Rescue Remedy—for shock
- 1 teaspoon St. John's wort flower tincture—for toothache, bruises, cuts, and trauma in general
- codeine—for pain killing
- 3 teaspoons coffee tincture—for alcohol poisoning and other situations in which a nerve stimulant is necessary; prickly ash bark tincture will work in a similar way
- colon capsules—both strong and mild

- slippery elm inner bark powder—for diarrhea, or use bentonite clay for serious diarrhea
- fresh juniper berries—for those unable to urinate
- 3 to 5 teaspoons of a formula of five parts hawthorn leaf tincture and one part cayenne tincture as a heart attack tonic
- 3 to 5 teaspoons of a formula of one part valerian root tincture and one part lobelia leaf—as a nerve sedative
- 5 teaspoons of a formula of 3 teaspoons chaste tree berry tincture and 2 teaspoons cramp bark tincture—for premenstrual symptoms, cramps, and so on

Lobelia and Cayenne Pepper

LOBELIA (*LOBELIA INFLATA*)

Lobelia (often known as Indian tobacco in the United States) is one of the most useful systemic relaxants available to us. It has a general depressant action on the central and autonomic nervous systems and on neuromuscular action. Lobelia contains alkaloids called pyridine and piperidine—these act to stimulate and then to block autonomic nervous activity. It is very useful in a first-aid situation for shock and trauma. It may be used in many conditions and in combination with other herbs to further its effectiveness.

It is specifically used for bronchial asthma and bronchitis. Lobelia is a powerful respiratory stimulant, while the chemical isolobelinine found in lobelia is an emetic and respiratory stimulant, which will stimulate catarrhal secretion and expectoration while relaxing the muscles of the respiratory system. The overall action is a truly holistic combination of stimulation and relaxation. It can be used for any internal or external situation, a few drops in most cases being sufficient. This dosage comes nowhere near the dose allowed by the FDA and MHRA; a little goes a long way.

CAYENNE PEPPER (*CAPSICUM ANNUUM*)

Cayenne pepper is unsurpassed in its effect on the circulatory system. Cayenne is a herb that everyone should have in tincture or powder form, in the kitchen, the bathroom, and the car. As a prime first-aid measure it will prevent fainting or loss of consciousness, as it keeps the blood supply constant; yet it will not allow damaged arteries to lose dangerous quantities of blood, as it also assists blood clotting in certain circumstances. Cayenne pepper stops bleeding immediately, and its high level of vitamins A and C also cleans and disinfects.

It may be used both internally and externally (though caution should be observed when causing pain to open wounds in shocked or fragile patients).

Other Items

Burn paste (also for sprains and wounds): made from herb powders of eight parts comfrey leaf and flower, four parts slippery elm inner bark, four parts lobelia leaf and pod, one part lavender leaf and flower, and one part bentonite clay. Store the ingredients separately and mix when needed in a base of equal parts honey, wheat germ oil, and aloe vera gel. Spread evenly over the area and leave on, simply adding more to it as required.

Digestive and travel tincture: combine equal parts of tinctures of ginger-root, fennel seed, and peppermint leaf. Take drops as needed.

Mallow and walnut ointment (Dr. Christopher's bone, flesh, and cartilage formula): made from powdered herbs of six parts oak bark, three parts gravel root, three parts mullein leaf, three parts marshmallow root, three parts black walnut bark and leaf, two parts wormwood leaf, one part lobelia leaf, one part skullcap leaf, and one part comfrey leaf. See "Ointments" in chapter 3. This formula is useful for regeneration of tendons, ligaments, bone, and flesh.

Dr. Christopher's B & B ear formula: made from equal parts of garlic bulb and mullein flower oil, blue cohosh root, black cohosh root, vervain leaf, skullcap leaf, and lobelia leaf. Fill an eyedropper with the formula and hold it under warm running water for one minute. Insert eight to twelve drops of the warmed oil into each ear at night. Then plug the ears with cotton balls. Keep the plugs in overnight. If you prefer, use the drops only occasionally, gradually building up to every night, or every other night. Flush the ears out with equal amounts of warm water and cider vinegar the morning after each treatment. If you continue the treatment for longer than five or six weeks without results, go to your doctor or to an outpatient clinic at a hospital and get a nurse to syringe your ears out professionally.

Dr. Christopher's antimiscarriage formula: made from three parts Solomon's seal root and one part lobelia leaf. Get plenty of bed rest and drink tea made from these herbs at regular intervals: drink half a cup of tea or take ten drops of tincture at hourly intervals until the bleeding stops. Follow with a half dose every two hours for the next twenty-four hours. Seek medical advice.

Dr. Schulze's deep tissue oil: made from wintergreen essential oil, menthol crystals, arnica flower, St. John's wort flower, chile oil, and marigold flower in a base of olive oil.

Marigold and comfrey ointment (general healing salve): made from equal parts (two ounces each) of marigold flower, comfrey root, lobelia leaf, plantain leaf, thyme leaf, lavender leaf and flower, and turmeric rhizome. Useful as a first-aid measure for cuts and abrasions. See "Ointments" in chapter 3.

Trauma oil or ointment: this contains arnica flower oil, St. John's wort flower, and marigold flower oil. Mix equal parts of each in a base of organic virgin cold-pressed olive oil.

Plantain and barberry ointment (eczema ointment): equal parts (two ounces each) black walnut hull, barberry root, chickweed leaf, plantain leaf, marigold flower, and lavender essential oil. Useful in the treatment of eczema and similar skin conditions; see "Ointments" in chapter 3.

Healing and antiseptic ointment: use barberry root, marigold flower, and thyme leaf or flowers, mixing equal parts in an olive oil and beeswax base. See "Ointments" in chapter 3.

Herbal cast or deep wound paste: made from equal parts of comfrey root, marshmallow root, slippery elm bark, and turmeric rhizome powders. Make into a workable paste with olive oil and lavender essential oil. Pack into the wound and bandage. Do not worry about cleaning out the paste; it will grow into and become the new tissue—simply add more if any comes away when bathing. See "Ointments" in chapter 3.

Herbal snuff: made from equal amounts of powdered bayberry root, mustard seed, horseradish root, lobelia leaf, turmeric root, and cayenne pod. For further details, see "Nose Problems" in chapter 10.

Insect repellent: made from two parts lemongrass, one part thyme leaf, one part lavender leaf and flower, and one part peppermint leaf mixed with wheat germ oil.

Lavender spray for burns and bites: one cup distilled water and half a teaspoon lavender essential oil.

Mouth gargle: use for a sore throat, inflamed mouth, painful tonsils, or abscesses. Gargle three times daily with a mixture of two cups springwater, with three-quarters cup each cranesbill tincture, barberry root bark tincture, fennel seed tincture, myrrh tincture, yarrow leaf tincture, and peppermint leaf tincture. Choose two or three of the following essential oils and add two or three drops of each: cinnamon, sweet fennel, sage, thyme, angelica, tea tree, myrrh, or rosemary. Only a qualified herbalist should make up this formula because of the oral use of essential oils. Store in a dark cupboard.

Pain and headache: a tincture of willow bark, wild lettuce juice, feverfew leaf, meadowsweet leaf and flower, St. John's wort flower, and lavender leaf and flower. Take one teaspoon hourly. California poppy tincture can also be added for extra pain relief.

Swollen glands: use three parts mullein leaf and one part lobelia leaf in tea, tincture, or powder form during or after the first bout of swollen glands; take one teaspoon three times daily. If the throat, in particular, is painful, use tinctures of four parts echinacea root, two parts red clover flower, two parts sage leaf, two parts barberry root bark, two parts myrrh resin, and one part Siberian ginseng root . Take one teaspoon, three times daily, for ten days.

Book List

The Encyclopedia of Medicinal Plants by Andrew Chevallier (London: Dorling Kindersley, 1996)

The Herbal Medicine-Maker's Handbook by James Green (Berkeley, California: The Crossing Press, 2000)

Tom Brown's Field Guide to Wilderness Survival by Tom Brown Jr. (New York: Berkeley Books, 1983)

⇥ Appendix 1 ⇤
English to Latin Translation and Parts of the Herb to Use

COMMON NAME	PART	BOTANICAL NAME
Agrimony	herb	*Agrimonia eupatoria*
Aloe	leaf, gel	*Aloe ferox, Aloe barbadensis*
Angelica	root	*Angelica archangelica*
Apple	pectin	*Malus pumila*
Arborvitae (thuja)	leaf, seed	*Thuja occidentalis*
Artichoke	leaf	*Cynara scolymus*
Astragalus (milk vetch)	root	*Astragalus* (various species)
Balm of Gilead	bud, resin	*Populus* (various species)
Barberry	root bark	*Berberis vulgaris*
Bearberry (manzanita)	leaf	*Arctostaphylos uva-ursi*
Black cohosh	root	*Actaea racemosa*
Black pepper	seed	*Piper nigrum*
Black walnut	hull, leaf	*Juglans nigra*
Bladder wrack	seaweed	*Fucus vesiculosus*
Blessed thistle (holy thistle)	leaf, flower	*Cnicus benedictus*
Boneset	leaf	*Eupatorium perfoliatum*
Buchu	leaf	*Agathosma betulina*
Bupleurum	root, leaf	*Bupleurum chinense*
Burdock	seed, root	*Arctium lappa*
Butternut	bark	*Juglans cinerea*
Cascara sagrada	aged bark	*Rhamnus purshiana*
Catnip (catmint)	leaf, flower	*Nepeta cataria*
Cayenne pepper	pod	*Capsicum annuum*
Celery	seed	*Apium graveolens*
Chamomile, German	flower	*Matricaria recutita*
Chamomile, Roman	flower	*Chamaemelum nobile* (formerly *Anthemis nobilis*)
Chaste tree (agnus castus)	berry	*Vitex agnus-castus*
Chickweed	leaf	*Stellaria media*
Cleavers	leaf	*Galium aparine*
Clove	bud	*Syzygium aromaticum*
Coltsfoot	leaf	*Tussilago farfara*

COMMON NAME	PART	BOTANICAL NAME
Comfrey	leaf	*Symphytum officinale*
Corn	silk	*Zea mays*
Cramp bark	bark	*Viburnum opulus*
Cranesbill (American true geranium)	root	*Geranium maculatum*
Damiana	leaf	*Turnera diffusa*
Dandelion	root, leaf, flower	*Taraxacum officinale*
Dong quai	root	*Angelica sinensis*
Echinacea	root, flower, leaf	*Echinacea angustifolia*
Elder	berry, flower, leaf, bark	*Sambucus nigra*
Elecampane	root, leaf, flower	*Inula helenium*
Eucalyptus	leaf	*Eucalyptus* (various species)
Eyebright	leaf, flower	*Euphrasia officinalis*
Fennel	seed	*Foeniculum vulgare*
Fenugreek	seed	*Trigonella foenum-graecum*
Feverfew	leaf	*Chrysanthemum parthenium*
Figwort	root	*Scrophularia nodosa*
Flax	seed	*Linum usitatissimum*
Gentian	root	*Gentiana lutea*
Ginger	rhizome	*Zingiber officinale*
Ginkgo	leaf	*Ginkgo biloba*
Ginseng, American	root	*Panax quinquefolius*
Ginseng, Chinese white (ren shen)	root	*Panax ginseng*
Goldenseal	root	*Hydrastis canadensis*
Gotu kola	herb	*Centella asiatica*
Gravel root (joe-pye weed)	root	*Eupatorium purpureum*
Hawthorn	berry, flower, leaf	*Crataegus laevigata*
Hibiscus	flower	*Hibiscus sabdaritta*
Hop	flower (strobilus)	*Humulus lupulus*
Horehound	flower, leaf	*Ballota nigra, Marrubium vulgare*
Horse chestnut	fruit, bark	*Aesculus hippocastanum*
Horseradish	root	*Armoracia rusticana*
Horsetail	leaf	*Equisetum arvense*
Hydrangea	root	*Hydrangea arborescens*

COMMON NAME	PART	BOTANICAL NAME
Juniper	leaf, berry	*Juniperus communis*
Kola	nut	*Cola acuminata*
Lady's-Mantle	leaf	*Alchemilla vulgaris*
Lavender	flower, leaf	*Lavandula angustifolia*
Lemon balm	leaf	*Melissa officinalis*
Licorice	root	*Glycyrrhiza glabra*
Licorice, Chinese	root	*Glycyrrhiza uralensis*
Lime tree, (linden)	flower	*Tilia europaea*
Lobelia (Indian tobacco)	flower, leaf, seed, pod	*Lobelia inflata*
Mahonia (Oregon grape)	root, root bark, berry	*Mahonia aquifolium*
Marigold	flower	*Calendula officinalis*
Marshmallow	root	*Althaea officinalis*
Meadowsweet	leaf, flower	*Filipendula ulmaria*
Milk thistle	seed	*Silybum marianum*
Mistletoe/American mistletoe	leaf, berry	*Viscum album/ Phoradendron serotinum*
Motherwort	leaf	*Leonurus cardiaca*
Mugwort	leaf	*Artemisia vulgaris*
Mullein	leaf, flower	*Verbascum thapsus* (and other species)
Mustard	seed	*Brassica hirta, Brassica nigra*
Myrrh	resin	*Commiphora myrrha*
Neem tree (nim)	seed, leaf	*Azadirachta indica*
Nettle	leaf, root	*Urtica dioica*
Oak	bark, gall, twig	*Quercus* (various species)
Olive	leaf, fruit	*Olea europaea*
Parsley	root, leaf	*Petroselinum crispum*
Pasqueflower	flower	*Anemone pulsatilla*
Passionflower	leaf, flower	*Passiflora incarnata*
Pau d'arco (lapacho)	inner bark	*Tabebuia impetiginosa*
Pennyroyal	leaf	*Mentha pulegium*
Peppermint/spearmint	leaf	*Mentha × piperita/Mentha spicata*
Pfaffia (suma)	root, bark	*Pfaffia paniculata*
Pine	resin, needle	*Pinus* (various species)
Plantain	leaf, juice	*Plantago major*
Pokeweed	root	*Phytolacca americana*

COMMON NAME	PART	BOTANICAL NAME
Prickly ash	berry, bark	*Zanthoxylum americanum*
Psyllium	husk	*Plantago psyllium*
Pumpkin	seed	*Cucurbita pepo*
Red clover	flower	*Trifolium pratense*
Red raspberry (framboise)	leaf	*Rubus idaeus*
Rehmannia	root	*Rehmannia glutinosa*
Rhubarb, Chinese	root	*Rheum palmatum*
Rosemary	leaf, flower	*Rosmarinus officinalis*
Sage	leaf	*Salvia officinalis*
St. John's wort	flower, top leaves	*Hypericum perforatum*
Sarsaparilla	root	*Smilax officinalis*
Saw palmetto	berry	*Serenoa repens*
Schisandra (magnolia vine)	berry	*Schisandra chinensis*
Senna	leaf, pod, root	*Cassia* (various species)
Siberian ginseng	root	*Eleutherococcus senticosus*
Skullcap	leaf	*Scutellaria lateriflora*
Slippery elm	inner bark	*Ulmus fulva*
Sphagnum moss	herb	*Sphagnum* (various species)
Squaw vine	leaf (and all aerial parts)	*Mitchella repens*
Tea tree	oil	*Melaleuca alternifolia* (and other species)
Thyme	leaf	*Thymus vulgaris*
Turmeric	rhizome	*Curcuma domestica* and *longa*
Usnea	whole plant	*Usnea longissima*
Valerian	root	*Valeriana officinalis*
Vervain	leaf, flower	*Verbena officinalis*
Wild cherry	bark	*Prunus serotina*
Wild lettuce	leaf	*Lactuca virosa*
Wild oats	seed, top leaves	*Avena sativa*
Wild yam	root	*Dioscorea villosa*
Willow	bark	*Salix alba*
Wood betony	leaf, flower	*Stachys officinalis*
Wormwood	leaf	*Artemisia absinthium*
Yarrow	leaf, flower	*Achillea millefolium*
Yellow dock	root	*Rumex crispus*

❧ Appendix 2 ❦
Latin to English Translation

BOTANICAL NAME	COMMON NAME
Achillea millefolium	Yarrow
Actaea racemosa	Black cohosh
Aesculus hippo castranum	Horse chestnut
Agathosma betulina	*Buchu*
Agrimonia eupatoria	Agrimony
Alchemilla vulgaris	Lady's-mantle
Aloe ferox, Aloe barbadensis	Aloe
Althea officinalis	Marshmallow
Anemone pulsatilla	Pasqueflower
Angelica archangelica	Angelica
Angelica sinensis	*Dong quai*
Apium graveolens	Celery
Arctium lappa	Burdock
Arctostaphylos uva-ursi	Bearberry (uva ursi, manzanita)
Armoracia rusticana	Horseradish
Artemisia absinthium	Wormwood
Artemisia vulgaris	Mugwort
Astragalus (various species)	Milk vetch
Avena sativa	Wild oats
Azadirachta indica	Neem tree (nim)
Ballota nigra	Black horehound
Berberis vulgaris	Barberry
Brassica hirta, Brassica nigra	Mustard
Bupleurum chinense	*Bupleurum*
Calendula officinalis	Marigold
Capsicum annuum	Cayenne pepper
Cassia (various species)	Senna
Centella asiatica	Gotu kola
Chamaemelum nobile	Chamomile, Roman
Chrysanthemum parthenium	Feverfew
Cnicus benedictus	Blessed thistle (holy thistle)
Cola acuminata	Kola
Commiphora myrrha	Myrrh

BOTANICAL NAME	COMMON NAME
Crataegus laevigata	Hawthorn
Cucurbita pepo	Pumpkin
Curcuma domestica and *longa*	Turmeric
Cynara scolymus	Artichoke
Dioscorea villosa	Wild yam
Echinacea angustifolia	Echinacea
Eleutherococcus senticosus	Siberian ginseng
Equisetum arvense	Horsetail
Eucalyptus (various species)	Eucalyptus
Eupatorium perfoliatum	Boneset
Eupatorium purpureum	Gravel root (joe-pye weed)
Euphrasia officinalis	Eyebright
Filipendula ulmaria	Meadowsweet
Foeniculum vulgare	Fennel
Fucus vesiculosus	Bladder wrack
Galium aparine	Cleavers
Gentiana lutea	Gentian
Geranium maculatum	Cranesbill (American true geranium)
Ginkgo biloba	Ginkgo
Glycyrrhiza glabra	Licorice
Glycyrrhiza uralensis	Licorice, Chinese
Hibiscus sabdaritta	Hibiscus
Humulus lupulus	Hop
Hydrangea arborescens	Hydrangea
Hydrastis canadensis	Goldenseal
Hypericum perforatum	St. John's wort
Inula helenium	Elecampane
Juglans cinerea	Butternut
Juglans nigra	Black walnut
Juniperus communis	Juniper
Lactuca virosa	Wild lettuce
Lavandula angustifolia	Lavender
Leonurus cardiaca	Motherwort
Linum usitatissimum	Flax
Lobelia inflata	Lobelia (Indian tobacco)
Mahonia aquifolium or *Berberis aquifolium*	Mahonia (Oregon grape)
Malus pumila	Apple

BOTANICAL NAME	COMMON NAME
Marrubium vulgare	White horehound
Matricaria recutita	Chamomile, German
Melaleuca alternifolia (and other species)	Tea tree
Melissa officinalis	Lemon balm
Mentha × piperita/Mentha spicata	Peppermint/spearmint
Mentha pulegium	Pennyroyal
Mitchella repens	Squaw vine
Nepeta cataria	Catnip (catmint)
Olea europaea	Olive
Panax ginseng	Ginseng, Chinese white (ren shen)
Panax quinquefolius	Ginseng, American
Passiflora incarnata	Passionflower
Petroselinum crispum	Parsley
Pfaffia paniculata	*Pfaffia* (suma)
Phytolacca americana	Pokeweed
Pinus (various species)	Pine
Piper nigrum	Black pepper
Plantago major	Plantain
Plantago psyllium	Psyllium
Populus (various species)	Balm of Gilead
Prunus serotina	Wild cherry
Quercus (various species)	Oak
Rehmannia glutinosa	*Rehmannia*
Rhamnus purshiana	Cascara sagrada
Rheum palmatum	Rhubarb, Chinese
Rosmarinus officinalis	Rosemary
Rubus idaeus	Red raspberry (framboise)
Rumex crispus	Yellow dock
Salix alba	Willow
Salvia officinalis	Sage
Sambucus nigra	Elder
Schisandra chinensis	*Schisandra* (magnolia vine)
Scutellaria lateriflora	Skullcap
Serenoa repens	Saw palmetto
Silybum marianum	Milk thistle
Smilax officinalis	Sarsaparilla
Sphagnum (various species)	Sphagnum Moss

BOTANICAL NAME	COMMON NAME
Stachys officinalis	Wood betony
Stellaria media	Chickweed
Symphytum officinale	Comfrey
Syzygium aromaticum	Clove
Tabebuia impetiginosa	*Pau d'arco*
Taraxacum officinale	Dandelion
Thuja occidentalis	Arborvitae (thuja)
Thymus vulgaris	Thyme
Tilia × *europea*	Lime tree (linden)
Trifolium pratense	Red clover
Trigonella foenum-graecum	Fenugreek
Turnera diffusa	Damiana
Tussilago farfara	Coltsfoot
Ulmus fulva	Slippery elm
Urtica dioica	Nettle
Usnea longissima	Usnea
Valeriana officinalis	Valerian
Verbascum thapsus (and other species)	Mullein
Verbena officinalis	Vervain
Viburnum opulus	Cramp bark
Vitex agnus-castus	Chaste tree (agnus castus)
Zanthoxylum americanum	Prickly ash
Zea mays	Corn
Zingiber officinale	Ginger

❧ Appendix 3 ❧
How to Make a Herbal Profile

Making a herbal profile of your own can be a worthwhile and enjoyable experience. It will ultimately give you a deep understanding of a dozen or so herbs that grow near your home. With them, you will be able to treat many commonly experienced diseases or, preferably, learn how to help resist their manifestation in the first place. Some ideal choices in Britain would be oak, apple, yarrow, plantain, nettle, hawthorn, red clover, dandelion, and burdock. Only choose the very common ones, or you will defeat the main purpose of the herbal profile.

A ring binder, with clear plastic sheaths to protect pictures and writing alike, will be useful. Photograph, paint, draw (using color), or freshly press the herb.

You can buy a flower press or make your own from particle board, rigid poles, and wing nuts with cardstock and blotting paper. A press is ideal for keeping at home, but too bulky to take out into the field, except by car. If you want to make your own large but more portable flower press, construct it to the herbarium size of approximately 17 by 11 inches, and make it with 1¼-inch squares using ¾-inch slatted wood. To create layers, you will require quantities of blotting paper with paper towel and cardstock. To tighten your press, you will need to use fixed Velcro luggage straps (or something like a horse girth with clasps, capable of expanding to any width, is ideal). Small or large numbers of plant specimens may have to be accommodated at times in the press, so this ability to open, close, tighten, and loosen is vital.

When you first harvest your plant, thank it, then shake off any excess water or dew. When it is dry, place it carefully and with consideration as to its arrangement on white paper towels, underneath which you have placed several layers of blotting paper, thick cardstock, and the base of the press. If leaves are overlapping each other, carefully spread them out, and if there are really too many, carefully pluck some out. Spread any flower petals out carefully so that they don't get crushed and distorted. Afterward, put a paper towel on top, then blotting paper, more cardstock, and finally the lid of the press. Until you become more dexterous, get another pair of hands to help you with all of this; the result will be better. Finally, tighten the press, but only gently—only as the water starts to leave the plants can you gradually tighten it more. Every day you should change the paper towels until the very wet stage is over. Also, tighten your straps or wing nuts a little more each day. The time taken to reach the dry-plant stage will vary according to the climate you are in and the lushness or density of the plant you are pressing. Once it is really dry and there is no longer any more water content, there will be far less risk of the color fading.

To mount your plant pressings, use a white background and glue. Label, using both the botanical name and the common name. If you can, list the kind of area and soil you found your plant growing in.

Take at least one year over your herbal profile—though two are often needed, and the pleasure doubled! It is important that you experience each season with the plants or trees of your choice. It can be fun to photograph the plant one season and paint it the next, or photograph the berries or flowers and paint the whole plant.

When writing a description of the plants, you may wish to use botanical language, but do so only if it means something to you. For instance, *palmate* is a botanical term for the visual description of a plant with leaves that resemble the outspread hand. Otherwise, simply describe the plant in language that means something to everybody, including yourself. Note the exact sensory details as seen, felt, and experienced by you, for instance, "the beautiful blue-gray bark is also smooth, shiny, and smelling faintly musky-sweet in summer, but hardly smelling at all in winter." Make sure you describe everything—the roots, stem, bark, height, breadth, color, shape, size, leaf shape and size, flowers, seeds, fruit, needles, and smells. Keep the information easy to read, adding subheadings like "Flowering Time" to help both the writer and the reader.

Dealing descriptively in this much detail involves spending many hours of intimate time with each plant. This could involve sleeping against your chosen tree or peering at it through a magnifying glass. Both approaches will be needed. Watching plants with so much sensitivity gives you pleasure and joy, with a sense of bonding to nature. Writing down the plant's active components and medicinal uses will be additionally helpful. You will gain much from knowing the action of a plant in relation to a particular body system as well as the actual diseases it treats.

Folklore will bring a sense of historical use into your quest, while modern scientific research will give you even more invaluable information.

Glossary

Acid-Alkaline — This is the pH scale of the residue ash that forms when a particular food is oxidized.

Acupuncture — The Chinese practice of inserting fine needles into the body at specific points, to energize, unblock, or reroute subtle energies, known as *chi*.

Agribusiness — Generic term referring to the business of agriculture and its associated politics.

Alkaline — see Acid-Alkaline.

Allicin — The active component of garlic.

Antioxidants — These substances, found commonly in high-chlorophyll plants, especially those high in flavonoids, protect cells from free-radical damage.

Antispasmodic — A herb that limits, corrects, or prevents excessive involuntary muscular contractions.

Aphrodisiac — Any herb that increases sexual desire and potency. Some herbs are gender-specific, and some are shared.

Ayurveda — The healing modality of ancient East India, based on the comprehension of constitutional typing into three basic *dashas* (or dispositions): *pitta* (fire), *vata* (air), and *kapha* (moisture).

Carminative — A herb that expels gas from the gastrointestinal tract through excitation of internal peristalsis.

CFCs — abbreviation of chlorofluorocarbons, any of various usually gaseous substances, commonly used in refrigeration, thought to be harmful to the ozone layer of the upper atmosphere.

Detoxification — This is the general term indicating a systematic cleansing of the body and mind in total or specific systems.

Endocrine System — Glands that govern and regulate bodily functions, comprising pituitary, thyroid, parathyroid, thymus, adrenals, liver, pancreas, testes, and ovaries.

Enzymes — Substances secreted in the body, and present in live foods, that aid digestion.

Estrogen — This is the female hormone whose production in the body is lessened during menopause.

Fecal — Pertaining to the physical material of the stool.

Fibroids — These are nonmalignant growths that form from muscle and connective tissue.

Flavonoids—Flavonoids are classified as antioxidant, as they are generally capable of free-radical scavenging.

High-Density Lipoproteins—These are the proteins containing a high ratio of protein to fat that carry cholesterol from tissue to the liver. Low-density lipoproteins are considered to be more harmful.

HIV—Human immunodeficiency virus, the retrovirus considered to be the precursor to AIDS.

Immunity—The capacity and function of the body to fend off foreign bodies (fungi, viruses, bacteria), or to disarm and eject them.

Lymphatic System—This is the system of glands that secretes white blood cells.

Maceration—A medicinal oil that has been made by infusing a base oil with a herb or a number of herbs over a period of time. A typical maceration would be of St. John's wort in olive oil, used for cuts and bruises.

Microflora—Tiny plant cells.

Mucilaginous—Having the quality of mucus, that is, viscous, thick, and sticky. Internally used to soothe raw membranes.

Mucous—The quality of thickness and stickiness in plant and flesh foods. Something described as mucous is said to be binding.

Organophosphates—Chemical fertilizers.

Oxygenators—Substances that bring oxygen into the system.

Phagocytosis—A mechanism by which a phagocyte unleashes chemicals that engulf and digest bacteria and other pathogens (and dead cells).

Polysaccharide—A large number of sugars linked together where energy is stored in living tissue.

Probiotics—Substances that increase the presence of "friendly" bacteria in the intestines.

Progesterone—The female hormone of the second phase of the menstrual cycle; it prepares for and supports pregnancy.

Rubefacient—A category of herb defined by its capacity to draw blood to the surface of the body, causing redness by stimulating capillary action; for instance, cayenne pepper.

Steroids—In the body, essential fatty acids are converted into hormonelike substances called prostaglandins; steroids block their production in order to relieve clotting and pain.

Stimulant—Any herb that increases energy and function in the body.

T Cells — Also called T lymphocytes, these are immune cells that play several roles in the body's defenses. T cells are so called because they mature in the thymus.

Uterine — Pertaining to the uterus.

Vibration — In the esoteric sciences, all beings are considered to have an energetic quality, known as their vibration.

Virus — Any of a group of minute infective and disease-producing agents consisting of a core of nucleic acid (DNA or RNA) enclosed in a protein shell. Viruses are acellular and able to function and reproduce only if they can invade a living cell to use the cell's system to replicate themselves. In the process they may disrupt or alter the host cell's own DNA.

Vitamin — Any of a number of organic compounds, essential in small quantities for the normal functioning of the body.

Index